Ophthalmology: Clinical Diagnosis and Treatment of Eye Disease

Ophthalmology: Clinical Diagnosis and Treatment of Eye Disease

Editor: Ray George

AMERICAN
MEDICAL PUBLISHERS
www.americanmedicalpublishers.com

AMERICAN
MEDICAL PUBLISHERS
www.americanmedicalpublishers.com

Cataloging-in-publication Data

Ophthalmology : clinical diagnosis and treatment of eye disease / edited by Ray George.
p. cm.
Includes bibliographical references and index.
ISBN 979-8-88740-353-3
1. Eye--Diseases. 2. Eye--Diseases--Diagnosis. 3. Eye--Diseases--Treatment.
4. Therapeutics, Ophthalmological. 5. Ophthalmology. I. George, Ray.
RE46 .O68 2023
617.7--dc23

American Medical Publishers,
41 Flatbush Avenue,
1st Floor, New York,
NY 11217, USA

ISBN 979-8-88740-353-3 (Hardback)

Contents

Preface VII

Chapter 1 **Application of Electron Paramagnetic Resonance Spectroscopy in Ophthalmology** 1
Magdalena Zdybel and Barbara Pilawa

Chapter 2 **Electronic Communication and Digital Images: Referral Pathways and Clinical Uses in Ophthalmology** 25
Hannah Timlin and Roshini Sanders

Chapter 3 **Retinopathy of Prematurity** 46
Vikas Tah, Walid Sharif, Imran Yusuf, Marcus Posner, Louise Ramskold, Farihah Tariq, Dev Mukhey and Zuhair Sharif

Chapter 4 **Fabry Disease - Ocular Manifestations and Visual Symptoms** 81
Pinakin Gunvant Davey

Chapter 5 **Excitotoxicity and Glaucoma** 90
Makoto Ishikawa, Takeshi Yoshitomi and Yukitoshi Izumi

Chapter 6 **Utilization of Portable Digital Camera for Detecting Cataract** 110
Retno Supriyanti, Hitoshi Habe and Masatsugu Kidode

Chapter 7 **Recent Advances in Ocular Nucleic Acid-Based Therapies: The Silent Era** 128
Covadonga Pañeda, Tamara Martínez, Natalia Wright and Ana Isabel Jimenez

Chapter 8 **Clinical Application of Photodisruptors in Ophthalmology** 158
Emina Alimanović Halilović

Chapter 9 **Nontuberculous Mycobacterial Keratitis** 174
Ana Lilia Pérez-Balbuena, David Arturo Ancona-Lezama, Lorena Gutiérrez-Sánchez and Virginia Vanzzini-Zago

Chapter 10 **Genetics and Environmental Stress Factor Contributions to Anterior Segment Malformations and Glaucoma** 199
Yoko A. Ito and Michael A. Walter

Permissions

List of Contributors

Index

Preface

Every book is a source of knowledge and this one is no exception. The idea that led to the conceptualization of this book was the fact that the world is advancing rapidly; which makes it crucial to document the progress in every field. I am aware that a lot of data is already available, yet, there is a lot more to learn. Hence, I accepted the responsibility of editing this book and contributing my knowledge to the community.

Ophthalmology is a medical specialty that focuses on diagnosing and treating eye disorders. Common eye disorders include refractive errors, cataracts, diabetic retinopathy (DR), age-related macular degeneration, glaucoma, amblyopia and strabismus. Red eyes, night blindness, headache, light sensitivity, floaters, flashes, dry eyes, excessive tearing, blurred or distorted vision, and swelling are the common symptoms of eye disorders. A range of tests can be performed to confirm an eye condition or establish the extent or severity of an eye disorder. Angiography, electroretinography, ultrasonography, pachymetry, optical coherence tomography (OCT), computed tomography (CT), and magnetic resonance imaging (MRI) are a few such tests. There are a variety of treatment options available for treating eye disorders depending upon the type of disorder and its extent. Conventional surgery, medicines, laser surgery, and artificial tears are some of the available treatment options. In the past few years, the use of artificial intelligence (AI) has become quite popular for screening, diagnosing, and treating eye diseases. This book unfolds the recent developments in the diagnosis and treatment of eye diseases. Medical professionals and students actively engaged in the field of ophthalmology will find it full of crucial and unexplored concepts.

While editing this book, I had multiple visions for it. Then I finally narrowed down to make every chapter a sole standing text explaining a particular topic, so that they can be used independently. However, the umbrella subject sinews them into a common theme. This makes the book a unique platform of knowledge.

I would like to give the major credit of this book to the experts from every corner of the world, who took the time to share their expertise with us. Also, I owe the completion of this book to the never-ending support of my family, who supported me throughout the project.

Editor

1

Application of Electron Paramagnetic Resonance Spectroscopy in Ophthalmology

Magdalena Zdybel and Barbara Pilawa

1. Introduction

Electron paramagnetic resonance (EPR) spectroscopy is the method of examination of free radicals and the others paramagnetic centers [1-22]. EPR measurements reveal applications in medicine [8-11, 23-34], biology [8-11], pharmacy [35-48], cosmetology [49, 50], biotechnology [51-54]. EPR method is useful to examination of tissues, cells, biopolimers, drugs, cosmetic substances, herbs, and biomaterials [8-11, 23-34]. Free radicals in such mentioned samples may be characterized by EPR spectra, and the influence of physical and chemical factors on them may be tested. The important information about light, oxygen, temperature, gamma irradiation on the biological or pharmacological objects may be obtain from analysis of their absorption signals [8-11, 23-54]. Free radical properties and concentration are determined by the use of electron paramagnetic resonance [1-8]. Applications of EPR method to determine the optimal conditions of photodynamic therapy [24-26], the best conditions of sterilization of drugs [35-48], herbs [22] and cosmetic substances [49, 50], was proposed.

1.1. Aim

The aim of this work is to present usefulness of EPR analysis in ophthalmology. EPR studies of free radicals and their interactions with tissues structures are described. Melanins, which contain o-semiquinone free radicals (S=1/2) and biradicals (S=1) exist in the eye. EPR studies of paramagnetic centers in melanin biopolymers are presented. The effect of light irradiation and temperature on free radicals in melanin biopolymer is shown. The effect of dia- and paramagnetic metal ions on free radicals in melanins is discussed. The effect of drugs on free radicals in melanins tested by EPR is presented. Different types of free radicals, their chemical and thermodynamic stability are compared. Free radicals and reactive oxygen species in ophthalmology are presented.

The effect of electron paramagnetic resonance as the absorption of electromagnetic waves by the sample located in magnetic field and the EPR spectrometer are described. The positive aspects of the EPR analysis in the technical meaning such are bring to light. EPR measurements are not destructive to the samples and only the low amount of the sample is needed. The types of EPR spectrometers and microwave frequencies are presented. EPR spectra of tissues may be multi-component and the frequency of microwaves influences the resolution of detection of EPR lines of different types of free radicals. The parameters of the EPR spectra: amplitudes, integral intensities, linewidths, g-factors, and both physical and practical meaning of them are shown. Amplitudes and integral intensities increase with increasing of free radical concentration in the sample [1-8]. Linewidth depends on molecular structure of the samples and magnetic interactions in the chemical units [1-6]. g-Values let us to determine the type of free radicals [1-3]. Free radical concentration determination and the references for these measurements are shown. The concentration is proportional to the area under the absorption lines [1-8]. The spin probes in EPR investigation to ophthalmology are presented. The professional spectroscopic programs are characterized.

Sample preparation to EPR measurements are presented. The measurements in the wide range of temperatures and microwave powers relative to their usefulness in ophthalmologic samples are discussed. The methods of differentiation of free radicals and biradicals in melanin biopolimers are presented.

2. Paramagnetic centers

2.1. Types of paramagnetic centers

Paramagnetic centers are the molecular units with unpaired electrons and they have characteristic behavior in magnetic field applied in EPR spectroscopy [1-8]. Paramagnetic centers are formed during photolysis, thermolysis, radiolysis, electrolysis, and the others chemical reactions [11]. Oxygen is very active in generation of paramagnetic centers [1, 11, 55]. The most known paramagnetic centers are free radicals, biradicals, paramagnetic metal ions, oxygen O_2 molecules in triplet ground state and paramagnetic conducting species [l, 5, 11]. Paramagnetic centers differ in spins and in stability. Free radicals have spin with the value of 1/2, biradicals and O_2 spins are equal of 1, paramagnetic ions mainly reveal spin of 1/2, delocalized electrons in conducting materials have spins of 1/2. Magnetic moments of paramagnetic centers result from their spins, and they are responsible for the orientations in magnetic field during their EPR detection.

Paramagnetic centers differ in lifetime [8, 11]. Stability of paramagnetic centers is connected with their chemical building and the external conditions in the environment. There is known stabile organic free radicals and labile reactive oxygen species. Samples in vacuum have usually free radicals for the longer times than the samples in air, where oxygen molecules O_2 in paramagnetic triplet states with spin S=1 exist [1, 11]. The reactions with oxygen is stronger in the higher temperatures [11]. The intensive reactions between paramagnetic centers become in the structures with the large amount of unpaired electrons.

2.2. Stable free radicals

Stabile free radicals with different localization of unpaired electrons exist in organic molecular units [10, 11, 55]. Thermodynamic stability of free radicals depend on their chemical structure [55]. The lifetime is longer for free radicals in aromatic units than in aliphatic units. The major types of free radicals exist in cells and tissues, because of differentiation on their building and composition. o-Semiquinone free radicals are the aromatic free radicals [55]. There is known the chain the aliphatic free radicals [55]. The exemplary popular free radicals in living organism are peroxyl radicals ($ROO^{\bullet}$) and alkoxyl radicals ($RO^{\bullet}$).

2.3. Reactive oxygen species

The group of reactive oxygen species consists of both paramagnetic free radicals and diamagnetic non-radical compounds [11, 55]. The reactive oxygen species are not stabile, they have the short lifetimes often lower than one second, and they easy react with others molecules. The exemplary paramagnetic reactive oxygen species are hydroxyl radical ($^{\bullet}OH$), hydroperoxyl radical ($HO_2^{\bullet}$), superoxide radical anion ($O_2^{\bullet}$), and nitric dioxide ($NO_2^{\bullet}$) [11]. Reactive oxygen species appear in inflammatory states in human organism [10, 11], irradiated tissues, in thermally [35-43] and gamma [44-48] sterilized drugs.

2.4. Paramagnetic centers in eye

Paramagnetic centers in eye exist mainly in melanin biopolymer [56]. Melanin is a natural pigment that is found in most organisms. In humans, melanin is found in skin, eyes, hair, leucocytes, *Substantia nigra, Locus coerules* and inner ear [31, 32, 57-60]. Through a process called melanogenesis, melanin is produced by melanocytes [32, 58].

There are three basic types of melanin: eumelanin, which is a brown and black, pheomelanin, which is red or yellow, and neuromelanin, which is present in the brain [33, 59].

Chemically, melanins are amorphous biopolymers consisting of various monomer units i.a. 5, 6-dihydroxy indole-2-carboxylic acid and 5, 6-dihydroxy indole [59, 60]. Chemical structures of eu-and pheomelanins are compared in Figure 1 [59]. Eumelanin contains carbon (C), oxygen (O), and nitrogen (N) atoms. Besides C, O, and N, sulphur (S) exists in pheomelanin [59, 60].

Melanins are found in the eye in higher concentrations than anywhere else in the human body [61]. In the eye, melanin content in the iris, ciliary body, choroid and retinal pigment epithelium (RPE) [60]. Cornea and lens don't have the pigment [60, 62].

Content of melanin differs in various ocular tissues [60, 62]. In humans, scleral melanin levels are higher than retina and central choroid-RPE. Besides, it is also different distribution of melanin in human eyes. The peripheral tissue pigment levels are generally higher compared to the central regions [60]. The melanin content of human RPE decreases with age [56, 62].

Differences in iris color are caused by three factors: the concentration of pigment within stromal melanocytes, light scattering and absorptive properties of extracellular components, and the pigment granules in the iris pigment epithelium (IPE) (located on the back of the iris) [63].

a)

b)

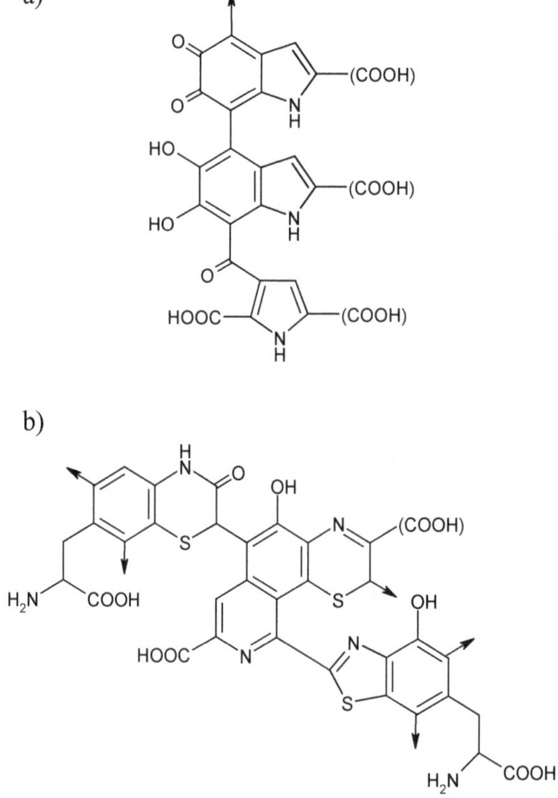

Figure 1. Chemical structure of eumelanin (a) and pheomelanin (b) [59].

Melanin from the IPE is essentially eumelanin, while melanin from IPE-scraped iris (consisting mainly of stroma plus anterior IPE) exhibiting content of both eumelanin and pheomelanin [63].

It is shown that the green iris appear to be more pheomelanic, whereas blue-green iris appear to be more eumelanic [63]. Blue eyes contain little of either pigment, while green-brown and brown irides feature a mixed pigment content [63].

Many drugs and metal ions bind to melanin [32, 52, 64-68]. The binding of drug to melanin is the result of physicochemical properties of the pigment [61]. Melanin protects the pigmented tissues through the absorption of many drugs and chemicals. On the other hand, this may lead to toxic accumulation of these substances in melanin, and consequently to the degradation of pigmented tissues [69, 70]. Differences in melanin content in ocular tissues might contribute to differences in drug binding and toxicity [60].

Melanin in the eyes helps protect them from ultraviolet and high-frequency visible light [34, 61, 70]. Besides, ocular melanin may also play a protective role against free radicals [61].

The main paramagnetic centers in melanin are the o-semiquinone free radicals with spin of 1/2 and with unpaired electrons localized on oxygen atoms [64-68]. Additionally it was spectroscopically proved that biradicals with spin of 1 also exist in melanins [71, 72]. o-Semiquinone free radicals and biradicals were also found in melanin complexes with copper(II) ions and drugs, as kanamycin [71] and netilmicin [72]. So far in eye melanin only o-semiquinone free radicals were studied [56].

3. The effect of electron paramagnetic resonance – Basic theory

Electron paramagnetic resonance (EPR) is the effect which appears in the paramagnetic samples exposed to microwaves in magnetic field [1-3]. Magnetic field causes Zeeman splitting of energy levels. After splitting the energy levels of unpaired electrons in magnetic field relate to different orientation of their magnetic moments, i.e. parallel and non parallel to the magnetic induction vector B. Both the magnetic moments in magnetic field and the magnetic spin quantum number M_S have 2S+1 values [1, 5, 8]. The energy level of unpaired electron with the magnetic spin quantum number M_S in magnetic field is splitted into 2S+1 levels. The unpaired electron may be excited by microwaves and it comes to the higher energy levels, when the frequency and the energy of microwaves are equal as is given in the resonance condition formula [1]:

$$h\nu = E_2 - E_1 = g\mu_B B_r \tag{1}$$

where h – Planck constant, ν – microwave frequency, g – spectroscopic factor, μ_B – Bohr magneton, B_r – resonance induction of magnetic field, E_2 – energy of the excited level of unpaired electron, E_1 – energy of the ground level of unpaired electron.

The energy E of unpaired electron with the magnetic spin number M_S in magnetic field with induction **B** is given as [1, 4]:

$$E(M_S) = M_S g\mu_B B_r \tag{2}$$

The electron paramagnetic resonance (EPR) effect is also called electron spin resonance (ESR), because unpaired electrons in the paramagnetic samples have unpaired spins [1-8]. The described above effect is the basis of EPR (ESR) spectroscopy, which is the experimental method of examination of paramagnetic species. Paramagnetic samples are located in magnetic field and they absorb microwaves with energies fulfill the resonance conditions (1) [1-8]. EPR spectroscopy use to analysis the absorption and the first derivative lines. The first derivative curves are very important for the samples with complex paramagnetic center system, when the several types of paramagnetic species exist [1]. The resolution of the multicomponent EPR spectra to the component lines is easier for the first derivatives than for the absorption curves.

For paramagnetic samples with free radicals, when the spin is S=1/2 the Zeeman splitting of the individual energy level in magnetic field causes the appearance of two levels [1, 3, 5]. The Zeeman splitting for free radicals in magnetic field is shown in Figure 2 [3]. Free radicals mainly exist in eye, so this example is the most important for ophthalmology. In the Figure 2 the energy levels of unpaired electrons of free radicals outside and in magnetic field are presented, and the absorption and the first derivative lines are shown.

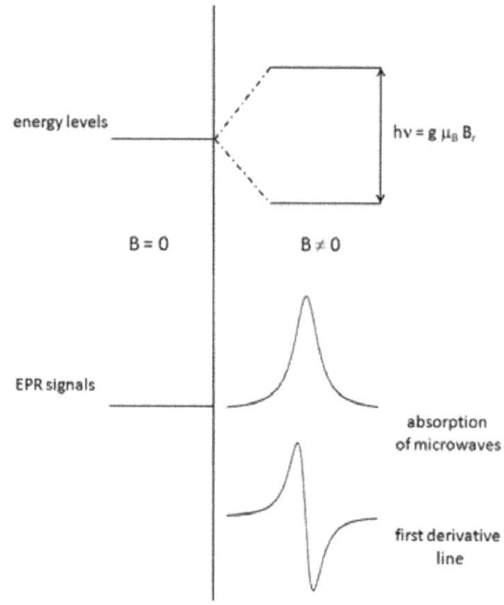

Figure 2. The Zeeman effect in magnetic field for free radicals with spin S=1/2. The absorption and the first absorption EPR curves are presented. B – induction of magnetic field, B_r – magnetic resonance induction, h – Planck constant, ν – microwave frequency, g – spectroscopic factor, μ_B – Bohr magneton, the resonance formula: $h\nu = g\mu_B B_r$. The scheme was prepared by the use of work [3].

4. EPR spectrometers useful in ophthalmology

4.1. The electronic blocks of the continuous microwave (CW) spectrometer

Electron paramagnetic spectrometer with continuous microwaves (CW-EPR) is the most useful apparatus for ophthalmology. For such type of the spectrometer samples are located in magnetic field and the microwaves are continuously send to the tested object [1, 3]. Unpaired electrons of the paramagnetic sample is continuously excited by microwaves and the spin-spin and spin-lattice relaxation processes occur [1, 3, 5, 8]. This spectrometer consists of microwave bridge, waveguides, resonance cavity, electromagnet, the modulation block, detector, and the amplifier. The source of microwaves and attenuator exist in microwave bridge. The attenuator is applied to change microwave power in the experiment. The popular source of microwaves is klystron. The microwave changes with attenuation according to the formula [4]:

$$attenuation\left[dB\right] = 10lg\left(M_o / M\right) \quad (3)$$

where M_o – the total microwave power produced by klystron, M – microwave power used during the measurement of EPR spectra.

The EPR spectra should be detect with low microwave power without the saturation effect to obtain the proper amounts of paramagnetic centers in the tested samples [1, 3]. The changes of microwave power and detection of EPR lines is used to characterize magnetic interactions in the samples.

Electromagnetic waves are send from microwave bridge via attenuator by waveguides to the resonance cavity [1-8]. The paramagnetic sample is located in the resonance cavity in the magnetic field produced by electromagnet. The absorption of the microwaves took place in the resonance cavity. Modulation of magnetic field is done by modulator and the signal is measured by detector. The receiver gain is used during the detection. Numerical detection of the EPR lines is done. Magnetic field is measured by NMR detector. Microwave frequency is usually measured, but sometimes the references are used. The measurement of the microwave frequency is necessary to accurately determine g-factor, which is important to study the type of paramagnetic centers in the samples.

The classic CW-EPR spectrometer of Bruker BioSpin GmbH is shown in Figure 3. The exemplary resonance cavity of Bruker BioSpin GmbH is presented in Figure 4. Electromagnet – the source of magnetic field is presented in Figure 5.

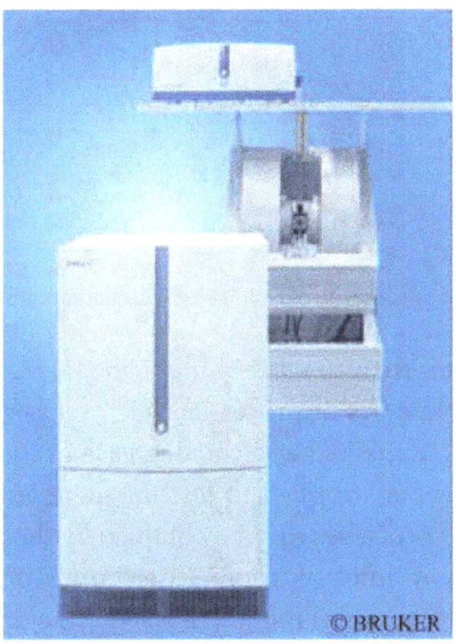

Figure 3. Continuous microwave EPR spectrometer EMXplus produced by Bruker BioSpin GmbH.

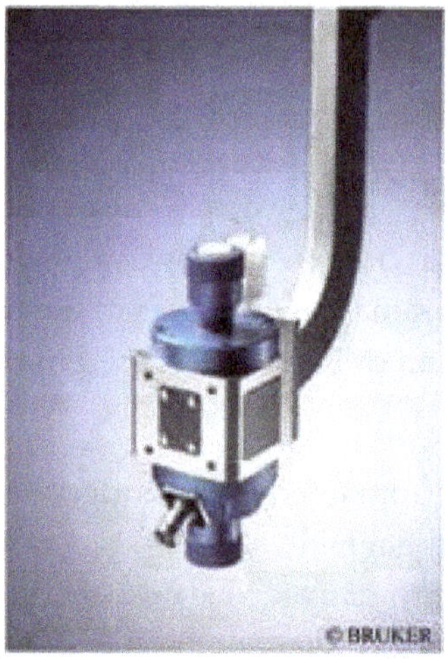

Figure 4. The resonance cavity of CW-EPR spectrometer of Bruker BioSpin GmbH.

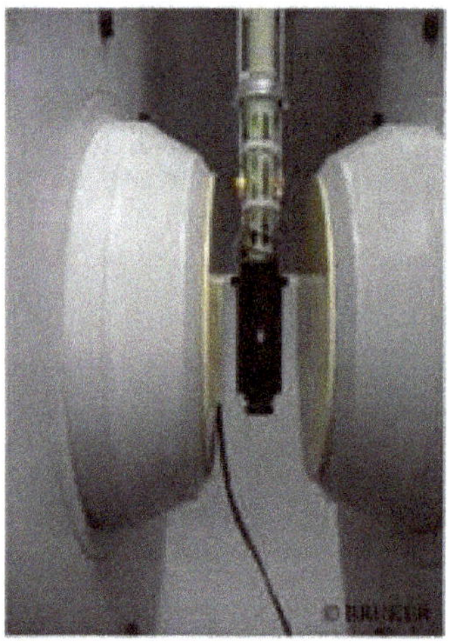

Figure 5. Electromagnet and the resonance cavity of CW-EPR spectrometer produced by Bruker BioSpin GmbH.

The pulsed EPR spectrometers are also used in medicine [1, 8]. These types of spectrometers are useful in examination of kinetics of processes. Microwaves are sent to the paramagnetic sample between poles of electromagnet and the decrease of the absorbed signal is detected. The pulsed EPR spectrometers are applied to test magnetic interactions in the samples [1]. Time of spin-lattice relaxation processes may be obtained by the pulsed method [1, 3, 5, 8]. The different spin-lattice relaxation times of unpaired electrons of major paramagnetic centers brings to light the component signals of them. It is used to determine the number of different types of paramagnetic centers in the samples. Determination of the number of component lines in the CW-EPR spectra is performed by fitting the resultant spectra by superposition of Gauss and Lorentz lines [1, 4].

4.2. Types of microwave bands in EPR spectrometers

Different microwave frequencies are used in the EPR spectrometers [1, 2]. The most popular is the frequency about 9.3 GHz (X-band). The typical microwave bands and corresponding frequencies of electromagnetic waves are presented in Table 1 [1, 2].

Microwave band	Microwave frequency [GHz]
L	1.5
S	3.0
C	6.0
X	**9.3**
K	23
Q	36
V	50
W	95

Table 1. Microwave bands used in EPR spectroscopy [1, 2].

5. EPR spectra

5.1. The parameters of EPR spectra and their practical meaning in studies of eye free radicals

The basic parameters of the first derivative EPR spectra give important information about type of paramagnetic centers in the sample, their amounts, and magnetic interactions which reflect chemical structure of the tested object [1-8]. The following parameters of EPR spectra: amplitudes (A), integral intensities (I), linewidths (ΔB_{pp}), and g-factors are usually analyzed. The parameters for the model eumelanin – DOPA-melanin (from SIGMA-ALDRICH) are shown in Figure 6. The first derivative EPR spectrum of DOPA-melanin is presented, because of the eumelanin mainly exists in eye.

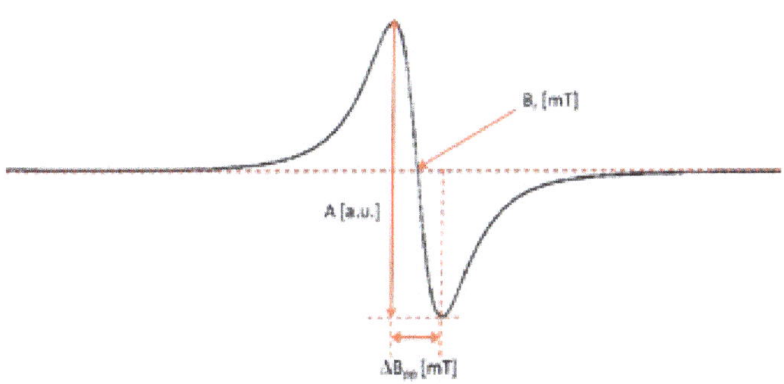

Figure 6. The first derivative EPR spectrum of the model eumelanin – DOPA-melanin and the basic parameters: amplitude (A), linewidth (ΔB_{pp}), and the resonance magnetic induction (B_r).

Amplitudes (A) and integral intensities (I) increase with the increasing of free radical concentration in the samples [1, 8]. The comparison of amplitudes (A) of EPR spectra of different samples from eye give information about the relative contents of free radicals in them. But the free radical concentration in the individual biological sample is determined by integral intensity (I), and it is proportional to the value of this parameter (I). Integral intensity (I) of the EPR spectra is the area under the absorption line, so for the first derivative EPR curve double integrations should be done. Linewidth (ΔB_{pp}) increases for the stronger dipolar interactions of free radicals in the samples [1, 8]. Dipolar interactions increases for decrease distances between free radicals [1, 8].

g-Values are calculated from the resonance condition according to the formula [1]:

$$g = h\nu / \mu_B B_r \quad (4)$$

where h – Planck constant, ν – microwave frequency, μ_B – Bohr magneton, B_r – induction of resonance magnetic field.

Determination of g-value is possible for known microwave frequency (ν) and resonance induction (B_r). Microwave frequency is detected by the recorder, and resonance induction is obtained from the EPR spectrum (Figure 6). g-Values characterize type of free radicals existing in the samples [1, 5]. The individual free radicals have EPR lines in the correspond to their chemical structures magnetic field. The resonance magnetic induction effect on the g-factor of free radicals (formula 4). g-Values are used in EPR spectroscopy to identification of the species which causes paramagnetic character of the sample.

5.2. EPR spectra of complex biological samples

Free radical system in biological samples, for example for species obtained from eye, is usually complex. In cells or tissues several groups of free radicals may exist [8]. The EPR spectra are then multi-component as the superposition of the lines of all the groups of free radicals. The information about the each group of free radicals is obtain by numerical fitting of the shape of the resultant EPR spectrum of the sample by sum of theoretical lines. The shape of the component lines is gaussian or lorentzian [1-4]. The percentage fraction of the individual component lines in the total EPR spectrum means the percentage fraction of their concentration in the sample [1]. Such numerical fitting were done for example for model neuromelanins [29, 30].

The analysis of shape of the EPR spectra and determination of their parameters are performed by spectroscopic programs. The known modern program to spectral analysis is WINEPR of Bruker, ORIGIN 6.0 of Microcal Software, LabVIEW 8.5 by National Instruments (Austin, Texas) or programs of JAGMAR (Kraków, Poland) and EPRAD (Poznań, Poland).

6. Application of EPR spectroscopy in ophthalmology

6.1. Sample preparation to the examination

EPR spectra can be measure for solid state, liquid and gaseous samples [1, 4, 8]. Solid state samples, for example melanin from eye, are examined in glass or quartz tubes with the diameters higher than for liquid samples. The mass of the solid samples located in the tubes should be determined to obtain the content of free radicals in one gram of the probe. The melanin in the glass tubes for spectroscopic studies is shown in Figure 7. The external diameter of the thin walled tube is 3 mm. The materials used in tubes should not reveal EPR signals for the measurement parameters used in the experiment. The EPR spectrum of DOPA-melanin is presented in Figure 8.

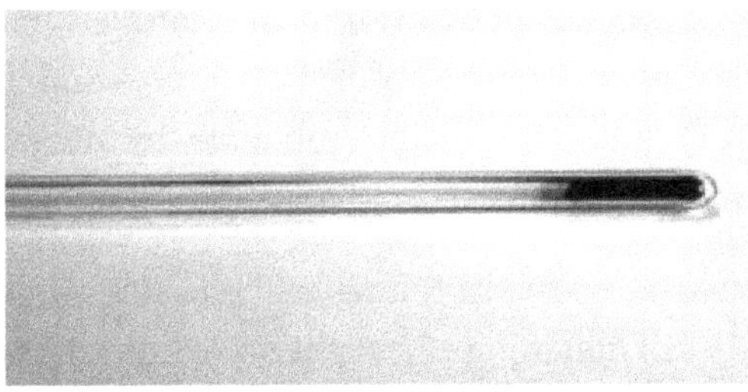

Figure 7. The model eumelanin – DOPA-melanin in the glass tube with diameter of 3 mm for EPR measurements.

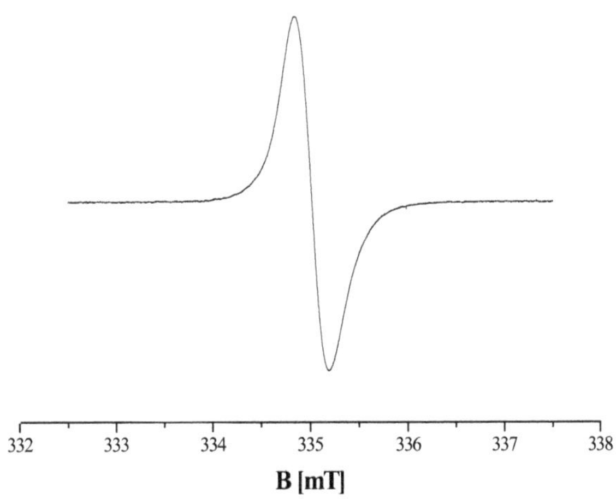

Figure 8. The EPR spectrum of model eumelanin – DOPA-melanin recorded at room temperature with low microwave power of 2.2 mW. B is the induction of magnetic field.

Liquid samples should be measure in the thin glass or quartz tubes with diameter below 1 mm. The special flat cells are also used. Water in the sample quenches EPR signals, so the large dimensions of wet samples are practically not used.

Paramagnetic gases in the environment usually decrease EPR lines of the paramagnetic samples. Such effects were observed for example for melanins [73, 74]. The samples susceptible to oxygen may be evacuated before the EPR measurements.

6.2. Determination of free radical concentration in the samples in ophthalmology

6.2.1. The measurement of the concentration

Free radicals concentrations in the samples are determined by the use of integral intensities of their EPR spectra and the spectra of the reference with the known amounts of paramagnetic centers [1, 3, 8]. Free radical concentrations (N) in the samples are determined as the value which is proportional to the area under the absorption curves and the integral intensity (I) [1, 3, 8]. Integral intensities (I) of the absorption line is obtained by integration of this curve. Double integration of the first-derivative EPR spectra give us the value of integral intensity (I).

To obtain free radical concentration the EPR lines of the tested samples and the references are measured. In our EPR studies of melanin polymers two references were used: ultramarine and the ruby crystal. Amplitudes of the EPR lines of the ruby crystal (A) located with the analyzed sample and ultramarine (A_u) in the resonance cavity were determined. The integral intensities (I) of the EPR spectra of the tested melanin samples and the reference-ultramarine (I_u) were compared.

The concentration of the free radicals (N) in the melanins was calculated as [3]:

$$N = N_u\left[(W_u A_u)/I_u\right]\left[I/(WAm)\right] \quad (5)$$

where N_u – the number of paramagnetic center in the ultramarine reference; W, W_u – the receiver gains for sample and the ultramarine; A, A_u – the amplitudes of ruby signal for the sample and the ultramarine; I, I_u – the integral intensities for the sample and ultramarine, m – the mass of the sample.

6.2.2. The paramagnetic references and their properties

The paramagnetic references should contain high amounts of stabile paramagnetic centers [1-8]. In our studies of melanin biopolymer from eye [56], others melanins [64-68, 71-78], cells [24-26, 68], drugs [35-48], ultramarine was used as the reference. In Figure 9 ultramarine in the glass tube is shown. The broad EPR line of ultramarine with paramagnetic centers with unpaired electrons located on sulfur atoms is presented in Figure 10.

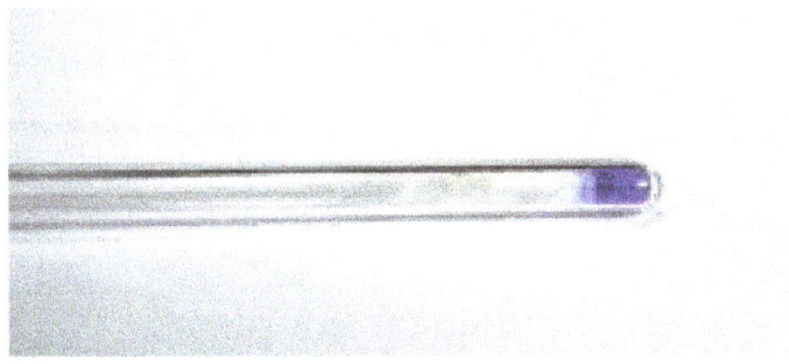

Figure 9. Ultramarine in the glass tube to EPR measurements.

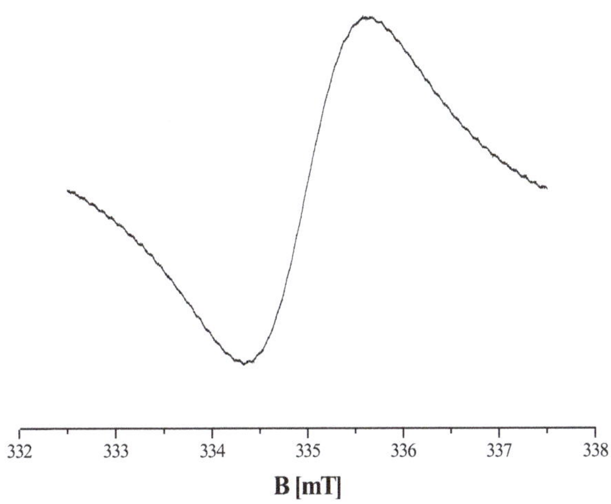

Figure 10. EPR spectrum of ultramarine – the reference for free radical concentration recorded with low microwave power of 2.2 mW. B is the induction of magnetic field.

The second reference – a ruby crystal (Al_2O_3: Cr^{3}) was permanently placed in a resonance cavity. For tested sample and for ultramarine the EPR line of a ruby crystal are measured. The ruby crystal is shown in Figure 11.

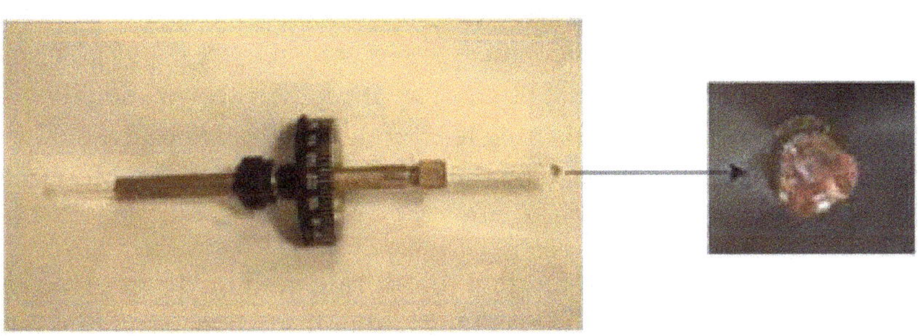

Figure 11. A ruby crystal.

The other reference for free radical concentration is DPPH (2, 2-diphenyl-1-picrylhydrazyl) [4]. Unpaired electron in DPPH is localized on nitrogen atom. DPPH is not so stabile such as ultramarine, because it is susceptible for oxygen. During storage of DPPH in air its free radical concentration decreases, so it should be evacuated.

6.3. Magnetic interactions in ophthalmological samples

Information about magnetic interactions between unpaired electrons in paramagnetic samples gives linewidth and changes of the spectra with microwave power [1-3]. The influence of microwave power (M) on the EPR spectra of the melanin samples from eye [56] and the others melanins [64-68] were examined. The changes of amplitudes (A) and linewidths (ΔB_{pp}) of EPR spectra with increasing of microwave power were analysed to determine type of broadening of EPR lines. The influence of microwave power (M) on amplitudes (A) and linewidths (ΔB_{pp}) of the EPR spectra depend on free radicals distribution (homogeneous or inhomogeneous) in the samples. For homogeneous broadened EPR lines the amplitude (A) increases with increasing of microwave power (M) and for the higher microwave powers it value decreases [1]. The increase of linewidth (ΔB_{pp}) with increasing of microwave power (M) is characteristic for the homogeneously broadened EPR lines [1]. For inhomogeneous broadening of spectral lines the amplitude (A) increases with increasing of microwave power (M) and for the higher microwave powers it value does not change [1]. Linewidth (ΔB_{pp}) of the inhomogeneously broadened EPR lines is unchanged with increasing of microwave power (M) [1].

Spin-lattice interactions in the samples may be characterized by observation of changes of amplitudes (A) of EPR lines with increasing of microwave power [1-3]. The slow and fast spin-lattice relaxation processes in the samples differ in microwave saturation of EPR lines [1-3]. The higher power of microwave saturation of EPR lines reveal the samples with the fast spin-lattice relaxation processes than the samples with the slow spin-lattice relaxation processes [1-4].

6.4. EPR investigation of melanin biopolymer in eye

6.4.1. Free radicals and biradicals in melanin biopolymer

The important paramagnetic structures existing in eye are melanin biopolymers [56, 60-63]. EPR examination of melanins from low temperature of liquid nitrogen to room temperature proved that two types of paramagnetic centers are located in them [71, 72]. The characteristic for both free radicals with spin S=1/2 and biradicals with spin S=1 correlations between integral intensities (I) of EPR lines and the measuring temperature (T) were observed. IT value for free radicals was constant independent on temperature, and the IT values for biradicals depended on the measuring temperature.

Free radicals and biradicals play an important role during binding drugs to melanins [71, 72]. The amounts of these paramagnetic centers changes after formation of complex melanin-drug. Such effects were observed for example for kanamycin [71] and netilmicin [72]. Paramagnetic copper(II) ions influence on free radicals and biradicals in melanin complexes with kanamycin and netlimicin was observed. It is expected that drugs applied in ophthalmology change free radicals and biradicals concentrations in melanin biopolymers in eye. So electron paramagnetic resonance spectroscopy seems to be very useful in examination of interactions of drugs with melanin in eye.

6.4.2. EPR results for melanin in eye

Electron paramagnetic resonance spectroscopy was used to examine free radicals in RPE melanosomes from different aged donors [56]. o-Semiquinone free radicals were identified in RPE melanosomes with the characteristic g-values and single broad EPR lines. Concentrations of free radicals in RPE melanosomes depend on the age of donors. The higher free radicals concentrations were obtained for donors aged > 45 years, than for donors aged < 22 years [56]. Free radicals concentrations in RPE melanosomes (~10^{17} spin/g) [56] were lower than the concentrations in model eumelanin – DOPA-melanin [56], A-375 melanoma cells [68], *Cladosporium cladosporioides* mycelium [52], and *Cladosporium herbarum* mycelium [53]. Free radical concentration in melanin changed after irradiation of eumelanin by visible light [34].

EPR spectra of RPE melanosomes were similar to those observed for DOPA-melanin (Figure 8), which is the synthetic model eumelanin. The unresolved hyperfine structure characteristic for pheomelanins was not observed for melanin of RPE. The exemplary complex shape of EPR spectra with signals of pheomelanin is shown in Figure 12 [52].

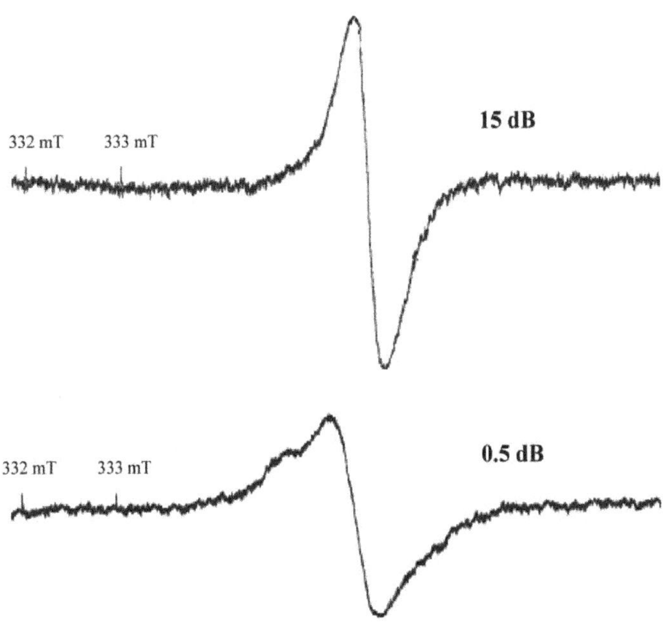

Figure 12. EPR spectra with signals of pheomelanin in *Cladosporium cladosporioides* recorded with different microwaves. The melanin samples were studied in paper [52].

Melanin in *Cladosporium cladosporioides* mycelium is the mixture of eu-and pheomelanin [52, 75-77]. The signal of pheomelanin is clearly visible in the EPR spectrum recorded with 0.5 dB attenuation, while it was not observed in the EPR spectrum measured with attenuation of 15 dB (Figure 12). It is proposed that the lower attenuation and higher microwave powers should be used to search pheomelanin in the biological samples.

6.4.3. EPR method proposed to examine free radicals in drugs in ophthalmology

EPR may be applied to examine of free radicals formed in ophthalmological drugs in process of their sterilization. Drugs used in ophthalmology should not contain microorganisms, and the sterilization is performed to remove or killed them [35-48]. Sterilization methods are gamma irradiation or thermal treatment of drugs [35-48]. Radiative and thermal sterilization should not produce free radicals in drugs, because changes of their interactions on eye as the result of modification of their chemical structure. Free radicals in sterilized optalmological drugs may be responsible for toxic effects during therapy.

Electron paramagnetic resonance spectroscopy was used to optimize sterilization procedure and conditions of antibiotics and the other drugs [35-48]. The methods of sterilization and temperatures for which the low amounts of free radicals are produced in drugs were searched. Similar examination of drugs may be proposed in ophthalmology.

6.4.4. EPR studies of antioxidant properties of drugs in ophthalmology

Electron paramagnetic resonance spectroscopy may be used in ophthalmology to examine antioxidant properties of drugs. The interactions of drugs with free radicals are tested with DPPH as the reference [79-81]. Chemical structure of DPPH is shown in Figure 13 [4]. DPPH is the model source of free radicals in this study. The EPR spectrum of DPPH is presented in Figure 14.

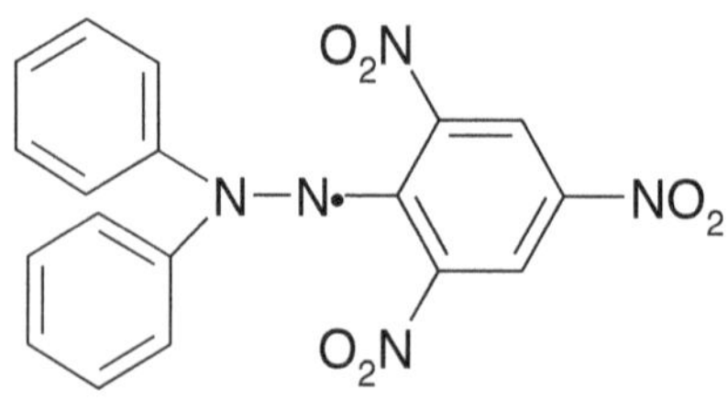

Figure 13. Chemical structure of DPPH [4].

The antioxidant properties of drugs reflects the decrease of amplitudes of the EPR line of DPPH after adding the tested samples to the solution [79-81]. The changes of integral intensities are also observed.

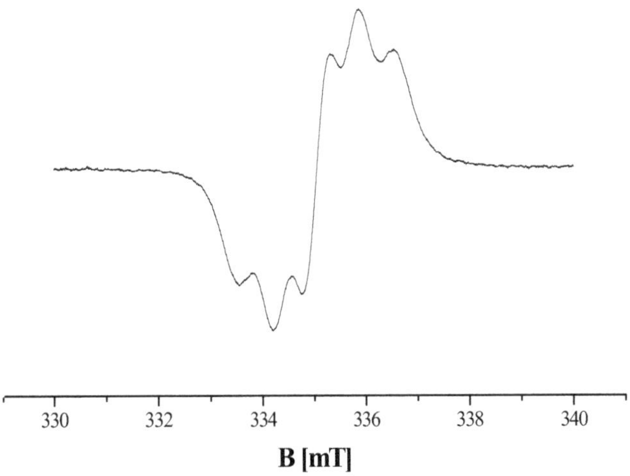

Figure 14. EPR spectrum of DPPH recorded with low microwave power of 2.2 mW. B is the induction of magnetic field.

7. Conclusions – Advantages of EPR measurements in ophthalmology

Electron paramagnetic resonance spectroscopy is the useful method to examine free radicals in eye, drugs and their interactions with free radicals (Table 2). Microbiological tests may be accompanied by EPR analysis to obtain the best conditions of sterilization process. Antioxidant properties of drugs may be determined by EPR measurements.

EPR IN OPHTHALMOLOGY	
Application	**Characteristics**
determination of free radical properties and concentrations in eye structures	type and chemical structure of free radicals, localization of unpaired electrons in free radicals, light and temperature effect on free radicals, oxygen molecules effect on free radicals, para- and diamagnetic metal ions effect on free radicals, changes in free radicals of eye melanin biopolymers after drug binding, spin-spin and spin-lattice interactions depend on chemical structures in eye
examination of biradicals in melanin biopolymers in eye	chemical structure and amounts of biradicals, effect of drugs and physical conditions on biradicals
studies of free radical interactions in eye	kinetics and products of free radicals

EPR IN OPHTHALMOLOGY	
Application	**Characteristics**
determination of antioxidants influence on free radicals in eye	decrease of the amount of free radicals in eye structures after interactions with antioxidant drugs and substances
use of spin-labels to examine biochemical units in eye	numerical analysis of shape of EPR lines of spin-labels to obtain information about chemical units in eyes
determination of antioxidant and free radical properties of ophthalmological drugs	analysis of quenching of free radicals by individual drugs, and study free radicals contents in pharmacological substances
optimization of thermal and radiative sterilization processes of ophthalmological drugs	searching temperatures or doses of irradiation, which do not produce high amounts of free radicals in drugs during heating or gamma irradiation
optimization of storage conditions of ophthalmological drugs	searching effects of light, temperature, and oxygen on free radical formation in drugs; the best conditions of drugs storage do not produce high amounts of free radicals in the samples

Table 2. Application of electron paramagnetic resonance (EPR) spectroscopy in ophthalmology [1-4, 11, 24-48, 52-56, 64-68, 70-81].

The most important advantages of EPR analysis in ophthalmology are the low amount of the samples necessary to test, the non destructive type of this analysis, the major information about free radicals. EPR spectra bring to light type and concentration of free radicals in eye, melanin biopolymer, and drugs.

Acknowledgements

The CW-EPR spectrometer (Figure 3), the resonance cavity (Figure 4), and electromagnet (Figure 5) are presented by courtesy of Bruker BioSpin GmbH. The cited EPR studies in medicine and pharmacy in Department of Biophysics are financially supported by Medical University of Silesia in Katowice (in 2013 grant number KNW-1-137/K/3/0).

Author details

Magdalena Zdybel* and Barbara Pilawa

*Address all correspondence to: mzdybel@sum.edu.pl

Medical University of Silesia in Katowice, School of Pharmacy with the Division of Laboratory Medicine, Department of Biophysics, Sosnowiec, Poland

References

[1] Wertz JE, Bolton JR. Electron Spin Resonance: Elementary Theory and Practical Applications. London: Chapman and Hall; 1986.

[2] Weil JA, Bolton JR. Electron Paramagnetic Resonance: Elementary Theory and Practical Applications. 2nd Edition. New York: John Wiley & Sons; 2007.

[3] Stankowski J, Hilczer W. Wstęp do spektroskopii rezonansów magnetycznych. Warszawa: PWN; 2005.

[4] Kęcki Z. Podstawy spektroskopii molekularnej. Warszawa: PWN; 1999.

[5] Morrish AH. Fizyczne podstawy magnetyzmu. Warszawa: PWN; 1970.

[6] Symons M. Spektroskopia EPR w chemii i biochemii. Warszawa: PWN; 1987.

[7] Kirmse R, Stach J. Spektroskopia EPR. Zastosowania w chemii. Kraków: Uniwersytet Jagielloński; 1994.

[8] Eaton GR, Eaton SS, Salikhov KM., eds. Foundations of Modern EPR. Singapore: World Scientific; 1998.

[9] Pryor W., editor. Free radicals in biology. New York: Acadmeic Press; 1976.

[10] Jaroszyk F., editor. Biofizyka. Warszawa: PZWL; 2008.

[11] Bartosz G. Druga twarz tlenu. Wolne rodniki w przyrodzie. Warszawa: PWN; 2006.

[12] Domagała W, Pilawa B, Lapkowski M. Quantitative in-situ EPR spectroelectrochemical studies of doping processes in poly(3, 4-alkylenedioxythiophene)s: Part 1: PEDOT. Electrochimica Acta 2008;53(13): 4580-4590.

[13] Zykwinska A, Domagala W, Czardybon A, Pilawa B, Lapkowski M. In situ EPR spectroelectrochemical studies of paramagnetic centres in poly(3, 4 ethylenedioxythiophene) (PEDOT) and poly(3, 4-butylenedioxythiophene) (PBuDOT) films. Chemical Physics 2003;292(1): 31-45.

[14] Moskwa T, Domagala W, Czardybon A, Pilawa B, Lapkowski M. ESR spectroelectrochemistry of functionalised long side chain derivatives of poly(3, 4-ethylenedioxythiophene). Synthetic Metals 2005;152(1-3): 189-192.

[15] Pilawa B, Więckowski AB, Trzebicka B. Numerical analysis of EPR spectra of coal, macerals and extraction products. Radiation Physics and Chemistry 1995;45(6): 899-908.

[16] Pilawa B, Więckowski AB. Comparative e. p. r. analysis of interactions between macerals and atmospheric oxygen. Fuel 1997;76(12): 1173-1177.

[17] Pilawa B, Więckowski AB, Pietrzak R, Wachowska H. Microwave saturation of EPR spectra of oxidised coal. Central European Journal of Chemistry 2007;5(1): 330-340.

[18] Pilawa B, Więckowski AB. Groups of paramagnetic center in coal samples with different carbon contents. Research on Chemical Intermediates 2007;33(8-9): 825-839.

[19] Pilawa B, Więckowski AB, Wachowska H, Kozłowski M. Effect of reduction and butylation on coal. Application of saturation of two-component EPR spectra. Applied Magnetic Resonance 2003;24: 73-83.

[20] Więckowski AB, Pilawa B, Lewandowski M, Wojtowicz W, Słowik G. Paramagnetic Centres in Exinite, Vitrinite and Inertinite. Applied Magnetic Resonance 1998;15(3-4): 489-501.

[21] Weszka J, Hajduk B, Zdybel M, Pilawa B. Dependence of EPR spectra on conditions of PPI thin films deposition. Paper presented at: Polymer on the Odra River; 6-7.07.2011; Opole.

[22] Pawłowska-Góral K, Ramos P, Pilawa B, Kurzeja E. Application of EPR spectroscopy to examination of the effect of sterilization process on free radicals in different herbs. Food Biophysics 2013;8(1): 60-68.

[23] Pawłowska-Góral K, Pilawa B. Detection of free radicals formed by in vitro metabolism of fluoride using EPR spectroscopy. Toxicology in Vitro 2011;25(7): 1269-1273.

[24] Pilawa B, Latocha M, Kościelniak M, Pietrzak R, Wachowska H. Oxygen effects in tumor cells during photodynamic therapy. Polish Journal of Environmental Studies 2006;15: 160-162.

[25] Latocha M, Pilawa B, Dudek J, Biniszkiewicz T, Kozdrowska L, Sieroń A, Wilczok T. Free radicals in melanotic human melanoma and human colon adenocarcinoma cells after photodynamic therapy. Physica Medica 2004;20(1): 61-63.

[26] Latocha M, Pilawa B, Zdybel M, Wilczok T. Effect of laser radiation on free radicals in human cancer G361 cells. Acta Physica Polonica A 2005;108(2): 409-412.

[27] Krzywda A, Petelenz E, Michalczyk D, Płonka PM. Sclerotia of the acellular (true) slime mould *Fuligo septica* as a model to study melanization and anabiosis. Cellular & Molecular Biology Letters 2008;13: 130-143.

[28] Okazaki M, Kuwata K, Miki Y, Shiga S, Shiga T. Electron spin relaxation of synthetic melanin and melanin-containing human tissues as studied by electron spin echo and electron spin resonance. Archives of Biochemistry and Biophysics 1985;242: 197-205.

[29] Zecca L, Costi P, Mecacci C, Ito S, Terreni M, Sonnino S. Interaction of human substantia nigra neuromelanin with lipids and peptides. Journal of Neurochemistry 2000;74: 1758-1765.

[30] Zucca FA, Giaveri G, Gallorini M, Albertini A, Toscani M, Pezzoli G, Lucius R, Wilms H, Sulzer D, Ito S, Wakamatsu K, Zecca L. The neuromelanin of human substantia nigra: physiological and pathogenic aspects. Pigment Cell Research 2004;17: 610-617.

[31] Plonka PM, Michalczyk D, Popik M, Handjiski B, Slominski A, Paus R. Splenic eumelanin differs from hair eumelanin in C57BL/6 mice. Acta Biochimica Polonica 2005;52: 433-441.

[32] Sarna T. Badanie struktury i właściwości centrów aktywnych melanin. Zagadnienia Biofizyki Współczesnej 1981;6: 201-219.

[33] Sealy RC, Hyde JS, Felix CC, Menon IA, Prota G. Eumelanins and pheomelanins: characterization by electron spin resonance spectroscopy. Science 1982;217: 545-547.

[34] Jung K, Seifert M, Herrling T, Fuchs J. UV-generated free radicals (FR) in skin: their prevention by sunscreens and their induction by self-tanning agents. Spectrochim Acta A 2008;69(5): 1423-1428.

[35] Zdybel M, Pilawa B, Kościelniak-Ziemniak M, Czyżyk D, Adamczyk J. Application of EPR spectroscopy to examination of free radicals in thermally sterilized chlortalidone. Farmaceutyczny Przegląd Naukowy 2010;7(2): 21-25.

[36] Ramos P, Pilawa B, Stroka E. EPR studies of free radicals in thermally sterilized famotidine. Nukleonika 2013;58(3): 413-418.

[37] Ramos P, Pilawa B, Wilczyński S, Czyż K, Adamczyk J. Effect of heating at 180°C on paramagnetic properties of diclofenac-EPR study. Engineering of Biomaterials 2009;12(87): 7-12.

[38] Skowrońska A, Wojciechowski M, Ramos P, Pilawa B, Kruk D. ESR studies of paramagnetic centers in pharmaceutical materials-Cefaclor and Clarithromycin as an example. Acta Physica Polonica A 2012;121(2): 514-517.

[39] Kościelniak-Ziemniak M, Pilawa B. Application of EPR Spectroscopy for Examination of Free Radical Formation in Thermally Sterilized Betamethasone, Clobetasol, and Dexamethasone. Applied Magnetic Resonance 2012;42(4): 519-530.

[40] Ramos P, Pepliński P, Pilawa B. Free radicals in thermally sterilized verapamil. Engineering of Biomaterials 2009;12(89-91): 162-164.

[41] Krztoń A, Liszka B, Ramos P, Pilawa B. FT-IR and EPR studies of changes of chemical structure of ampicyline during thermal sterilization. Engineering of Biomaterials 2009;12(89-91): 153-156.

[42] Ramos P, Pilawa B, Krztoń A, Liszka B. Free radicals in the thermally sterilized aminoglycoside antibiotics. Pharmaceutica Analytica Acta 2012;3(9): 1-13.

[43] Ramos P, Pilawa P. Effect of temperature and time of thermal sterilization on formation of free radicals in isosorbide. Farmaceutyczny Przegląd Naukowy 2010;7(5): 28-33.

[44] Wilczyński S, Lekki J, Kwiatek W, Chodurek E, Pilawa B. Formation of paramagnetic centers in sterilized gentamicin and neomycin irradiated by protons. Polish Journal of Environmental Studies 2006;15(4): 216-218.

[45] Wilczyński S, Pilawa B, Koprowski R, Wróbel Z, Ptaszkiewicz M, Swakoń J, Olko P. EPR studies of free radical decay and survival in gamma irradiated aminoglycoside antibiotics: sisomicin, tobramycin and paromomycin. European Journal of Pharmaceutical Sciences 2012;45: 251-262.

[46] Wilczyński S, Ptaszkiewicz M, Pierzchała E, Pilawa B, Swakoń J, Olko P. Electron paramagnetic resonance studies of gamma irradiated azithromycin. Current Topics in Biophysics 2008;31: 1-4.

[47] Wilczyński S, Ramos P, Pilawa B, Ptaszkiewicz M, Swakoń J, Olko P. Comparison of free radicals properties in radiosterilized and thermally sterilized streptomycin. Engineering of Biomaterials 2009;12(89-91): 170-172.

[48] Wilczyński S, Pilawa B, Ptaszkiewicz M, Swakoń J, Olko P. Free radicals properties of gamma irradiated solid forms of drugs. Engineering of Biomaterials 2008;11(81-84): 52-54.

[49] Deda A, Wilczyński S, Zdybel M, Pierzchała E, Pilawa B. Zastosowanie spektroskopii elektronowego rezonansu paramagnetycznego (EPR) w kosmetologii. Dermatologia Estetyczna 2010;12(4): 220-225.

[50] Deda A, Pierzchała E, Wilczyński S, Zdybel M, Pilawa B. Badania wolnych rodników w kosmetologii metodą elektronowego rezonansu paramagnetycznego (EPR). Zeszyty Naukowe Wyższej Szkoły Nauk Społecznych z siedzibą w Lublinie – Kosmetologia 2010;1: 11-22.

[51] Pilawa B, Pietrzak R, Wachowska H, Babeł K. EPR studies of carbonized cellulose – oxygen interactions. Acta Physica Polonica A 2005;108(2): 151-154.

[52] Pilawa B, Zdybel M, Buszman E, Witoszyńska T, Cieśla H. Effect of flucytosine on paramagnetic properties of Cladosporium cladosporioides. Engineering of Biomaterials 2009;12(89-91): 167-169.

[53] Zdybel M, Pilawa B, Buszman E, Witoszyńska T, Brotoń B. Paramagnetism of pigmented soil fungi of Cladosporium herbarum. Engineering of Biomaterials 2009;12(89-91): 172-174.

[54] Pawłowska-Góral K, Kurzeja E, Pilawa B, Ramos P. EPR studies of Rhizoma calami. Engineering of Biomaterials 2009;12(89-91): 159-161.

[55] Rozancew EG, Szolle WD. Chemia organiczna wolnych rodników. Warszawa: PWN; 1985.

[56] Bilińska B, Pilawa B, Zawada Z, Wylegala E, Wilczok T, Dontsov AE, Sakina NL, Ostrovsky MA, Ilyasova VB. Electron spin resonance investigations of human retinal pigment epithelium melanosomes from young and old donors. Spectrochimica Acta Part A 2002;58: 2257-2264.

[57] Tran ML, Powell BJ, Meredith P. Chemical and structural disorder in eumelanins: a possible explanation for broadband absorbance. Biophysical Journal 2006;90: 743-752.

[58] Ito S, Wakamatsu K, Ozeki H. Chemical analysis of melanins and its application to the study of regulation of melanogenesis. Pigment Cell Research 2000;13: 103-109.

[59] Wakamatsu K, Ito S. Advanced chemical methods in melanin determination. Pigment Cell Research 2002;15: 174-183.

[60] Durairaj C, Chastain JE, Kompella UB. Intraocular distribution of melanin in human, monkey, rabbit, minipig and dog eyes. Experimental Eye Research 2012;98: 23-27.

[61] Leblanc B, Jezequel S, Davies T, Hanton G, Taradach C. Binding of drugs to eye melanin is not predictive of ocular toxicity. Regulatory Toxicology and Pharmacology 1998;28(2): 124-132.

[62] Schmidt SY, Peisch RD. Melanin concentration in normal human retinal pigment epithelium. Regional variation and age-related reduction. Investigative Ophthalmology & Visual Science 1986;27(7): 1063-1067.

[63] Prota G, Hu DN, Vincensi MR, McCormick SA, Napolitano A. Characterization of melanins in human irides and cultured uveal melanocytes from eyes of different colors. Experimental Eye Research 1998;67(3): 293-299.

[64] Pilawa B, Chodurek E, Wilczok T. Types of paramagnetic centres in Cu^{2+}complexes with model neuromelanins. Applied Magnetic Resonance 2003;24: 417-422.

[65] Beberok A, Buszman E, Zdybel M, Pilawa B, Wrześniok D. EPR examination of free radical properties of DOPA-melanin complexes with ciprofloxacin, lomefloxacin, norfloxacin and sparfloxacin. Chemical Physics Letters 2010;497(1-3): 115-122.

[66] Najder-Kozdrowska L, Pilawa B, Więckowski AB, Buszman E, Wrześniok D. Influence of copper(II) ions on radicals in DOPA-melanin. Applied Magnetic Resonance 2009;36(1): 81-88.

[67] Buszman E, Pilawa B, Zdybel M, Wrześniok D, Grzegorczyk A, Wilczok T. EPR examination of $Zn^{2+}$and Cu^{2+}effect on free radicals in DOPA-melanin-netilmicin complexes. Chemical Physics Letters 2005;403(1-3): 22-28.

[68] Chodurek E, Zdybel M, Pilawa B, Dzierżewicz Z. Examination by EPR spectroscopy of free radicals in melanins isolated from A-375 cells exposed on valproic acid and cisplatin. Acta Poloniae Pharmaceutica – Drug Research 2012;69: 1334-1341.

[69] Hu DN, Savage HE, Roberts JE. Uveal melanocytes, ocular pigment epithelium, and Müller cells in culture: in vitro toxicology. International Journal of Toxicology 2002;21: 465-472.

[70] Sarna T. Properties and function of the ocular melanin-A photobiophysical view. Journal of Photochemistry and Photobiology B: Biology 1992;12: 215-258.

[71] Najder-Kozdrowska L, Pilawa B, Buszman E, Więckowski AB, Świątkowska L, Wrześniok D, Wojtowicz W. Triplet states in DOPA-melanin and in its complexes with kanamycin and copper Cu(II) ions. Acta Physica Polonica A 2010;118(4): 613-618.

[72] Zdybel M. Multi-component system of paramagnetic centers in DOPA-melanin complexes with netilmicin, zinc(II) and copper(II) ions. PhD thesis. Medical University of Silesia in Katowice; 2008.

[73] Zdybel M, Pilawa B, Buszman E, Wrześniok D. Effect of oxygen on free radicals in DOPA-melanin complexes with netilmicin, diamagnetic Zn(II), and paramagnetic Cu(II). Chemical Physics Letters 2013;556: 278-286.

[74] Pilawa B, Latocha M, Buszman E, Wilczok T. Effect of oxygen on spin-spin and spin-lattice relaxation in DOPA-melanin. Complexes with chloroquine and metal ions. Applied Magnetic Resonance 2003;25: 105-111.

[75] Zdybel M, Pilawa B, Buszman E, Witoszyńska T. EPR studies Cladosporium cladosporioides complexes with amphotericin B. Nukleonika 2013;58(3): 401-405.

[76] Matuszczyk M, Buszman E, Pilawa B, Witoszyńska T, Wilczok T. Cd^{2+}effect on free radicals in Cladosporium cladosporioides-melanin tested by EPR spectroscopy. Chemical Physics Letters 2004;394(4-6): 366-371.

[77] Pilawa B, Buszman E, Gondzik A, Wilczyński S, Zdybel M, Witoszyńska T, Wilczok T. Effect of pH on paramagnetic centers in Cladosporium cladosporioides. Acta Physica Polonica A 2005;108(1): 147-150.

[78] Buszman E, Pilawa B, Latocha M, Wilczok T, Tyrawska-Spychałowa D, Bajan C, Bijak A, Bilińska B. Spectroscopic studies of melanins isolated from pigmented soil fungi of the Karkonosze Mountains. Current Topics in Biophysics 1998;22: 21-24.

[79] Kurzeja E, Stec M, Ramos P, Pilawa B, Pawłowska-Góral K. The influence of sterilization on free-radical generation, discoloration and the antioxidant properties of certain spice herbs. Italian Journal of Food Science 2012;24(3): 254-261.

[80] Kurzeja E, Stec M, Ramos P, Pilawa B, Pawłowska-Góral K. Antioxidant properties of water extracts of sterilized and unsterilized Morus Alba L. leaves. International Journal of Food Properties 2013;16(4): 723-737.

[81] Rzepecka-Stojko A, Pilawa B, Ramos P, Stojko J. Antioxidative properties of bee pollen extracts examined by EPR spectroscopy. Journal of Apicultural Science 2012;56(1): 23-31.

2

Electronic Communication and Digital Images: Referral Pathways and Clinical Uses in Ophthalmology

Hannah Timlin and Roshini Sanders

1. Introduction

Our eyes are the only place in the body where abnormalities such as blocked blood vessels and pale atrophied nerves can be directly visualised and subsequently diagnosed without further invasive tests. This is due to the transparent properties of the cornea, aqueous humour, lens and vitreous. This unique property of the eye lends itself well to being photographed. We now have the technology to image all the structures of the eye, all the way from the cornea, through the lens to the retina, choroid and optic nerve. This even includes anterior chamber cells and flair. We now live in a world where the average camera has superseded the resolution of the human eye, allowing the ability to visualise small retinal lesions such as exudates only when digital imaging and zooming is performed. Additionally, technology which uses optical coherence tomography and scanning lasers produce images, which show information and data on the layers of the retina and nerve fibre thickness which cannot be visualised by the ophthalmologists' examination. This chapter aims to describe how digital images and internet connections, including the roll out of 3G and 4G mobile networks, are utilised to aid ophthalmologists and benefit patients around the world.

Internet connections have grown exponentially over the last 20 years, connecting rural areas to cities, and developing countries to developed countries. The rapid adoption of smartphones has also helped to increase the number of doctors and patients who have easy access to the internet. This rapid adoption of smartphone internet access is particularly apparent in developing countries, who previously had little internet access due to a sparse fixed line telecommunication infrastructure. The cost of smartphone handsets and mobile data prices are dropping and thus becoming more affordable for many. Broadband, 3G and 4G connections allow these digital images to be sent anywhere around the world within seconds. Thus, eye conditions can be diagnosed in patients who are remote to the doctor, in both place and time.

Ophthalmology departments worldwide are under intensifying pressure to reduce referral waiting times and work at a faster pace to deliver new sight saving treatments. Studies increasingly demonstrate that treatment of potentially blinding conditions, such as wet age related macular degeneration (ARMD) and retinal vein occlusion are most efficacious in preventing sight loss when treatment is commenced promptly [1]. This strain on ophthalmology departments has been compounded by the exponential growth of wet ARMD in an aging population where life expectancy is increasing. This means that traditional systems for referring patients and reviewing them in clinics many weeks later need to be updated to adapt to these time pressures. Digital electronic communication, if embraced, can have a significant impact on ophthalmic service. Digital image referrals can be reviewed within seconds and can avoid an unnecessary wait for the clinic review before investigation or treatment can begin.

2. Benefits of electronic digital diagnosis

Electronic digital diagnoses in ophthalmology mean that the patient and the doctor do not have to meet face to face, nor at the same time. These two basic principles have widespread benefits for the patient, non-ophthalmic clinicians and ophthalmologists;

- The patient doesn't have to travel long distances to see the doctor, benefiting patients' time and reducing cost.
- The patient can be seen in a location and at a time which suits them best.
- The patient's images can be seen by the most appropriate subspecialty doctor, rather than the doctor in the hospital on the day that the patient visits, who may not be an expert in that subspecialty.
- It facilitates rapid discussion of difficult cases between multiple doctors around the world, rather than the patient travelling to different hospitals for multiple opinions.
- It facilitates the screening of referrals, leading to some patients not requiring hospital review.
- The patient can be triaged, ensuring that conditions requiring urgent review and treatment are given priority clinics.
- Doctors can monitor patients' progress through self-photographing and emailing to their consultant.

There are many examples of how Ophthalmology departments worldwide are starting to use digital images to aid with telemedicine, for diagnosis, triage and follow up communication with other ophthalmologists or non-ophthalmic clinicians. Additionally digital images are enhancing communication between patients and their ophthalmologist. Some of these are described below.

3. Anterior segment

3.1. Periocular skin abnormalities

There are many differential diagnoses to eyelid lumps, which may pose diagnostic difficulty for General Practitioners. These lesions are easily amenable to photography with either a standard camera at the GP practice or a slit lamp mounted camera at the optometry practice. The most important thing is to differentiate between benign and malignant lesions. Most benign lesions such as cysts, naevae, chalazia, molluscum contagiosum and xanthelasma need not be seen by an ophthalmologist, whereas malignant lesions require soon review and treatment in an appropriate oculoplastic oncology clinic. The most common eyelid tumour is a basal cell carcinoma, which can be diagnosed in many cases by an ophthalmologist from a photograph though signs such as a skin lump with rolled pearly edges, ulceration, crusting or loss of lashes. However, care must be taken with morphoeic basal cell carcinomas or sebaceous cell carcinomas as these have subtle signs and are often misdiagnosed as scarring or blepharitis from photographs or clinical examination. Patients with an obvious malignant lesion on a referral photograph can be directly booked into a one-stop minor procedure clinic. This misses out the assessment clinic step, thus reducing the time from referral to treatment.

It is important to estimate the size of a malignant lesion so that appropriate reconstruction can be planned in the correct location, such as theatre if the lesion is large rather than a clinical procedure room if the lesion is small. This can be difficult to do on digital images and we have found it extremely useful for referrers to place a ruler within the photograph.

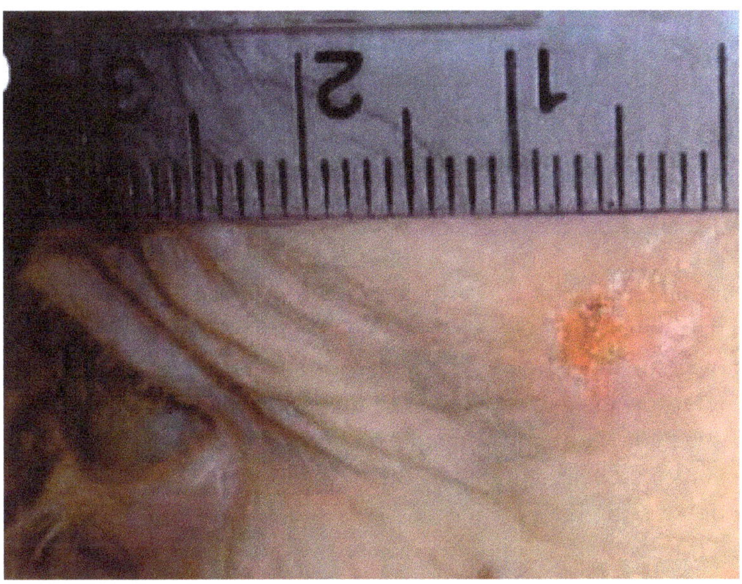

Figure 1. Photograph of a 10mm Periocular Basal Cell Carcinoma referred by an optometrist. This shows the classic signs of rolled pearly edges with central ulceration. This patient was booked directly into a minor procedure list for excision and rhomboid flap reconstruction.

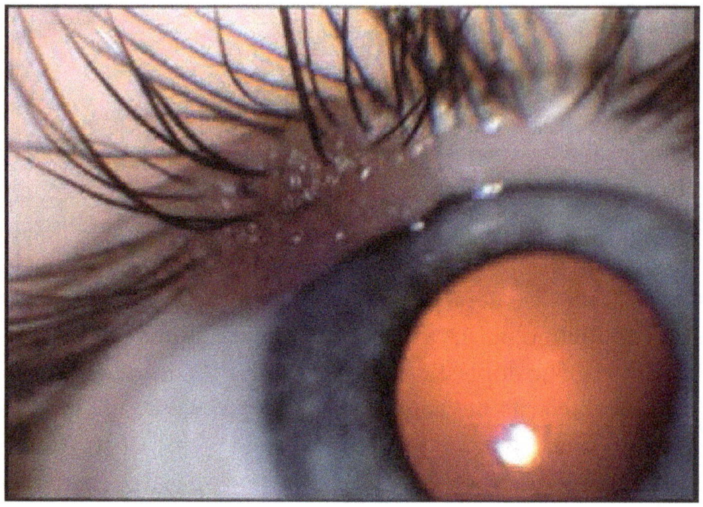

Figure 2. Photograph of an eyelid naevus, demonstrating normal growth of lashes though the benign lesion

3.1.1. Patient communication examples

Although there is limited published evidence of the use of electronic digital diagnosis in the periocular area of the skin by ophthalmologists, we can utilize the experience from dermatologists. In Brisbane, patient generated photographs of melanocytic skin lesions from camera phones showed 69% diagnostic concordance with face to face diagnosis, suggesting potential for remote diagnosis [2]. In Dundee, referrals of suspected malignant skin lesions from GPs which included digital images had reduced time to diagnosis by 81% and time to treatment by 30%, with diagnostic accuracy comparable to face to face diagnosis [3].

Digital images can also be useful for monitoring progress following skin surgery. In Heidelberg, plastic surgeons monitor post-operative skin flaps using smart phone images sent from the patient at home. Compared to traditional in-person clinic review, the response time to re-exploration was significantly shorter [4]. In Taiwan, this method enabled rapid and thus successful re-exploration [5].

It is relatively simple for patients to use their own phone to photograph themselves and email the image within a few seconds, without having to get off their sofa. This can be planned every day postoperatively, or as and when the patient has concerns. It is easy to foresee how this enables rapid detection of problems when compared with a planned one week follow up hospital appointment. It is not unimaginable that patients following ptosis surgery or periocular reconstruction could be monitored by their consultant through smartphone images, with a hospital visit only required if an abnormality is seen on the photographs such as erythema and discharge. Other potential examples of their use are; a patient emailing in a photograph showing over correction of a ptosis could be advised to perform lash traction over an email without needing to attend the hospital, or a patient emailing in a camera phone image of a graft showing contraction and ectropion can be advised to perform firm massage without having to attend the hospital.

3.2. Corneal, conjunctival and anterior chamber abnormalities

Many corneal and conjunctival images are amenable to digital imaging for example pterygium, pinguecula, conjunctival pigmentation, corneal scarring, corneal vascularisation, ulcers and hypopion. Larger lesions can be photographed with a standard camera, whereas smaller lesions, particularly of the cornea are best imaged using a slit lamp camera. Various illumination techniques commonly used by the ophthalmologist can be used for the slit lamp camera also. Direct diffuse illumination is most commonly used. However, more information can be gained by using the fine slit direct illumination or retroillumination using the red reflex from the fundus. Indirect and scleral scatter can be harder to photograph.

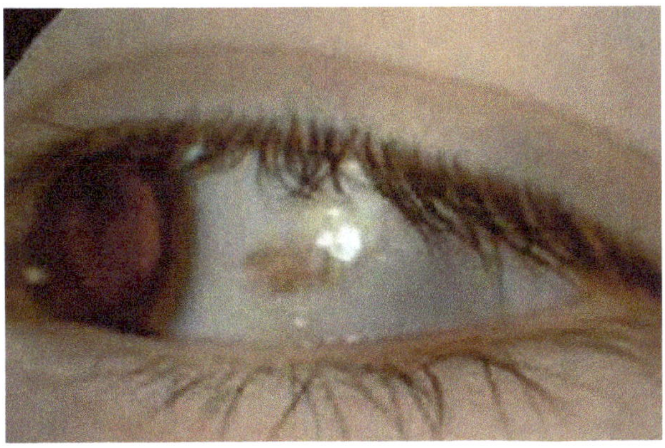

Figure 3. Photograph of a benign pigmented conjunctival naevus in a child

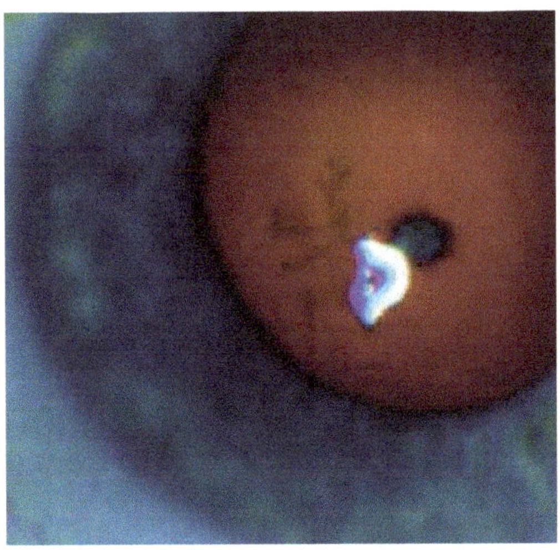

Figure 4. Slit lamp photograph of a dendritic ulcer seen with retroillumination, using the red reflex of the fundus to illuminate the corneal epithelial lesion.

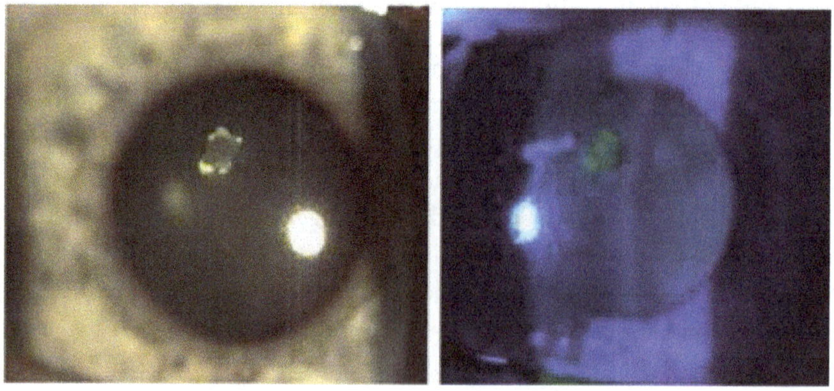

Figure 5. Slit lamp photographs using white light with no filter and cobalt blue filter showing a white foreign body on the cornea which stains with fluorescence.

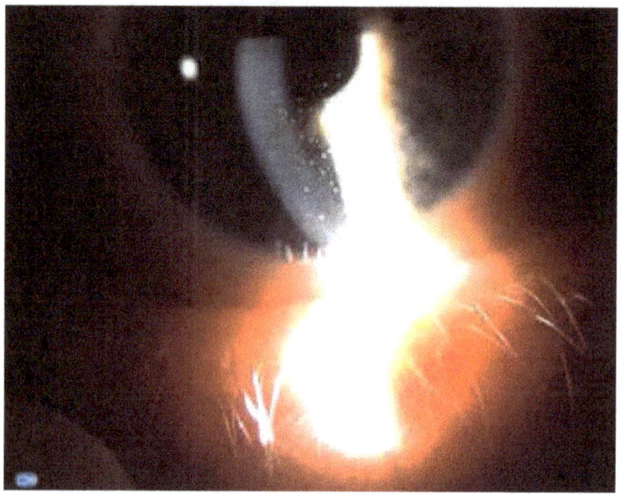

Figure 6. Slit lamp photograph using a broad beam of light showing keratic precipitates on the endothelium

3.2.1. Non-ophthalmic clinician communication example

In Perth, Western Australia, a portable hand held slit lamp camera has been created to be small, portable and simple to operate by health care workers across the large geographical area of Western Australia. They have demonstrated that this instrument had good correlation to slit lamp anterior segment image diagnoses [6].

3.2.2. Patient communication example

Perhaps ophthalmologists could learn from dermatologists in Austria, whose patients on biologics for psoriasis send in weekly camera phone images for monitoring [7]. This could potentially be used for conditions such as mucous membrane pemphigoid, where frequent images over years can perhaps be made into a time-lapse video, which could potentially show clearer evidence of disease progression than clinical drawings. This technology is currently used in natural history programmes to demonstrate slowly changing environments such as sand dunes, within a few seconds of film, and could be easily adapted into the ophthalmic domain.

4. Posterior segment

4.1. Glaucoma

Glaucoma is a massive worldwide problem. The problem with open angle glaucoma is the lack of symptoms perceived by the patient. This means that patients will only self-present with end-stage glaucoma once central vision is being lost, when treatment is less effective. In poorer communities, most of the population is not examined regularly by an optometrist or ophthalmologist. In these places, the issue is the lack of diagnosis, which could be assisted with the use of health care assistants with camera phones, sending the images over the internet to a distant ophthalmologist for diagnosis.

In more affluent communities, optometrists are trained to rigorously screen for any sign or suspicion of glaucoma and refer to a hospital assessment e.g. raised intraocular pressure, field loss and abnormal optic disc appearance including thinned rim, change in cup disc ratio and disc haemorrhage. The main issues here are that of a high rate of false positives (the worried well) and the large volume of patients requiring long term hospital follow up. Many of these glaucoma suspects require hospital review over a few years only to then be discharged without requiring any treatment. Additionally, many ocular hypertensives are detected and require long term follow up without ever developing any field loss. These two examples constitute a large volume of patients seen in hospital eye services, and who would benefit from a digital electronic virtual clinic. All the data required by the consultant for the patients' management can be viewed digitally with computerised field of vision data sheets, intraocular pressure documentation and optic disc images with or without further ancillary glaucoma tests including red free photographs of the nerve fibre layer, optic disc Ocular Coherence Tomography, Heidelberg Retina Tomography and Scanning Laser Polarimetry. Thus large numbers of patients can be monitored by the consultant ophthalmologist virtually.

There is an obvious difference between slit lamp disc examination of the optic disc, which is binocular and thus 3D, and a standard fundus image which is 2D. The optic disc rim shape and cup disc ratio in 2D images are often interpreted using the colour change from the peach coloured optic rim to the whiter coloured optic cup and the distortion of blood vessels, rather than depth perception. This can lead to inaccurate interpretation of the optic disc. However, this can be accommodated for to some extent using serial photographs to identify subtle anatomical change over time and with stereo images where two photographs of the optic disc are taken from slightly different angles and viewed on a screen either side by side and viewed with specially designed goggles or displayed alternately with a fast flicker, where no goggles are required.

4.1.1. Allied ophthalmic professionals communication examples

Data from Virtual Glaucoma Clinics in Portsmouth have been published. These virtual clinics involve the glaucoma consultant electronically reviewing digital disc images, Humphrey visual field tests and Goldman intraocular pressure results to assess new glaucoma referrals without meeting the patients. 94% of disc photographs were gradable and only 32% of patients required to be accepted into the hospital eye clinic, thus saving 1400 clinic appointments per year [8]. Swansea performed a virtual glaucoma clinic trial using scanning laser ophthalmoscopy. Although 22% of images were unable to be graded, the remaining had 94% sensitivity and 87% specificity when compared to clinical assessment, with no case of glaucoma being misdiagnosed [9]. These two examples demonstrate how digital images can enable a consultant to review more glaucoma referrals in a shorter period of time than if examining the patient themselves thus saving money.

In these two published virtual glaucoma clinics, the patients still attended the hospital but were seen directly by photographers, nurses and hospital optometrists. There is potential for the tests to be performed at the patients' local optometry practice to save on travel time and costs. However, this would be limited by the costs of purchasing investigative equipment such as computerised field of vision analysers and fundus cameras.

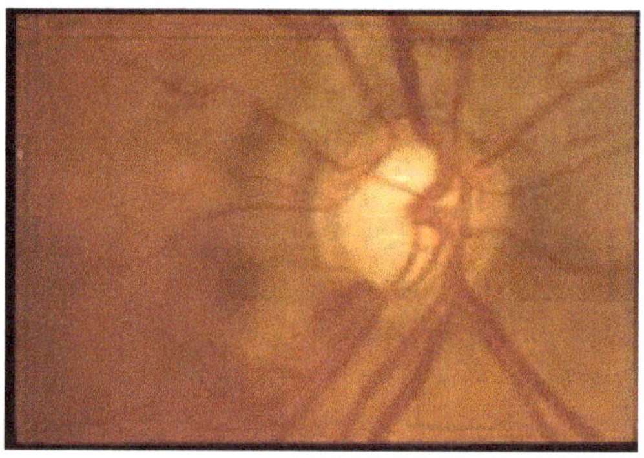

Figure 7. Right optic disc photograph taken by an optometrist at a local practise. This shows inferior temporal disc haemorrhage and rim thinning. This rim thinning is seen on this 2D image by the location of both the colour change and blood vessel distortion. This patient was given a glaucoma assessment clinic and diagnosed with glaucoma.

4.2. Disc anomalies

Normal optic discs have a huge range of appearances. Thus there is a large grey area where an unusual looking disc can either be at one end of the normal range or be showing pathology. Pattern recognition plays a large part in determining a diagnosis in these patients. Optometrists and General Practitioners see large volumes of normal optic discs and thus find it difficult to distinguish between disease and normal range. The main condition which causes concern in this area is bilateral swollen discs with diagnosis of possible raised intracranial pressure. This can trigger referral for a CT scan and lumbar puncture, both of which have side effects. Actual diagnoses are often myopic discs, where the large peripapillary atrophy is misinterpreted as disc oedema and swelling when performing a uniocular examination through a direct ophthalmoscope by a non-ophthalmologist, or optic disc drusen which can give a lumpy raised appearance and scalloped margins with anomalous vascular branching. Digital imaging and an ophthalmologist's opinion can negate the need for these unnecessary tests in many within a few seconds of seeing the image.

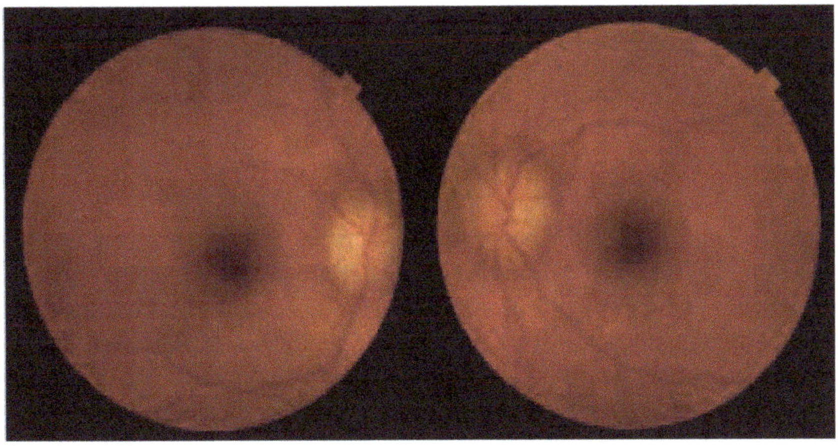

Figure 8. Fundus photographs of a child, taken at their local optometry practice showing bilateral disc swelling. This is characterised on digital 2D image as blurred disc margin due to oedema, curving of blood vessels over the swollen nerve with an angle as the vessel flattens onto the retina, reduced or no colour change from optic disc rim to cup due to swelling. The digital electronic referral of these images was seen within minutes by a consultant ophthalmologist who was able to arrange a CT scan and paediatric admission to the patient's local hospital all of which was performed within 2 hours, without the need for long travel and time delay to the regional Emergency Eye Clinic. The patient was diagnosed with a brain tumour and raised intracranial pressure.

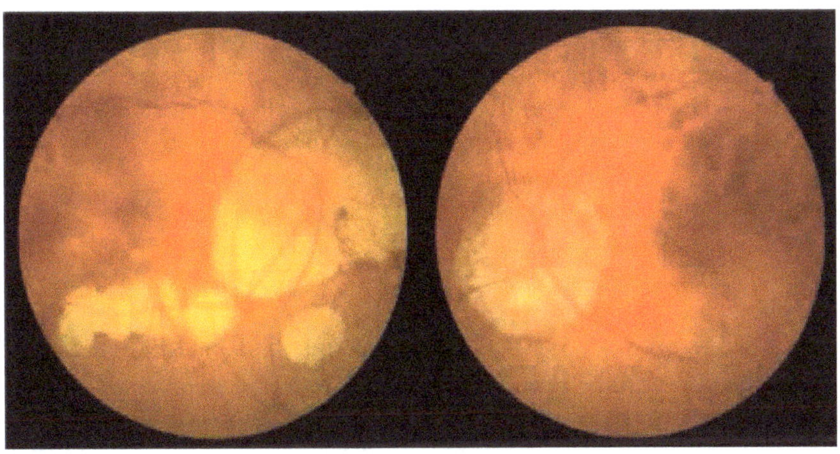

Figure 9. Fundus photographs of a patient with myopic discs. This patient was misdiagnosed as swollen discs due to the 'large' pale discs with no visible cup. An ophthalmologist can see in the photo that this is significant peripapillary atrophy and reassure the referrer. The digital image electronic referral means that a diagnosis is made quickly and the patient does not need to travel to the eye department or undergo CT scans or lumbar punctures.

4.3. Retinopathy of prematurity

Retinopathy of prematurity guidelines recommend fundus screening to be performed 1 to 2 weekly in babies of <32 weeks gestation or <=1.5kg at birth [10]. Physical examination with an indirect ophthalmoscope and indentation is a difficult skill to master and is thus done by very experienced ophthalmologists. Additionally, the process of examination can be distressing for the baby and often affects their vital signs. The guidelines recommend grading retinopathy according to the area of retina where normal vascular development has occurred as well as the extent of abnormal vessels that have grown, along with their sequelae. These grades dictate whether treatment of the peripheral retina with laser is recommended, which is done by an expert usually in a tertiary referral centre [10].

4.3.1. Non-ophthalmic clinician communication examples

However, these premature babies have multiple other comorbidities making transfer over long distances to tertiary hospitals precarious for their health and life. Studies have shown that only 6% of these babies actually develop sight threatening disease [10] and require treatment by a specialist ophthalmologist. Thus, this condition is ideally suited to digital image screening where babies in peripheral hospitals have their fundus photographs taken by trained nurses. These are then emailed to the specialist ophthalmologist in the distant tertiary centre for grading. This method of viewing the fundus is also potentially less distressing for the baby. For some time, the wide field 120 degrees camera Retcam has been used for this purpose, producing clear images and reliable grading [11-16]. The use of this digital screening system means that most babies can stay in their hospital surroundings without the instability of a transfer. The only babies requiring transfer are those 6% requiring laser treatment, without which vision loss and blindness can develop. More recently, the noncontact ultra-widefield Optos dual wavelength scanning laser ophthalmoscope Optomap is being used for this purpose in Oxford [17].

Recent advances in neonatology have led to an increase in the number of premature babies at risk of sight loss. However, the frequency of sight threatening retinopathy is low, meaning that experts in the field are small in number and often covering a large geographic area. In poorer, remote populations, these fundus cameras could allow robust and effective retinopathy of prematurity screening, where there had previously been none.

4.4. Diabetic retinopathy

4.4.1. Non-clinical personnel communication examples (medical photographers)

A national screening programme for diabetic retinopathy has been set up in the UK [18] with the use of mobile non-mydriatic fundus cameras operated by technicians. This programme enables all diabetic patients to have a fundus examination close to their home. These fundus images are graded electronically, with patients only needing to travel to the hospital ophthalmology clinic if there are signs of sight threatening retinopathy or maculopathy. In some regions, Optical Coherence Tomography images are also taken to screen for macula oedema, thus further reducing the number of patients requiring hospital appointments. The attendance rate is likely to be higher if the patients have to give up less time and money for travelling, thus screening occurs in multiple locations with mobile cameras. Teleretinal screening data for diabetic retinopathy has also been published from the USA [19,20], Bahrain [21], Canada [22,23] and France [24].

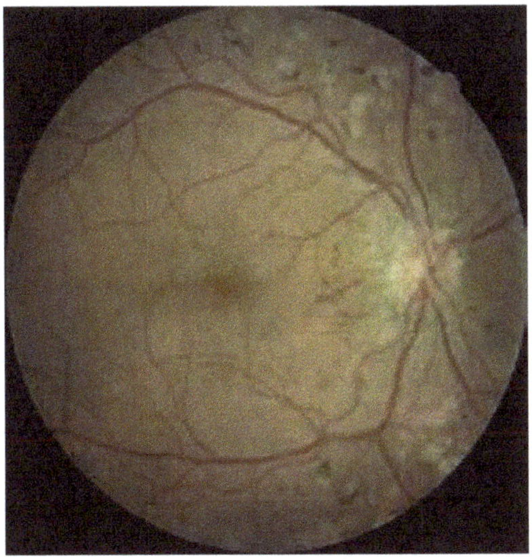

Figure 10. Diabetic Retinopathy screening photograph taken with a non-mydriatic fundus camera showing proliferative diabetic retinopathy with new vessels visible and previous pigmented pan retinal photocoagulation scars.

4.5. Wet age related macular degeneration

Age Related Macular Degeneration is a common condition causing visual loss. Unfortunately, only the less common wet subtype is treatable. Unnecessary referral and review of patients with the dry subtype are common and results in a large number of unnecessary hospital appointments. The wet type results from abnormal growth of vessels from the choroidal circulation into the retina and is identified clinically by intraretinal fluid and / or haemorrhage. Intraretinal fluid is best seen as retinal thickening when examining binocularly on the slit lamp, which cannot be perceived on a fundus photograph. However, photographic signs of fluid identifiable are a grey appearance, loss of focus of fine detail of the retina and distortion of blood vessels. Additionally Optical Coherence Tomography machines are becoming more widely available. These are now used routinely in the macular degeneration clinics as they can show even very small pockets of fluid within the retina which are not perceivable on slit lamp examination of the fundus. Use of these fundus and OCT images with referrals, has the scope to avoid the unnecessary hospital visit of a patient with dry age related macular degeneration.

4.5.1. Allied ophthalmic professionals communication examples

Evaluating colour retinal images of patients referred with suspected wet age related macular degeneration has been reported to have high sensitivity and specificity and facilitate more timely treatment [25]. In York, there is a Mobile Community Eye Care Clinic with OCT machines. This is relocated overnight on a 4 weekly location cycle around the region, with fundus and OCT images viewed at the central hospital [26]. In Salford, an optometry practise with an OCT machine refers in patient details with the OCT image via nhsmail, meaning that patients can attend directly for a treatment clinic [26]. Thus the patient's number of visits to the hospital is reduced.

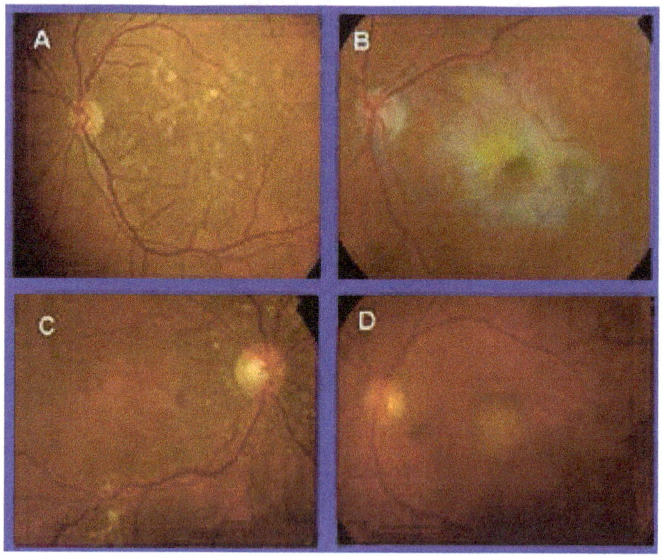

Figure 11. Four fundus photographs of patients referred by optometrists with macular degeneration, illustrating the benefit of fundus photographs when triaging hospital referrals. Figure 11A shows dry age related macular degeneration, which does not require hospital review. Figure 11B shows scaring from advanced wet age related macular degeneration with vision worse than 6/96, who can be directed to the low vision services. Figure 11C shows wet age related macular degeneration, which can be triaged to an urgent wet ARMD treatment clinic. Figure 11D shows a pigment epithelial detachment, which needs triage into an assessment clinic within 2 weeks. This last image illustrates the limitations of using images. In this case, the patient requires an Optical Coherence Tomography image, which their local optometrist did not have and thus required to be done at a hospital visit, in order to detect any intraretinal fluid that would require treatment.

Treatment of wet age related macular degeneration requires multiple intravitreal injections of anti vascular endothelial growth factor often over many years. Best visual outcomes occur when treatment is given within the first two weeks of disease onset. However, the number of wet age related macular degeneration patients are already greater than capacity, and with an aging population this is set to worsen. One solution to this crisis is a virtual clinic, which can be used to follow up patients who have been treated. Electronic Patient Databases have been shown to facilitate virtual wet age related macular degeneration diagnosis and monitoring by consultants, who can view a patient's vision, fundus image and OCT without face to face contact. This increases the number of patients monitored by a consultant within the same session [26].

4.6. Retinal vein occlusion

Central and branch retinal vein occlusions are common causes of reduced vision. The vast majority of cases do not require treatment. However, patients need to be monitored for the growth of new vessels, which requires laser treatment. More recently, treatment with intravitreal steroid or anti vascular endothelial growth factor have shown benefit in patients with macular oedema. Additionally, manufacturers report better visual outcomes if treatment is commenced promptly. Therefore patients with a vein occlusion would benefit from a digital electronic referral from the optometrist in a similar way to those with wet age related macular degeneration, where the referral is made via a fundus image email along with an Optical Coherence Tomography image when available to demonstrate the macular oedema. This would enable rapid triage for a soon appointment directly into a treatment clinic when macular oedema is seen.

4.7. Retinal lesions

Abnormal pigmentary changes are commonly detected by optometrists at routine review in asymptomatic patients. Common lesions detected are choroidal naevae, chorioretinal scars, congenital hypertrophy of retinal pigmented epithelium, laser scars and myelinated nerve fibres. None of these lesions are visually significant and thus are best managed in the community with digital imaging. The digital image acts firstly as a referral to an ophthalmologist who will often be happy to diagnose the condition on the image alone. Secondly, the image acts as a record for long term monitoring. If a choroidal naevus shows even a small growth from one image to the next, then referral for investigation for melanoma is required. Subtle changes in lesion appearance are much easier to detect when comparing image to image, rather than fundus examination to a drawing. Thus digital imaging enables rapid diagnosis and accurate monitoring for malignant signs.

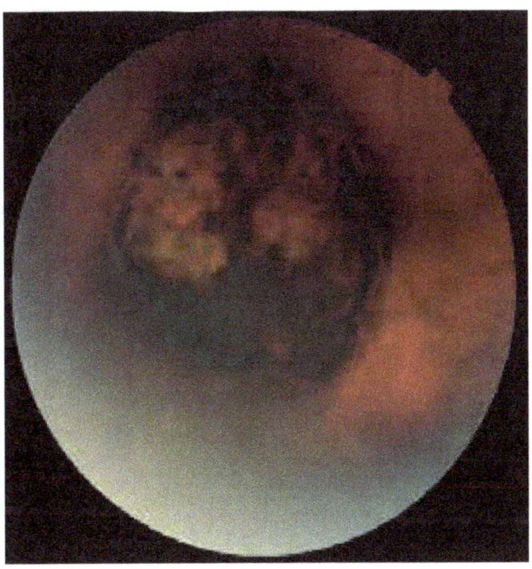

Figure 12. Fundus image showing pigmented chorioretinal scar. This is most likely a longstanding scar as the lesion has sharp pigmentary boundaries and no acute signs of haemorrhage or exudation. Therefore, the patient does not require hospital review.

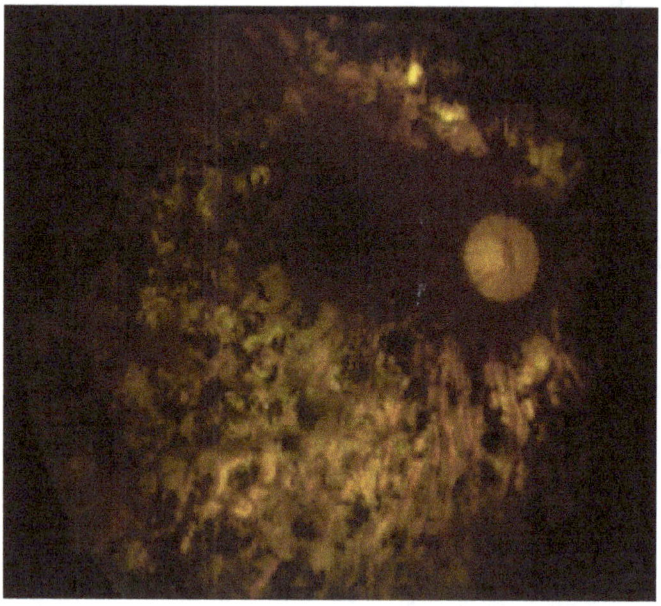

Figure 13. Fundus image showing heavy pan retinal photocoagulation, not requiring hospital review

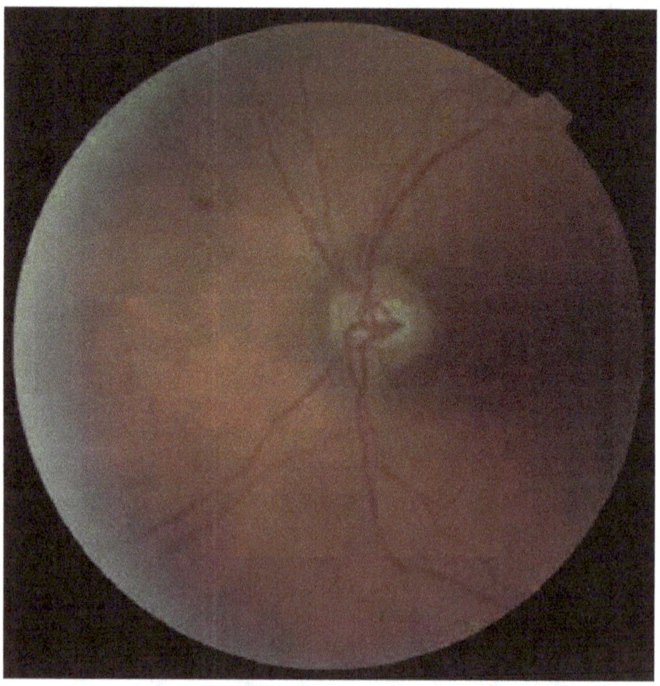

Figure 14. Fundus image showing an isolated small blot haemorrhage

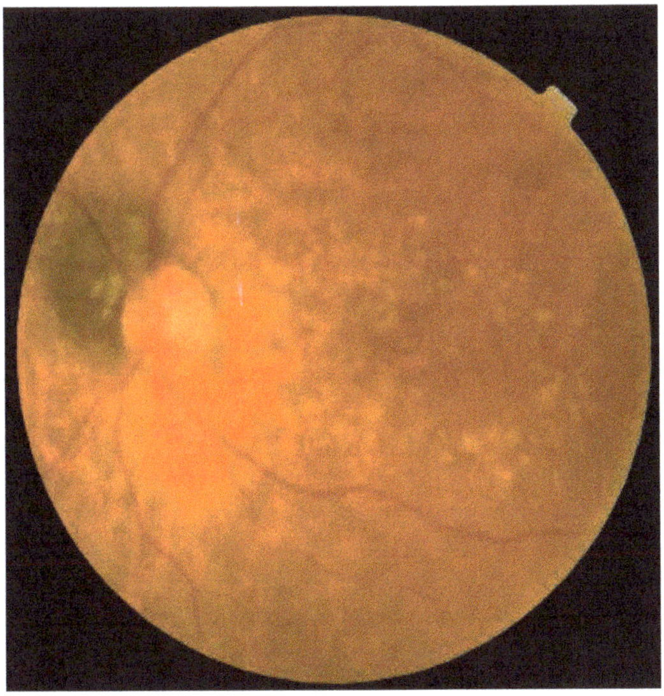

Figure 15. Fundus image showing a choroidal naevus at the disc and drusen. Careful monitoring is required and changes in the lesion are best detected by comparing fundus image to fundus image side by side.

4.8. Optos

One of the limitations of standard fundus imaging is the small field of view of 45 degrees, making it difficult to capture the mid peripheral and peripheral retina. Optos have developed the optomap ultra-widefield scanning laser ophthalmoscope which produces a pseudo-colour image [27].This is a significant addition to the current ophthalmic imaging tools. It has a 200 degree field of view enabling peripheral lesion imaging whilst simultaneously imaging the disc and macula, which enables the location of the lesion in relation to them. This is especially useful for picking up retinal detachments by non-ophthalmologists or documenting peripheral choroidal naevae or melanomas for long term follow up. The two main benefits to this system are that dilation is not required, and that it requires very little training to perform enabling a non-ophthalmologist to view large areas of the retina and share electronically via email.

4.8.1. Non clinical personnel example (medical photographers)

Studies in an emergency eye clinic have shown the Optos limitations at picking up only 33% of peripheral retinal tears and holes [28], although interestingly, this was the same accuracy as their casualty doctor's examination. However, it accurately photographed retinal detachments, which are commonly missed on conventional fundus imaging.

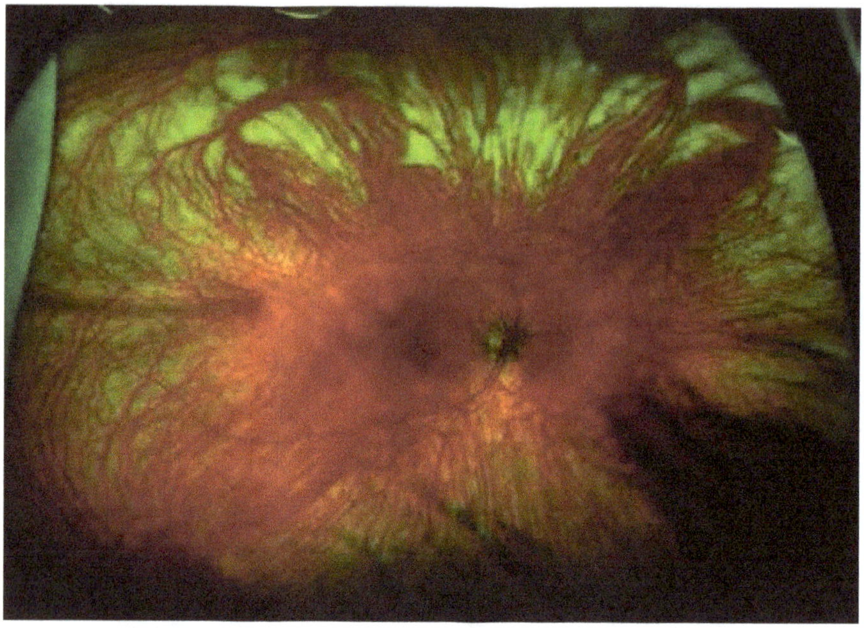

Figure 16. Optomap fundus image of a patient with ocular albinism showing more peripheral changes than can be visualised with standard fundus cameras.

5. Video conferencing

Live video conferencing facilitates live consultation between either doctor and patient or doctor and the doctor/optometrist/nurse currently examining a patient. It requires a faster internet connection than that needed for sending images via email, which is becoming increasingly available in more rural areas. Skype and FaceTime are commonly used software which are user friendly and regularly used non-professionally by the internet generation to communicate to friends and family. Thus it is an acceptable and non-frightening means of communication for both patients and doctors.

5.1. Non-ophthalmic clinicians example

Telemedicine video conferencing has been utilised in Western Australia, in a remote hospital where an ophthalmologist from Perth only visits twice a year. The average video conference length was 30 minutes and reduced emergency air evacuations to Perth from seven per year to none. This lead to a huge cost saving, better utilisation of air transfer staff and potentially increased patient satisfaction at remaining in their own home [29].

This is clearly a valuable resource in locations where there is no local ophthalmologist. Perhaps there will be increased access in Accident and Emergency Departments worldwide, which would most likely be utilised at night when ophthalmologists are on duty from home.

Video Technology is useful for conditions such as nystagmus and pupil abnormalities, which are difficult to capture with photographs.

6. Referrals to the hospital eye service

Trying to encompass all ophthalmic telemedical digital imaging techniques is the Central Ophthalmic electronic Referral Unit (COeRU) in Fife, Scotland. Here, patients have benefited from a Government financed set up of broadband connection from all community optometrists to the hospital. All referrals to the hospital Ophthalmology Department are done electronically by the local optometrist with electronic images from any machinery attached. It has demonstrated a global benefit to the hospital department of; a reduction in waiting times from 14 to 4 weeks, a reduction in the number of patients seen in the emergency clinic, and a reduction in 'Did Not Attend' patients [30]. This has had enormous benefit from patients who are now seen rapidly, especially patients with wet ARMD who are rapidly seen and treated.

The pilot study was set up in 2005 on 350 consecutive patients who were electronically referred with attached digital images by their community optometrists to the hospital using NHS mail [31]. The results were encouraging and showed that sight threatening disease could be identified early and that 37% of referral images allowed an electronic diagnosis which did not require a hospital appointment. Following the success of the pilot, the scheme was rolled out to the entire region in 2007 and a central ophthalmic electronic referral unit (COeRU) was created. In 2011, the five year data was studied, which analysed over 40,000 patient episodes [30]. The new electronic pathway meant that waiting times were reduced, which was mainly because the old tortuous paper referral pathway was bypassed by emailing the referral directly to the ophthalmology department and simultaneously copying in the GP. Significant changes to service delivery were achieved with all sight threatening disease seen within days rather than weeks, 15% of new patient referrals retained in the community and between 20 – 25% reduction in both the casualty attendance and DNA (did not attend) rate.

The Fife service data following implementation of COeRU was compelling and fed into three business case submissions to the Scottish government between 2009 – 2010 for electronic connection between community optometrists and hospital ophthalmic departments across the whole of Scotland.

In 2010 the Scottish government health department (SGHD) committed 6.6 million pounds for electronic connections between the community and the hospitals and in 2011 the Eyecare Integration Project was formed. The group has representation from Eyecare Scotland (all Scottish lead clinicians), Optometry Scotland, general practice (GP) and the Royal National Institute for the Blind. There is also representation from subdivisions of the SGHD that support the project to include the Practitioner Services Division (PSD), eHealth, SCI Gateway, ISD (information and statistics division) and National Information Systems Groups (NISG). The goals of this project are to provide a nationally supported electronic link between every community optometry practice and hospital ophthalmic department, which will enable electronic referrals with attached digital images. Concurrently the PSD are working on electronic software that will connect with the optometry practices' IT management systems to enable electronic payment verification [32].

The effect of this Scotland wide implementation of digital image referral is much awaited by other regions of the UK and worldwide.

7. Limitations of diagnoses with digital imaging

One of the main limitations of digital images is that they are 2D rather than the 3D image seen when using the slit lamp or indirect ophthalmoscope binocularly. This can make it difficult to identify oedema or raised suspicious choroidal naevae. However, the Optical Coherence Tomography images can help to overcome this concern, by providing a cross sectional view of the retina. Another difficulty in using digital images is the difficulty in imaging the peripheral retina, which is the common location of retinal tears. The Optomap ultrawide field images have improved peripheral retinal visualisation on images and have been shown to pick up lesions posterior to the equator with high specificity. However, they do not pick up all lesions anterior to the equator [33].

8. Conclusion

With the widespread access to camera phones in both developed and developing countries, imaging of eyes by patients and health carers becomes more accessible. Additionally, accessories have been designed to fit onto phone cameras to act as non mydriatic fundus cameras [34]. The new Portable Eye Examination Kit (PEEK) [35] is a smartphone App that enables health carers to perform detailed eye examinations including vision, fields, lens and fundus imaging in extremely rural homes with only a £300 iPhone and clip on camera hardware with little training. The diagnoses and management plans are then made remotely in the UK from the electronic data and images. Patients can then be located for treatment via the GPS coordinates of their home, which is automatically attached to smartphone photographs at the time of image capture.

The future of ophthalmology will undoubtedly involve more virtual clinics and perhaps more digital imaging from patients themselves. Perhaps there will be a time where all diabetics have a fundus camera phone accessory to photograph their own fundi and email their images to the hospital graders themselves.

In summary, electronic communication with digital images and teleconferencing has huge potential for eye care service delivery. It has the ability to overcome geographical barriers and pick up sight threatening disease at the earliest opportunity. With the exponential growth in global electronic communication there is no doubt that this will be incorporated into several health service delivery models. We have outlined the existing models within ophthalmology and have also outlined the future growth areas.

Author details

Hannah Timlin and Roshini Sanders

*Address all correspondence to: hannahtimlin@nhs.net.uk

Cataract Unit, Queen Margaret Hospital, Dunfermline, NHS Fife, UK

References

[1] Matthe E, Sandner D. Early treatment of exudative age-related macular degeneration with ranibizumab: the key to success. Ophthalmologe. 2011;108(3):237-43.

[2] Boyce Z, Gilmore S, Xu C, Soyer HP. The remote assessment of melanocytic skin lesions: a viable alternative to face-face consultation. Dermatology 2011;223(3):244-50.

[3] Tadros A, Murdoch R, Stevenson JH. Digital image referral for suspected skin malignancy – A pilot study of 300 patients. Journal of Plastic, Reconstructive & Aesthetic Surgery 2009;62:1048-1053.

[4] Engel H, Huang JJ, Tsao CK, Lin CY, Chou PY, Brey EM, Henry SL, Cheng MH. Remote real-time monitoring of free flaps via smartphone photography and 3G wireless Internet: a prospective study evidencing diagnostic accuracy. Microsurgery 2011;31(8):589-95.

[5] Varkey P, Tan NC, Girotto R, Tang WR, Liu YT, Chen HC. A picture speaks a thousand words: the use of digital photography and the internet as a cost-effective tool in monitoring free flaps. Annals of Plastic Surgery 2008;60(1):45-8.

[6] Kumar S, Yogesan K, Constable IJ. Telemedical diagnosis of anterior segment eye disease: validation of digital slit-lamp still images. Eye 2009;23(3):652-60.

[7] Koller S, Hofmann-Wellenhof R, Hayn D, Weger W, Kastner P, Schreier G, Salmhofer W. Acta Dermato-Venereologica 2011;91(6):680-5.

[8] Trikha S, Macgregor C, Jeffery, Kirwan J. The Portsmouth-based glaucoma refinement scheme: a role for virtual clinics in the future. Eye 2012;26(10):1288-94.

[9] Rathod D, Win T, Pickering S, Austin M. Incorporation of a virtual assessment into a care pathway for initial glaucoma management: feasibility study. Clinical & Experimental Ophthalmology 2008;36(6):543-6.

[10] Guidelines for the screening and treatment of retinopathy of prematurity. May 2008. Royal college of ophthalmologists and Royal college of Paediatrics and Child Health.

[11] Lorenz B, Spasovska K, Elflein H, Schneider N. Wide-field digital imaging based telemedicine for screening for acute retinopathy of prematurity. Six-year results of a

multicentre field study. Graefes Archive for Clinical & Experimental Ophthalmology 2009;247(9):1251-62.

[12] Weaver DT, Murdock TJ. Telemedicine detection of type 1 ROP in a distant neonatal intensive care unit. Journal of Aapos: American Association for Pediatric Ophthalmology & Strabismus 2012;16(3):229-33.

[13] Salcone EM, Johnston S, Vanderveen D. Review of the use of digital imaging in retinopathy of prematurity screening. Seminars in Ophthalmology 2010;25(5-6):214-7.

[14] Dai S, Chow K, Vincent A. Efficacy of wide-field digital retinal imaging for retinopathy of prematurity screening. Clinical & Experimental Ophthalmology 2011;39(1): 23-9.

[15] Ells AL, Holmes JM, Astle WF, Williams G, Leske DA, Fielden M, Uphill B, Jennett P, Hebert M. Telemedicine approach to screening for severe retinopathy of prematurity: a pilot study. Ophthalmology 2003;110(11):2113-7.

[16] Schwartz SD, Harrison SA, Ferrone PJ, Trese MT. Telemedical evaluation and management of retinopathy of prematurity using a fiberoptic digital fundus camera. Ophthalmology 2000;107(1):25-8.

[17] Patel CK, Fung THM, Muqit MMK, Mordant DJ, Brett J, Smith L, Adams E. Non-contact ultra-widefield imaging of retinopathy of prematurity using the Optos dual wavelength scanning laser ophthalmoscope. Eye 2013;27:589-596.

[18] www.diabeticeye.screening.nhs.uk/national

[19] Ogunyemi O, Terrien E, Eccles A, Patty L, George S, Fish A, Teklehaimanot S, Ilapakurthi R, Aimiuwu O, Baker R. Teleretinal screening for diabetic retinopathy in six Los Angeles urban safety-net clinics: Initial findings. AMIA Annual Symposium Proceedings / AMIA Symposium 2011:1027-35.

[20] Li Z, Wu C, Olayiwola JN, Hilaire DS, Huang JJ. Conneticut Medicine 2012;76(2): 85-90.

[21] Al alawi E, Ahmed AA. Screening for diabetic retinopathy: the first telemedicine approach in a primary care setting in Bahrain. Middle East African Journal of Ophthalmology 2012;19(3):295-8.

[22] Boucher MC, Nguyen QT, Angioi K. Mass Community Screening for diabetic retinopathy using a nonmydriatic camera with telemedicine. Canadian Journal of Ophthalmology 2005;40(6):734-42.

[23] Choremis J, Chow DR. Use of telemedicine in screening for diabetic retinopathy. Canadian Journal of Ophthalmology 2003;38(7):575-9.

[24] Massin P, Aubert JP, Erginay A, Bourovitch JC, Benmehidi A, Audran G, Bernit B, Jamet M, Collet C, Laloi-Michelin M, Guillausseau PJ, Gaudric A, Marre M. Screen-

ing for diabetic retinopathy: the first telemedical approach in a primary care setting in France. Diabetes & Metabolism 2004;30(5):451-7.

[25] Maberley DAL, Isbister C, MacKenzie P, Aralar A. An evaluation of photographic screening for neovascular age-related macular degeneration. Eye 2005;19:611-616.

[26] Amoaku W, Blakeney S, Freeman M, Gale R, Johnston R, Kelly SP, McLauglan, Sahu D, Varma D, Action on AMD Group. Action on AMD. Optimising patient management: act now to ensure current and continual delivery of best possible patient care. Eye 201; 26(S1)S2-S21.

[27] www.optos.com

[28] Khandhadia S, Madhusudhana KC, Kostakou A, Forrester JV, Newsom RSB. Use of optomap for retinal screening within an eye casualty setting. British Journal of Ophthalmology 2009;93(1):52-55.

[29] Kumar S, Yogesan K, Hudson B, Tay-Kearney ML, Constable IJ. Emergency eye care in rural Australia: role of internet. Eye 2006;20(12):1342-4.

[30] Borooah S, Grant B, Blaikie A, Styles C, Sutherland S, Forrest G, Curry P, Legg J, Walker A, Sanders R. Using electronic referral with digital imaging between primary and secondary ophthalmic services: a long term prospective analysis of regional service redesign. Eye 2013;27:392-397.

[31] Cameron JR, Ahmed S, Curry P, Forrest G, Sanders R. Impact of direct electronic referral with ocular imaging to a hospital eye service. Eye 2009;23:1134-1140

[32] Timlin H, Styles C, McPherson S, Sanders R. Eyecare Integration Project (Scotland); Electronic connections between primary and secondary sectors. Eye News 2013;20(1); 6-10.

[33] Mackenzie PJ, Russell M, Ma PE, Isbister CM, Maberley DA. Sensitivity and specificity of the optos optomap for detecting peripheral retinal lesions. Retina 2007;27(8): 1119-24.

[34] Lamirel C, Bruce BB, Wright DW, Newman, NJ, Biousse V. Nonmydriatic digital ocular fundus photography on the iPhone 3G: the FOTO-ED study. Archives of Ophthalmology 2012;130(7):939-40.

[35] www.peekvision.org

3

Retinopathy of Prematurity

Vikas Tah, Walid Sharif, Imran Yusuf,
Marcus Posner, Louise Ramskold, Farihah Tariq,
Dev Mukhey and Zuhair Sharif

1. Introduction

Retinopathy of prematurity (ROP) is a disease of premature infants and a leading worldwide cause of child blindness [1]. An epidemic of ROP occurred between 1941 and 1953, when an estimated 12,000 infants in affluent countries suffered visual loss from ROP. The first case of ROP, known then as retrolental fibroplasia (RLF), was identified in 1942 [2] with likely total retinal detachment [1]. However, RLF is currently applied to describe later stage cicatricial (severe retinal scarring) disease with retinal detachment and formation of retrolental fibroplastic membrane [2]. It is likely that the severe, advanced disease stage of RLF would have been more readily identifiable in 1942, in the absence of technological advancements that have added precision and clarity to ophthalmic diagnosis· Cases of ROP were reported throughout the developed world over the following decade. Intensive oxygen therapy as the key determinant of ROP was not known until the early 1950s when the suggestion of oxygen toxicity in ROP was made.

ROP is a biphasic condition comprising an initial phase of vessel growth retardation followed by a second phase of vessel proliferation characterised by abnormal retinal vasculature development [2]. Broadly it is thought to be caused by disorganised blood vessel growth that may result in scarring of the retina and retinal detachment.

The precise aetiology of ROP remains unclear [1]. Onset is associated with immaturity. The three factors that have shown a consistently significant association with retinopathy of prematurity are low birth weight, low gestational age and prolonged supplementary oxygen exposure after delivery [3].

The pathological process includes several risk factors that impact on each other. These include premature birth, multiple gestation, prenatal complications, genetic factors, immature pulmonary function, intraventricular haemorrhage, sepis, anaemia, patent ductus arteriosus, growth factors, prostaglandin synthetase inhibitors, vitamin E deficiency, lactic acidosis [1,23], vasoactive substances development of retinal vessels, maturation of retinal cells with subsequent growth of metabolic demands and the state of the antioxidant system. The exact role of these remains undetermined [3].

ROP is one of the few preventable causes of childhood visual impairment [5]. Early identification and treatment prevent blindness and offer the affected child better visual development [6]. Thus, new, innovative evidence-based approaches to the investigation, screening, prevention and treatment of ROP are still required [1].

2. Epidemiology

Increases in the incidence and prevalence of ROP became recognised as specialists began to theorise that oxygen toxicity might be a contributory factor in pathology among premature babies [1,23] this leading to a perceived 'epidemic' of ROP. Two epidemics of ROP have occurred in the last 70 years in the developed world. The first occurred in 1941-53. This was thought to be related to hyperoxia from incubators[7].

Subsequent research has confirmed that high blood level oxygen causes obliteration of retinal vessels [24-26]. Based on this, recommendations to lower oxygen supply were undertaken and the levels of ROP declined dramatically. Consequently, incubator oxygen concentrations, frequency of administration and duration of oxygen therapy became reduced in many neonatal units throughout the developed world [31].

In the 1970-80s, despite closer oxygen supply monitoring, a second epidemic was recorded, with more extreme low birth weight infants surviving in developed countries [8].

Currently it is thought a possible third epidemic is occurring in industrial medium-developed countries, with several explanations attributable [9-10]. Firstly, there is a higher ratio of premature born to newborns owing to progress in neonatology. The survival of extremely low birth weight infants has increased from 5% to 65% in the last 40 years. Whilst compulsory screening is available in some countries like those of the UK, this is no longer the case in other western countries owing to lack of resources and adequate training. This means that there are a higher number of advanced ROP cases in immature and mature children.

The incidence of the disease was first reviewed in the Cryotherapy for Retinopathy of Prematurity Cooperative Group (CRYO-ROP) study, based on a multicentre trial in the United States. 9751 infants from 23 centres were recruited, and 65.8% of those premature babies with a birthweight less than 1251 grams were noted to have some form of ROP. 18% developed stage 3 disease and 6% were treated [11].

The Early Treatment of ROP study (ET-ROP) study [12] looked at 317 newborns from 26 different centres with birth weight less than 1251 grams. The incidence was very similar at

68%, and was noted to decrease sharply with increasing birth weight and gestational age. Other trials have been undertaken, but have used different criteria (notable birth weight) to these trials listed, meaning a direct comparison is futile. These trials are listed in the table 1 below [13-19].

author	age (weeks of gestation)	weight (grams)	incidence %
Al Amro2003	<37	<2000	3.4
Hussan1999		<1500	21.3
Fortes, 2007	<36	<1000	48.9
		<1500	16.2
Good 2005		<1251	68
Shah 2005		<1500	29.2
Martin Begué 2003		<1501	29.2
Rehka, 1996	<34	<1500	46%

Table 1. Trials undertaken for incidence retinopathy of prematurity looking at the gestational age and weight

3. Classification

The International Classification of Retinopathy of Prematurity (ICROP) was devised by expert ophthalmologists in the field from 11 countries to help more suitably describe the observations of the disease. This was designed to help clarify what stage of disease was being treated, and to help audit results of treatment. The original ICROP was devised in 1984 [20], with subsequent minor revision in 1987 [21] and with enhanced imaging techniques further modification in 2005 [22].

The classification system has always been based on 3 basic paradigms; *location, extent* and *staging* of the disease.

3.1. Location

The original classification in 1984 describes 3 concentric zones of retinal involvement to define the antero-posterior location of the retinopathy. Each zone is centered on the optic disc rather than the macula, since normal retinal growth proceeds forward from the optic disc towards the ora serrata in a systematic fashion (although it is observed that the extent of retinal vascularisation and ROP may be observed closer to the optic disc nasally than temporally).

Zone I (posterior pole or inner zone consists of a circle), the radius of which extends from the centre of the optic disc to twice the distance from the centre of the optic disc to the centre of the macula. The radius of this zone subtends an angle of 30 degrees. The limits of the zone are consequently defined as twice the disc-foveal distance in all directions from the optic disc; an arc of 60 degrees.

Zone II is the area extending from the edge of zone I peripherally to a point tangential to the nasal ora serrata (at the 3 o clock position in the right eye and the 9 o clock position in the left eye. The temporal edge of zone II cannot be more accurately defined as the anatomic landmarks needed to identify the equator in premature infants are obscured.

Zone III is the residual crescent of retina anterior to zone II. By convention zones I and II are considered mutually exclusive. Retinopathy of prematurity should be considered in zone II until it can be confirmed that the nasal most 2 clock hours are vascularised to the ora serrata.

For the clinician as a practical approach, using a 25D or 28 diopter (D) condensing lens can help to determine the approximate temporal extent of zone I. The limit of zone I is at the temporal field of view by placing the nasal edge of the optic disc at one edge of the field of view.

3.2. Extent

The extent of the disease specified as the hours of the clock or as 30 degree sectors. As the observer looks at each eye, the 3o'clock position is to the right and nasal in the right eye and temporal in the left eye. The 9 o'clock position is to the left and temporal in the right eye and nasal in the right eye.

3.3. Staging of the disease

This refers to the amount of abnormal vascular response observed. Prior to ROP development in the premature infant, vascularisation of the retina is incomplete. There are now 5 stages used to describe the abnormal vascular response at the junction of the vascularised and avascular retina. Initially the ICROP had 4 stages, but this has been modified to 5 stages for the eye as a whole, based on the most severe manifestation present since more than one ROP stage may be present in the same eye. For the purpose of recording the examination, each stage is defined and the extent of clock hours is recorded.

Stage 1: Demarcation line

This is a thin but destructive structure separating the avascular anteriorly and vascular retina posteriorly. There is abnormal arcading or branching of vessels leading up to the demarcation line that is relatively flat, white, and lies within the plane of the retina. Vascular changes can be apparent prior to the development of the demarcation line, such as dilatation rather than tapering of the peripheral retinal vessels, but these changes are subtle and different to quantify, inadequate for diagnosing early ROP.

Stage 2: Ridge

This is the hallmark of stage 2 ROP. It arises in the region of the demarcation line that has now grown, has height and width, and extends above the plane of the retina. The ridge may change colour from white to pink and vessels may leave the plane of the retina to enter it. Small isolated tufts of new vessels lying on the surface of the retina may be seen posterior to this ridge structure. They do not make part of the growth necessary for stage 3. These small isolated tufts are commonly referred to as 'popcorn'.

Stage 3: Extraretinal fibrovascular proliferation

In stage 3 extraretinal fibrovascular retinal proliferation tissue develops from the ridge and extends into the vitreous. This extraretinal proliferating tissue is has 3 characteristics; first it is continuous with the posterior aspect of the ridge, causing a ragged appearance as the proliferation becomes more extensive. Second, it is immediately posterior to the ridge but not always appearing to be connected with it. Third it projects theinto the vitreous perpendicular to the retinal plane. The severity of a stage 3 disease can be subdivided into mild, moderate or severe depending on the extent of the extraretinal fibrovascular tissue infiltrating the vitreous.

Stage 4: Partial Retinal Detachment

Stage 4 is divided into extrafoveal (stage 4A) and foveal (stage 4B) partial retinal detachments. This may be caused by exudative effusion of fluid, traction or both. These are generally concave and most tend to be circumferentially orientated. The extent of retinal detachment depends on the number of clock hours of fibrovascular traction and their degree of contraction. Typically, retinal detachments begin at the point of fibrovacular attachment to the vascularised retina. In progressive cases, the fibrous tissue continues to contract and the tractional retinal detachment increases in height, extending both anteriorly and posteriorly. Radial detachments and more complex configurations of retinal detachments are less common.

Stage 5: Total Retinal Detachment

Typically retinal detachments are tractional, but may occasionally be exudative. They are usually funnel shaped. Funnel configuration permits a subdivision of this stage. The funnel is divided into anterior and posterior parts. When open, both anteriorly and posteriorly the detachment often has a concave configuration to the optic disc. A second frequent configuration is one where the funnel is narrow in both the anterior and posterior aspects, and the detached retina is located just behind the lens. A third less common type is where the funnel is open anteriorly but narrowed posteriorly. Least common is a funnel that is narrow anteriorly and open posteriorly.

'Threshold' and 'Pre-threshold' categories of ROP severity were also developed as a result of the CRY-ROP findings [35,36]. 'Threshold ROP', as a subdivision of ROP Stage 3, was associated with an approximate 50% risk of blindness if untreated. These definitions have prognostic importance, as 47% of threshold ROP categorisations culminated in retinal detachment [37].

3.4. "Plus" and "Pre-Plus" disease

The terms 'Pre-plus and Plus disease' denote increased venous dilation and arteriolar tortuosity of the posterior retinal vessels, which often lead to increased ROP severity [35-38]. These may be accompanied by vitreous haze, iris vascular engorgement and inadequate dilation of pupils

3.4.1. "Plus" disease

Progressive vascular incompetence occurring along with the change at the edge of the abnormally developing retinal vasculature may have additional signs indicating the severity of active ROP that can occur. These include venous dilatation and arteriolar tortuosity of the posterior retinal vessels and may later increase in severity to include iris vascular engorgement, poor papillary dilatation and vitreous haze. This group of supplementary signs was referred to as 'plus' disease in the ICROP original classification. Subsequent refinement from clinical trials has resulted in diagnosis of plus disease that can be made if sufficient vascular dilatation and tortuosity are present in at least 2 quadrants of the eye. A+sign is added to the ROP stage number where there is plus disease present. For example stage 3 ROP combined with posterior vascular dilatation is written as 'stage 3+ROP'. Progression may be rapid where ROP is located in zone I or posterior zone II with plus disease present.

In the CRY-ROP study, significant retinal venous dilation and arteriolar tortuosity in all 4 vascular arcade quadrants served as diagnostic criteria for 'Plus disease'[35-38]. However. currently, changes in at least 2 quadrants are required for the diagnosis of 'plus disease' [51] representing a terminological modification with implications for screening and treatment decisions.

3.4.2. "Pre-Plus" disease

This has been a more recent addition to classification. Abnormal dilatation and tortuosity of posterior pole vessels that demonstrate more than normal arterial and venous tortuosity, but are insufficient for the diagnosis of plus disease is termed 'preplus' disease [8,51]. These changes may over time progress to plus disease as vessels dilate and become more tortuous.

Despite absence of simultaneous manifestation, these symptoms are likely indicators of ROP progression and the 'Pre-plus disease' category may be a useful indicator of sudden increases in ROP activity.

3.5. Aggressive Posterior ROP (AP-ROP)

This is an uncommon rapidly progressing severe form of ROP, termed AP-ROP. Not included in the original ICROP classification, it has recently been defined by ICROP revisited as aggressive posterior ROP and is noted for its rapid progression to stage 5 ROP if not treated [34]. It has been referred to as type II ROP and Rush disease. The characteristic features of this type of ROP are the posterior location, prominence of plus disease and ill defined nature of the retinopathy.

AP-ROP is observed most commonly in zone I, but can occur in posterior zone II. Early in the development of AP-ROP, the posterior pole vessels show increased vascular dilatation and tortuosity in all 4 quadrants that is out of proportion to the degree of retinopathy peripherally. These changes progess rapidly. Shunting does not occur soley at the junction of the avascular and vascular retina but occurs from vessel to vessel within the retina. This can make AP-ROP difficult to distinguish arterioles and venules owing to significant dilatation of both vessel types. There may also be haemorrhages at the junction of the vascular and avascular retina.

AP-ROP is deceptively featureless and does not usually progress through the classic stages 1-3 [40,9], appearing as a flat network of neovascularisation at the junction between the vascularisaed and nonvascularised retina. It typically extends circumferentially and is often accompanied by a circuimferential vessel. The use of a 20-D condensing lens instead of a 25-D lens in indirect ophthalmoscopy may help distinguish the featureless neovascularisation.

On the basis of this evidence it was concluded that when the characteristics of rapidly progressing disease are observed, or when aggressive posterior ROP is present, the baby should be monitored closely and screening should be undertaken at least weekly [39].

4. Investigations of retinopathy of prematurity: A chronological overview of change, development and future directions

Effective investigation of ROP is dependent on reliable classification. However, as we have mentioned, ROP classification is not a static entity and is subject to evolutionary change resulting from research findings, modifications to practice, technological advances and terminological refinements. Accordingly, standard screening should be performed more frequently, perhaps on a weekly basis [8,39].

Determining and maintaining optimal oxygen saturation levels in preterm infants has remained something of a challenge because data regarding early mortality and long-term neuro-developmental outcomes resulting from effects of different oxygen saturation ranges are lacking [23,33]. The CRYO-ROP study found that the rate of progression of ROP (mean ± standard error) was faster in eyes with an unfavourable outcome (8.2 ± 1.2 days between first observation of ROP to pre-threshold) compared with those with a favourable outcome (12.3 ± 1.2 days), suggesting that in some situations even twice-weekly examinations are not frequent enough [36,37].

The findings from a meta-analysis of infants with postmenstrual ages of < or=32 week published in 2010 indicated an association between early low levels of oxygen saturation and reduced risk for severe ROP among and late high oxygen saturation the effect of oxygen on the development and progression of ROP is not straight forward. Ongoing investigation is necessary to understand the relationships among oxygen concentration, variability in oxygen concentration, and timing of oxygen delivery. Low oxygen saturation appears to decrease the risk of severe ROP in preterm newborns when administered during the first few weeks after birth. High oxygen saturation seems to reduce the risk at later postmenstrual ages [32]. However, individual clinical studies have not been conclusive.

A recent study by the Benefits of Oxygen Saturation Targeting (BOOST) Collaborative Group, evaluated the effects of targeting an oxygen saturation of 85 to 89%, as compared with a range of 91 to 95%, on disability-free survival at 2 years in 2,448 infants born before 28 weeks' gestation in three international randomized, controlled trials [8]. Halfway through the trials, the oximeter-calibration algorithm was revised. Recruitment was stopped early when an interim analysis showed an increased rate of death at 36 weeks in the group with a lower oxygen saturation [8]. The rate of death was significantly higher in the lower-target group than in the higher-target group (23.1% vs. 15.9%; relative risk in the lower-target group, 1.45; 95%

confidence interval (CI), 1.15 to 1.84; P=0.002) [8]. Oxygen saturation levels below 90% in extremely preterm infants was associated with an increased risk of death [8]. Although the lower targeted saturation group had a significantly reduced incidence of ROP, the infants also had a significant increase in the rate of developing necrotizing enterocolitis [8].

5. Evidence to inform investigations

The first evidence of successful treatment came from the multi-centre CRYO-ROP study reported in 1988 [35]. The CRYO-ROP study reported findings after 3 months, then at 1, 3.5, 5.5, 10 and 15 years. Unfavourable outcomes (defined by ROP in the posterior retina and retinal detachment) were less in the treated group than in the untreated group at every time point [35-38].

The percentage of eyes with unfavourable outcomes increased over time in both groups from 25.1% at one year to 30.0% at 15 years for treated eyes, compared with 44.7% vs 51.9% for untreated eyes [35-38]. CRYO-OP study data, describing the natural history of ROP, are probably the most comprehensive, with current understanding of ROP based largely on the findings of this study. Indeed, it is apparent that the CRYO-ROP study findings have influenced redefinition of ROP classification and as noted, this has implications for investigations, screening and treatment as well as identification of risk factors, clinical course of ROP and outcomes.

However, while outcomes of treatment in the CRYO-ROP study were superior to the untreated controls, they are perceived less than ideal [42]. Outcomes among treated patients were frequently poor, with 21.8% progression to macular distortion or retinal detachment and long-term loss of vision. Cryotherapy did not benefit neonates with stage 4 ROP with partial retinal detachment [42]. Over the longer term, even eyes with favorable anatomic outcomes still had poor vision. ROP located in Zone 1, young gestational age, multiple births, birth outside hospital, low birth weight, white race, plus disease (based on 4 affected eye quadrants), stage 3, >6 clock hour stage 3, and iris vessel dilatation were associated with an unfavorable anatomic outcome [42].

Subsequent to the theory that supplemental oxygen therapy was an important factor in the causal chain of ROP, randomized controlled trial findings indicated that restricting oxygen might result in a lower incidence of severe ROP [43,44], but at a cost of increased mortality [41]. Indeed, current evidence suggests that it is unadvisable to target oxygen-saturation concentrations below 90% in infants born prior to 28 weeks' gestation [46]. However, after seven decades of investigation, knowledge regarding optimal concentrations of oxygen required to balance risk in favor of avoiding adverse effects of both hyperoxia and hypoxia remains inadequate with no 'safe' level of supplementation identified [1] the clinically appropriate range for oxygen saturation in preterm infants remains unknown. In the absence of complete consensus over the oxygen issue, including a definition of optimal oxygen concentration' [39], it is apparent that new approaches to the investigation and prevention of ROP are required [45-48].

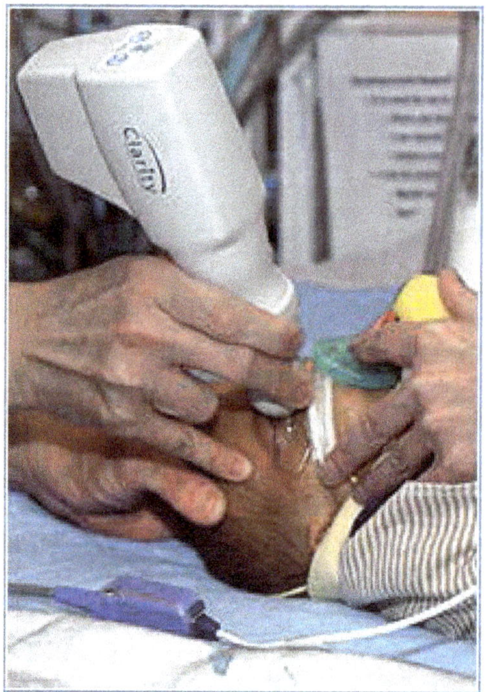

Figure 1. Courtesy of Hoag Levins. Clarity Medical Solutions. [72]

6. Current screening for ROP

An audit of UK ophthalmologists in 1999 established that although many of the 1995 Guideline recommendations were followed, practice varied in relation to when screening should stop and at what stage ROP should be treated [49]. Concerns were also expressed that the recommendations in the 1995 Guideline resulted in too many babies being screened, causing a heavy workload for ophthalmologists and distress to babies receiving unnecessary retinal examinations [33-35].

Key recommendations for good practice in the UK were published in 2008 by the Royal College of Paediatrics and Child Health and Royal College of Ophthalmologists [49].These were based largely on ICROP revisited publication [34], findings from the CRY-OP study [38] and the Early Treatment for Retinopathy of Prematurity study [53].

Babies of less than 32 weeks gestational age (up to 31 weeks and 6 days) or less than 1501g birth weight should be screened for ROP [49]. One criterion to be met for inclusion [49]: Babies of less than 31 weeks gestational age (up to 30 weeks and 6 days) or less than 1251g birth weight must be screened for ROP. Ophthalmological notes should be made after each ROP examination, detailing zone, stage, and extent in terms of clock hours of any ROP and the presence of any pre-plus or plus disease [49]. These notes should include a recommendation for the timing of the next examination (if any) and be kept with the baby's medical record [32]. Comfort care techniques (e.g. administering sucrose solution, nesting, swaddling and use of a pacifier) during the screening examination may be considered [49]. Babies with aggressive ROP (as defined in ICROP revisited) should be treated as soon as possible and within 48 hours. ROP requiring treatment but which is not aggressive posterior ROP should normally be treated within 48-72 hours [49].

The current screening guideline of ROP in the United States calls for dilated fundus examination by indirect ophthalmoscopy for all premature infants below 30 week gestational age or less than 1500g birth weight with the first examination performed by 31 week postmenstrual age or by 4 weeks chronologic age, with additional examinations performed repeatedly thereafter to detect late stage ROP requiring treatment [54]. Additional screening for older or larger babies is recommended at the discretion of the attending neonatologist [54].

Risk of sight-threatening ROP developing is considered to be minimal beyond 37 weeks postmenstrual age although any decision to cease screening certain babies before this point in time must be considered with caution. Examination of data from the CRYO-ROP study indicated that babies developing stage 1 or 2 ROP in zone III were at very low risk of developing sight-threatening ROP [55,56]. Investigations for serious ROP should be between 33 and 39 weeks post-conceptional age, while realizing that there is a degree of individual variability in the development of retinal vasculature [56].

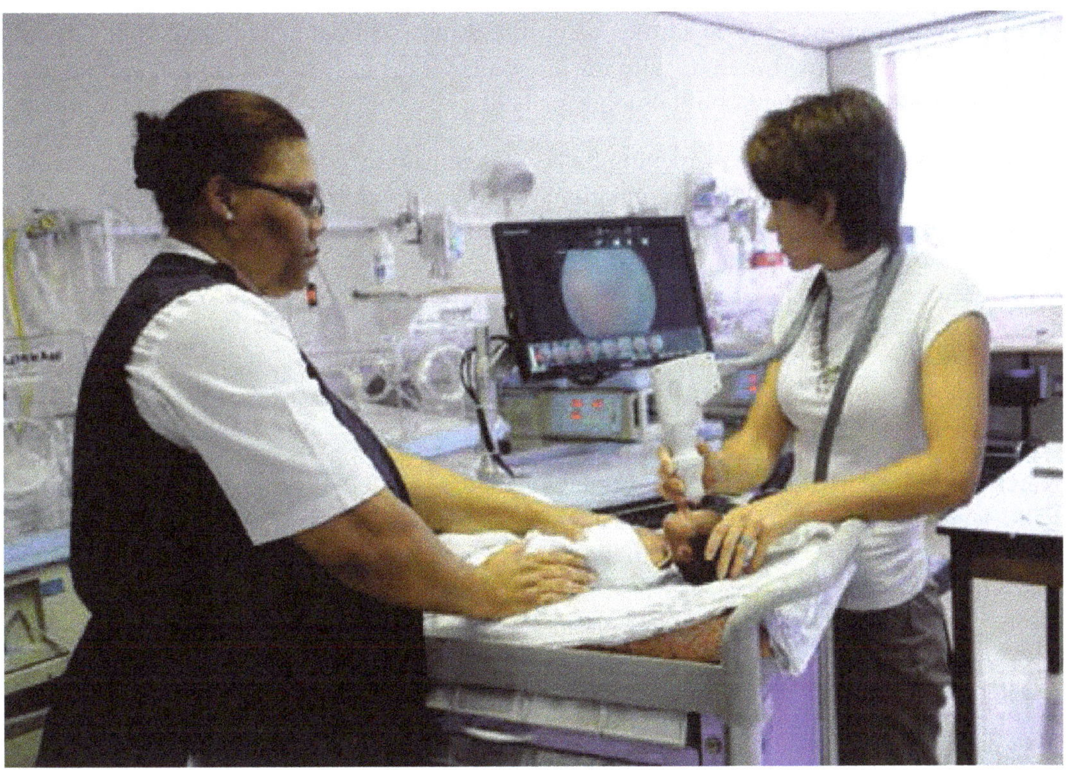

Figure 2. Courtesy of Tygerberg Children's Hospital. [71]

Risk of sight defect is regarded as minimal when regression occurs in babies with moderate ROP, with vascularisation of the retina spreading into zone III. However, it was shown that in 3% of babies, regression and zone III vascularisation had still not occurred by 3 months post term [56]. Therefore, the UK Guideline Development Group decided criteria for termination of screening should be when signs of regression of active ROP are apparent as opposed to vascularisation [49]. Signs of ROP regression have been defined by the ICROP revisited publication as lack of increase in severity, complete or partial resolution, reduction of pre-plus/ plus disease, transgression of vessels through the demarcation line and the commencement of the process of replacement of active ROP lesions by scar tissue [51]. The signs of regression should be confirmed by at least two examinations [49]. In babies without ROP, eye examinations may be stopped when vascularisation has extended into zone III, usually after 36 weeks post-conceptional age [57].

Babies with ROP that did not require treatment can have screening stopped when clear regression is seen on 2 successive examinations [57]. Babies that required treatment for ROP and babies diagnosed with stage 3 ROP, which resolved spontaneously, require ophthalmic review at least until 5 years of age [57]. Babies with stages 1 or 2 ROP can have routine vision screening, unless there is specific concern [49]. It should be noted that the process of regression may differ between individuals and ophthalmologists should err on the side of caution when they believe that there is still the possibility of sight-threatening ROP [49].

Until recently, universally accepted treatment criteria of 'threshold' ROP have been used and there is a requirement for new studies using pre-threshold treatment criteria [49]. The UK recommendations were drawn up with the intention not to negate use of clinical judgment by experienced and competent ophthalmologists [49].

As with the classification, the screening for ROP is constantly evolving. Screening investigations include frequent retinal examinations of at-risk preterm infants [57]. Delaying or postponing a screening examination could mean that the window of opportunity for treatment is missed [58,62].

7. Future screening

Newly developed ROP screening and prediction methods based on post-natal weight gain and IGF-1 levels can predict infants who are at high risk for ROP. These infants may be monitored more closely while those identified to be at low risk may be spared unnecessary diagnostic procedures. ROP evaluations and weekly weight measurements from birth to postmenstrual week 36 were entered into a computer-based surveillance system.

A prospective study of 50 preterm infants with a mean gestational age of 26 weeks was conducted to validate a surveillance algorithm for detecting infants at risk for proliferative ROP [59]. Weekly measures of body weight and (IGF-I) level from birth until postmenstrual age 36 weeks were compared using the Weight, insulin like growth factor I (IGF-1), Neonatal Retinopathy of Prematurity (WINROP) algorithm [59]. Gestational age, birth weight, and IGF

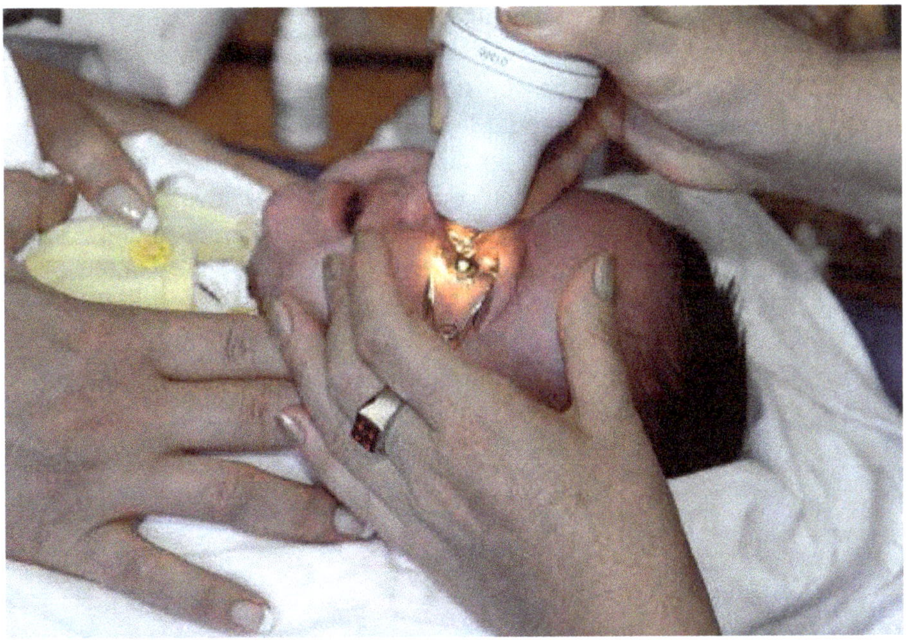

Figure 3. Courtesy of Minas Hambardzumyan. [73]

binding protein 3 level are entered. An alarm is raised if any of the variables indicate a certain degree of negative deviation [59]. The WINROP algorithm identified all infants (100% sensitivity) who were diagnosed with proliferative ROP 1. No infants with no alarm or with alarm at low risk developed proliferative ROP. Alarm at high risk before postmenstrual age 32 weeks was raised for 22 of 50 infants (44%); 9 of these infants developed proliferative ROP (54% specificity), of whom 8 were treated [60]. It was concluded that the WINROP algorithm may be a useful modification for ROP screening [59].

In another study using WINROP a total of 1706 infants with a median gestational age of 28 weeks (range, 22-31 weeks) and median birth weight of 1016 g (range, 378-2240 g) were included in the study analysis [60]. An alarm occurred in 1101 infants (64.5%), with a median time from birth to alarm of 3 weeks (range, 0-12 weeks) and from alarm to treatment of 8 weeks (range, 1 day to 22 weeks). The sensitivity of WINROP was 98.6% and the negative predictive value was 99.7%. Two infants with type 1 ROP requiring treatment after 40 weeks' postmenstrual age did not receive an alarm [60].

In a Mexican patient population, the WINROP algorithm correctly predicted severe retinopathy of prematurity in 84.7% of extremely preterm infants and correctly identified only 26.6% of infants in whom severe retinopathy of prematurity did not develop [61]. These findings suggest that potential differences exist among preterm infants with retinopathy of prematurity in different regions of the world.

The WINROP algorithm was recently tested using a retrospective cohort study in the South East of Scotland [63]. Anonymised clinical data were uploaded to the online WINROP site, and infants at risk of developing severe ROP were identified. The results using WINROP were compared with the actual ROP screening outcomes. Infants with incomplete weight data were included in the whole group, but were excluded from a subgroup analysis of infants with complete weight data. In addition, data were manipulated to test whether missing weight data points in the early neonatal period would lead to loss of sensitivity of the algorithm. The WINROP algorithm had 73% sensitivity for detecting infants at risk of severe ROP when all infants were included and 87% when the complete weight data subgroup was analysed. Manipulation of data from the complete weight data subgroup demonstrated that one or two missing weight data points in the early postnatal period lead to loss of sensitivity performance by WINROP [63]. It was concluded that the WINROP program offers a non-invasive method of identifying infants at high risk of severe ROP and also identifying those not at risk. However, for WINROP to function optimally, it has to be used as recommended and designed, namely weekly body weight measurements are required [63].

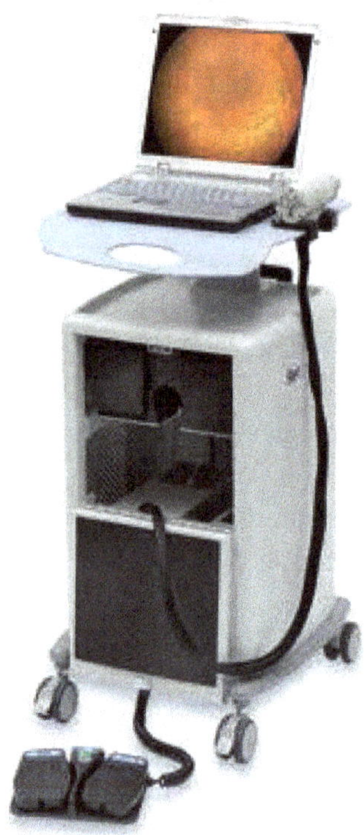

Figure 4. Courtesy of BIOPHOTONICS [74].

8. Digital imaging

Interpretation of digital images have been found to have good inter/intra-reader reliability [64,65] which enhances its potential for use in what is termed 'telemedicine' [49]. The use of digital photographic retinal images that are captured and sent for remote interpretation is a developing approach to ROP screening however, outcomes comparison between large-scale operational digital-imaging systems with remote interpretation versus binocular indirect ophthalmoscopy have not been published.

While there is not sufficient research evidence to demonstrate that wide field digital fundus photography is as effective as the indirect ophthalmoscope for ROP screening, some UK screeners already the technique 'RetCam' is of choice although the cost is likely to remain a deterrent for many units [49]. However, training of operators is an important issue and no studies have yet demonstrated that cameras operated by non-ophthalmologists are as sensitive at detecting ROP as the indirect ophthalmoscope in the hands of a skilled ophthalmologist [66].

Accurate assessment of ROP is essential in ensuring correct and timely treatment of this potentially blinding condition [67,68]. Current modes of assessment are based upon clinical grading by expert examination of retinal changes. However, this may be subjective, unreliable and difficult and there has been significant interest in alternative means of measurement. These have been made possible through technological advancements in image capture and analysis as well as progress in clinical research, highlighting the specific importance of the plus disease category in ROP [68]. Progress in these two fields has highlighted the potential for digital image analysis of plus disease to be used as an objective, reliable and valid measurement of ROP. However, with the potential benefits, there are significant challenges such as in image capture, segmentation, measurement of vessel width and tortuosity [68].

The standard method for diagnosis of ROP has been bedside indirect ophthalmoscopy for both routine clinical care and clinical trials. With this approach, the examiner's interpretations of the clinical findings are transcribed onto grading sheets, rather than a photographic record of the actual retinal features. One limitation to this approach is that the examiner's interpretation of fundus findings is presumed to be correct without opportunity for review. Photographic documentation would serve to confirm diagnosis and distinguish true therapeutic failure from poor outcome caused by incomplete treatment [68]. Thus, telemedicine may offer a solution to many of the current geographic and resource problems preventing a comprehensive ROP screening program throughout the world. Future additions to telemedicine could comprise weight-gain algorithms combined with other reliable quantitative data such as IGF-1 levels.

Furthermore, computer-based image analysis using quantitative methods has the potential to improve the objectivity of plus disease diagnosis [69]. Plus disease diagnosis is critical for decision-making in ROP, as it is necessary for threshold disease and sufficient for type 1 ROP. Plus disease is defined as abnormal arteriolar tortuorsity and venular dilation in the posterior pole greater than that of a standard published photograph, which was selected by expert consensus for the CRYO-ROP study and is still widely used [69]. During the past 10 years, several computer-based systems have been developed for ROP, particularly for detection of plus disease. This has potential to improve clinical ROP management [69,70]. However, more large-scale, robust clinical trials are still required to provide the necessary evidence to inform optimum investigation and screening for all aspects of ROP.

RISA analysis:

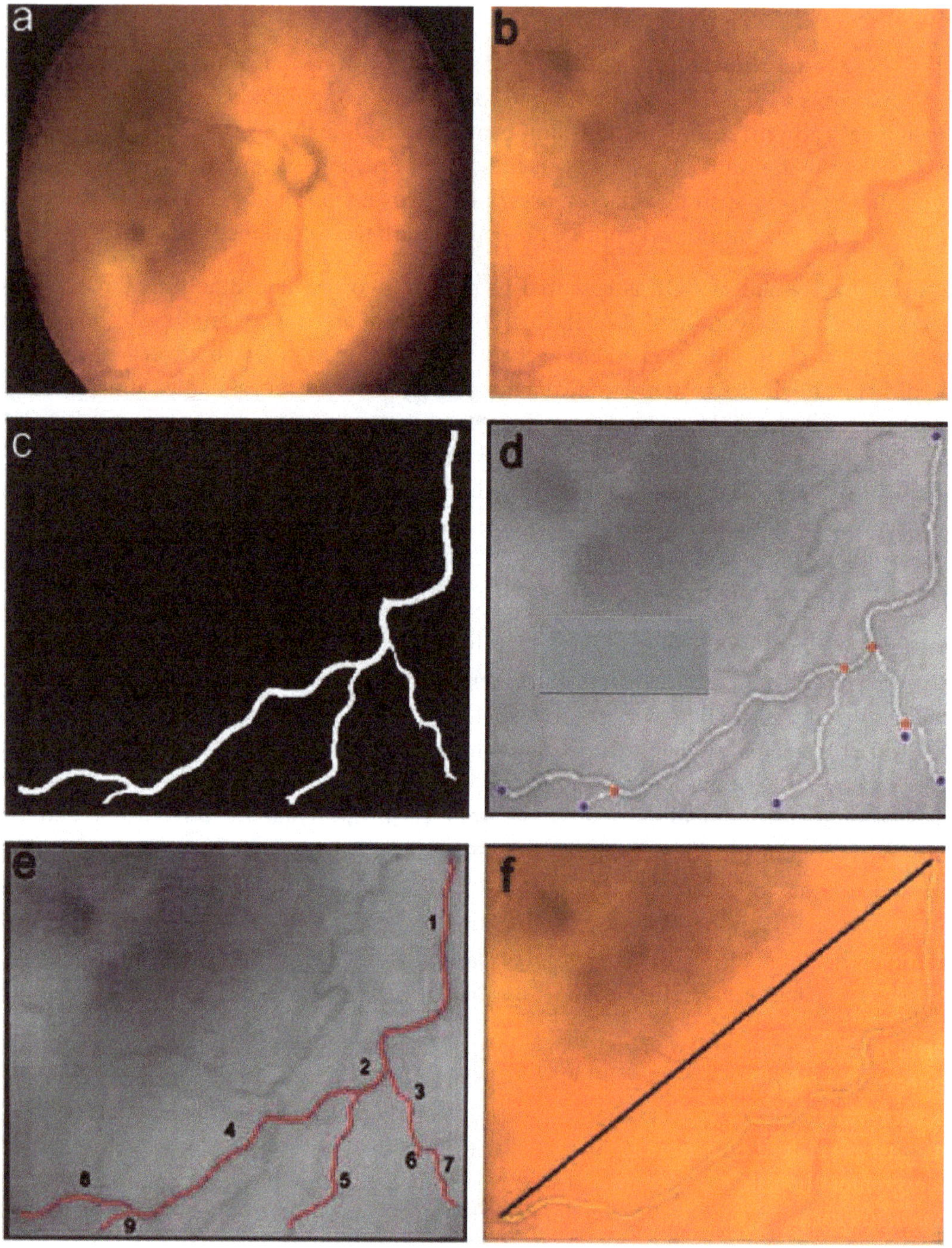

Figure 5. Image documented via RETCAM from (*Gelman et al., 2005*) [70] : a).(a) Retina (b) Choose the vessel. (c) Highlight the vessel. (d) & (e) Mark the vessel. (f) Tortuosity index :Measure actual vessel length, measure the length of point 1 to point 9, divide actual length by length of points 1&9

9. Management of retinopathy of prematurity medical management

9.1. Optimising oxygen therapy

Although incubators for infants had been developed around the mid-nineteenth century, it was not until the 1920s that neonates were grouped together for specialist care in early neonatal intensive care units. Special Care Baby Units became established in many hospitals in the 1940s, although incubators were expensive, oxygen, heat, humidity were considered desirable but influence of such parameters on clinical outcomes were anecdotal – hard clinical data were lacking.

The development of neonatal care, technology and research has reduced gestational age compatible with life to less than 24 weeks with additional challenges in the prevention of ROP. Identifying a safe level of oxygen therapy to prevent the development of ROP in such babies without increasing mortality has been the subject of numerous clinical trials [45, 76-82].

The efficacy and safety of supplemental oxygen therapy for premature infants with pre-threshold ROP was evaluated in the STOP-ROP trial [43]. Infants with oxygen saturations maintained at less than 94% with pre-threshold ROP were assigned to conventional oxygen of 89-94%, or supplemental oxygen with target saturations 96-99%. Supplemental oxygen did not increase progression to threshold ROP or reduce the numbers of infants requiring laser photocoagulation or cryotherapy. There was some suggestion in post-hoc subgroup analysis that infants without plus disease may be more responsive to supplemental oxygen therapy [43].

The HOPE study analysed data from the STOP-ROP trial, including infants who were excluded from STOP ROP with oxygen saturations >94% prior to enrolment [83]. The HOPE-ROP cohort were of a higher gestational age, progressing to threshold ROP in 25% of cases, compared to 46% of the STOP-ROP cohort. Logistic regression analysis identified oxygen saturation at the time of pre-threshold diagnosis to be of borderline significance once gestational age, race, post-menstrual age at diagnosis, zone I disease, and plus disease had been accounted for [83].

The NeOProM study is a prospective meta-analysis collaboration seeking to recruit 5,000 extremely premature neonates to detect rates of death and disability, including visual outcomes from ROP measured at 18 months gestation [85]. Results are expected from this study in 2014.

Increasing neonatal mortality with oxygen restriction suggests that ROP cannot be prevented by oxygen restriction alone in premature infants.

9.2. ROP: When to treat

The "ET-ROP" was a landmark study evaluating the *timing* of treatment of ROP [86], with some concern that a proportion of neonates would receive treatment for ROP that would regress spontaneously and therefore carry an excess risk of surgical complications. The ET-ROP trial was a nationally funded, prospective, randomized, controlled clinical trial that sought to identify clinical criteria to predict those neonates who had the highest risk for an adverse visual or structural outcome [86], and evaluate the implications for timing of ablative treatment for ROP. Natural history data of ROP from the CRYO-ROP study was used to formulate an algorithm, randomization occurred when the risk was calculated to be 15% or greater (high risk pre-threshold), either to early ablative treatment or observation until threshold or regression. Functional outcomes were assessed by grating visual acuity at 9 months gestation, and structural outcomes were evaluated through fundus examination with unfavourable outcome defined as retinal fold involving the macula, retinal detachment involving the macula, retrolental tissue obscuring posterior pole.

499 high risk pre-threshold neonates with ROP were randomized. The ET-ROP study identified that peripheral retinal ablation should be considered in any eye with zone I ROP with plus disease (any stage), zone I ROP stage 3 with or without plus, or zone II stage 2 or 3 ROP with plus disease (two quadrants, or six clock hours). Those neonates with type II ROP should be considered for treatment when progression to threshold or any of the above criteria are met. These treatment criteria have been influential and are incorporated into many national standards for ROP screening, defining thresholds for treatment [86,87].

9.3. ROP: How to treat

9.3.1. Cryotherapy

Reduction of VEGF production may be achieved with peripheral retinal ablation using cryotherapy. The (CRYO-ROP) studies evaluated the safety and efficacy of cryotherapy for stage 3 ROP. A randomised, controlled clinical trial evaluated 9,751 neonates, 291 of whom developed severe ROP. Cryotherapy reduced the incidence of unfavourable outcomes and improved functional outcomes in neonates with threshold ROP [88]. No intraoperative, or immediate post-operative complications were identified, and no deaths were attributed to cryotherapy treatment [89]. Risk reduction was found to be around 50% [35,36], and consequently recommendations were made for cryotherapy treatment to both eyes of neonates with stage 3 ROP in zone I [36]. The CRYO-ROP study was terminated prematurely due to significant treatment benefit with cryotherapy at the 3 month interim analysis [89,90]. A structural and functional benefit of cryotherapy was demonstrated after evaluation 3 years post-intervention [91]. 10 year follow-up revealed a clear protective effect of cryotherapy in ROP in the long-term in neonates with ROP [92]. New retinal detachments were identified in 15 year follow up [93].

The CRYO-ROP study provided numerous insights into the natural history of ROP, risk factors [94] and racial predilection [95], predictors of disease severity [96], prognosis [37,56,97], symmetry or concordance of disease between eyes [98], functional outcomes [99-101], involutional change [56], myopia [102], strabismus [103] and ocular comesis [104]. Cryotherapy did not benefit neonates with stage 4 ROP with partial retinal detachment [105]. The CRYO-ROP study identified a small loss of peripheral field around 6.4 degrees compared to controls [106] in eyes with severe ROP [107], and an increased incidence of myopia [108].

9.3.2. *Laser photocoagulation*

9.3.2.1. *Anterior to the ridge laser photocoagulation (Avascular retina)*

Zone I ROP owing to posterior location and area of ischaemic or avascular retina cannot be treated with cryotherapy alone. Diode laser photocoagulation anterior to the neovascular ridge in neonates with threshold zone I ROP has been demonstrated effective treatment, in contrast to cryoablation [109]. Further studies have demonstrated diode laser photocoagulation for stage 3 ROP to be at least as effective as cryotherapy treatment, with 40 of 42 eyes of eyes regressing after a single laser treatment; only 1 eye progressed to stage 4 ROP.

A study of 48 eyes found argon laser photocoagulation to be effective in the management of threshold ROP in zone I or posterior zone II with confluent laser to the avascular retina, with only 7 eyes progressing to stage 4A retina or beyond, without any recorded complications attributable to laser itself [110]. The mechanism of argon laser photocoagulation in stage 3 ROP is thought to be through reduced peripheral retinal oxygen consumption and reduction of VEGF.

Laser photocoagulation may be achieved with scattered laser; near-confluent [111] or confluent laser burns [112]. Confluent laser burns anterior to the ridge through 360 degrees in threshold ROP demonstrated low rates of progression to stage 4 or 5 ROP (6%), with mean spherical equivalent of-3.80DS in infants [112]. Near confluent laser photocoagulation anterior to the neovascular ridge prevented progression in 4 of 7 eyes with zone I ROP, and all with zone II ROP [111]. A larger combined retrospective and prospective study evaluated 107 neonates with threshold ROP compared near-confluent with scatter diode laser, finding that near-confluent laser photocoagulation was superior to scatter laser in reducing progression in eyes with both zone I and zone 2 ROP [113]. However, randomized trials of anterior to the ridge laser photocoagulation have not been conducted to evaluate the relative efficacy of burn distribution; it is likely that large studies are required to detect a difference as rate of progression to stage 4 and 5 ROP are low.

9.3.2.2. *Ridge laser photocoagulation*

A randomized, interventional comparative study evaluated the efficacy of argon laser photocoagulation to the neovascular ridge and anterior avascular retina versus laser to the avascular retina only [114] in neonates with threshold ROP. No immediate benefit of ridge laser photocoagulation was apparent, but longterm analysis is awaited. A retrospective study of anterior and ridge laser photocoagulation for threshold ROP with a favourable anatomical outcome in 96% of eyes, although long-term sequalae were not reported [115]. No vitreous haemorrhage was reported in this series. The additional benefit of direct laser photocoagulation of the neovascular ridge in ROP remains unproven [116].

9.3.2.3. *Posterior to the ridge laser (Vascular retina)*

Posterior to the ridge argon laser photocoagulation is a surgical approach that considers the presence of ischaemic retina posterior to the neovascular ridge, with or without confirmation of ischaemia with fluorescein angiography. Posterior to the ridge laser has been demonstrated in a non-comparative case series (no control arm) to be effective in the management of stage 3 ROP in zone II, where only 2 of 18 eyes progressed to stage 4A ROP. None developed stage 4B [117]. Aggressive posterior ROP (AP-ROP) may benefit from posterior argon laser photocoagulation in neonates with late stage 3 or stage 4A ROP following unsuccessful treatment to the avascular retina in threshold stage 3 disease [109]. The benefit of FFA guided posterior to the ridge laser has not been evaluated.

9.3.3. Anti-VEGF agents

9.3.3.1. Bevacizumab

Bevacizumab (Avastin) is a humanized monoclonal antibody raised against vascular endothelial growth factor (VEGF) isoform A, directly inhibiting angiogenesis. Avastin was originally developed and licensed for treatment of metastatic colorectal cancer, non-small cell lung cancer, renal carcinoma and glioblastoma multiforme. Avastin has been used off-label for the treatment of choroidal neovascularisation secondary to age-related macular degeneration, degenerative myopia, retinal vein occlusion, diabetic macular oedema and other disorders characterised by retinal or choroidal vascular abnormalities.

Retinopathy of prematurity is associated with high levels of VEGF within the vitreous and the rationale of administering intravitreal biologic drugs to inactivate it was considered as early as 2008. Avastin for stage 3 ROP with plus disease in zone I or posterior zone II was shown in a limited, non-comparative series to prevent progression of ROP with a single intravitreal injection of Avastin [118]. The BEAT-ROP study was the first prospective, randomized controlled trial comparing laser photocoagulation with intravitreal Avastin for zone I or posterior zone II stage 3+ROP, finding a significant benefit for zone I disease with Avastin, with continued vascularisation compared with conventional laser photocoagulation [119]. Laser photocoagulation for Zone I ROP involves extensive retinal ablation, with increased risk of visual field loss and secondary myopia.

Some studies have evaluated the outcome of combined laser and bevacizumab (0.25mg) for zone I ROP, finding all 18 study eyes demonstrated regression of plus disease without recurrence and vascularisation retina in zone I in all patients. The authors argue that a lower dose of bevacizumab may be used if combined with laser photocoagulation, reduced recurrence than with monotherapy and preservation of central field [120]. Others demonstrate the use bevacizumab as monotherapy (0.625mg), demonstrating efficacy in zone I stage 3 ROP [119,121]. Other groups demonstrate efficacy with rescue intravitreal bevacizumab following laser photocoagulation in aggressive posterior ROP [122]. The optimal dosage for ROP remains to be determined [123]. Late recurrence of ROP in has been reported with subsequent late tractional retinal detachment following initial regression of ROP [124]. Bevacizumab is associated with less significant myopia and astigmatism compared to laser [125].

Systemic absorption of bevacizumab is of concern, and although short-term follow-up studies and surveillance has not demonstrated any attributable systemic morbidity or mortality, this remains unproven. Fellow eyes demonstrate response to contralateral bevacizumab in ROP, suggesting significant systemic absorption of the drug [126].

9.3.3.2. Ranibizumab

Ranibizumab (Lucentis) is a monoclonal antibody directed against all isoforms of VEGF. It has been used off-label in retinopathy of prematurity, although data is more limited compared to that of bevacizumab. Experience from studies with ranibizumab in adult disorders, particularly neovascular age-related macular degeneration, has demonstrated fractionally increased systemic risk with bevacizumab versus ranibizumab but not enough to reach statistical significance. Logic would therefore consider ranibizumab in the treatment of ROP, particularly zone I ROP in which the ETROP study demonstrated a 55% treatment failure rate.

Combined laser-ranibizumab in this patient group has demonstrated promising control of stage 3 zone I ROP with regression in all cases, in a non-comparative series of 34 eyes [127]. Combination laser-ranibizumab has been demonstrated effective in the treatment of aggressive, posterior ROP, although this was a limited series of two neonates [128]. Three year outcomes with ranibizumab monotherapy in a series of six eyes with high-risk pre-threshold or threshold ROP with plus disease demonstrated complete regression of neovascularisation with a single treatment and continued vascularisation [129]. No attributable ocular or systemic side-effects were recorded [129]. Single case series of efficacy add limited evidence in favour of ranibizumab in ROP [130] Late retinal detachment in stage 3 zone I ROP has been reported similar to bevacizumab after initial neovascular regression [131].

Different pharmacokinetic and pharmacodynamic properties of ranibizumab and bevacizumab require randomized clinical studies to compare the efficacy in AP-ROP, threshold ROP. Ocular effects and systemic absorption, and non-inferiority demonstrated between ranibizumab and bevacizumab in neovascular AMD cannot be extrapolated to neonates with ROP. Long-term surveillance is required to document systemic outcomes in neonates treated with anti-VEGF agents for ROP to detect late adverse effects not currently encompassed in short-term published trial data.

9.3.3.3. Pegaptinib

Pegaptinib (Macugen, 0.3mg in 0.02mls) has been evaluated for stage 3+ROP with adjunctive laser photocoagulation in a randomized controlled clinical trial found to be more efficacious than laser alone [132]. Recurrence of neovascularisation was noted at 14.4 weeks with bevacizumab, at 15.1 weeks with pegaptinib with laser, and 5.9 weeks with laser alone [133]. Risk factors for recurrence, the interval for follow-up examination, and length of time required for follow-up is unknown [133].

10. Surgical management

Surgical intervention is necessary for patient with stage 4 partial retinal detachments, which may or may not involve the fovea, or those with open or closed funnel retinal detachments. Surgical approaches include scleral buckle, vitrectomy and combined vitrectomy-lensectomy.

Factors affecting surgical outcome of stage 4 and 5 ROP have been examined and a poorer surgical outcome may be associated with vitreous haze, active neovascularisation and plus disease [134]. Plus disease was identified as the most significant factor associated with failed retinal reattachment; additional surgery or intravitreal anti-VEGF agents may be considered pre-operatively to improve outcome in this group [134].

Outcomes from neonates from the ET-ROP study who stage 4 or 5 ROP were generally poor. Vitreoretinal surgery was associated with macular attachment in 16 of 48 eyes (33%). Normal acuity was maintained in 21% of eyes after 4a retinal detachment. Stage 5 ROP was associated with good anatomical but poor functional outcome [135].

10.1. Scleral buckling

Stage 4 ROP, partial retinal detachment with or without foveal involvement (stage 4a/ stage 4b respectively) may be treated with lens-sparing vitrectomy with or without the use of external tamponade with a scleral buckle. Studies on the outcome of scleral buckles for stage 4 ROP are limited, and limited study numbers, without randomization make conclusions on the efficacy of scleral buckles difficult. Variability in surgical experience and expertise with scleral buckles in stage 4 ROP makes comparison between studies difficult. Long-term outcome in patients from the ETROP trial with retinal detachments (stage 4a/4b/5 ROP) were reported [87]. Vitrectomy with or without scleral buckle resulted in macular attachment in 17 of 50 eyes, scleral buckle only achieved macular attachment in 6 of 9 eyes after 7 years. This data was from multiple centres and surgeons, and not randomized making cross comparison difficult. A high proportion of retinal detachments (20%) were not classified [87].

A small retrospective interventional case series identified 21 eyes with stage 4 ROP, comparing anatomical outcomes of lens-sparing vitrectomy versus combined lens-sparing vitrectomy and scleral buckle [135]; 12 undergoing combined LSV and SB, and 9 LSV alone. The authors conclude that scleral buckle adds little to the success or failure of LSV with similar outcomes in each group [135], but this small series may not have been adequately powered to detect a difference in treatment outcome. Another retrospective series of 16 eyes who underwent scleral buckling for stage 4 ROP reported anatomical success of 100% in stage 4a and 50% in stage 4b ROP [136]. The buckle was removed in 11 of 12 infants, and mean refraction was-8.68 diopters. There was no control group in this study, but evidence was offered of reducing progression to stage 5 ROP [136].

A further single-surgeon series of 8 neonates who underwent scleral buckling for stage 4a ROP conclude efficacy in preventing progression of retinal detachment, although this study was non-comparative [137].

Scleral buckling requires further procedures under general anaesthetic to reduce the tension of the buckle, or remove it altogether. The tension created by the buckle causes axial myopia (reduced by 5.5 dioptres after division of the buckle), and removal or adjustment of tension necessitates repeat refraction to prevent ametropic amblyopia [138]. Removal of scleral buckle has been demonstrated without resulting retinal detachment or vitreous traction [139].

Anatomical success in patients with repair of stage 4 or 5 ROP may not equate simply to visual improvement in such studies [134]. This is supported by evidence from a systematic review of outcomes of surgical intervention for ROP [140], which demonstrated poor vision in many patients regardless of retinal attachment status. There is difficulty in many studies of measuring low visual acuity in infants; this may not be achieved by grating acuity that is often used as an output in many ROP series.

Large, multicentre, long term studies with randomization are required to determine the efficacy of scleral buckling, but variations in surgical expertise and preference may be prohibitive. It is unlikely that meta-analysis will be valid for this reason. A systematic review of anatomical and visual function outcomes in ROP with vitrectomy and scleral buckle identified a wide variation of retinal reattachment rates between centres of 0.8 to 90% [140]. Earlier surgery was associated with a superior retinal reattachment rate, although longer follow-up was associated with increasing anatomical failure [140].

10.2. Vitrectomy

Evaluating surgical outcomes in ROP is difficult due to the long interval between intervention and reliable recording of monocular visual acuities, variability in surgical technique and experience, and the effect of neurological co-morbidity in clinical evaluation. Many studies are retrospective case series with non-standardised follow-up intervals, and no control arms which limits inferences of efficacy.

Early data from the CRYO-ROP study evaluated the functional outcome of neonates with stage 5 ROP (total retinal detachment) who underwent lensectomy-vitrectomy procedures before one year of age, comparing this cohort with infants who did not. Almost all infants had visual acuity of light perception or worse at 5 years [141].

Further studies demonstrate more promising results. A single-centre retrospective case series reported 37 eyes treated with LSV for stage 4A and 4B ROP, with follow up of 5 years. 63% had measureable visual acuity, 18% had form vision, and 19% had light perception vision or worse [142]. Further similar series evaluated LSV in the setting of progressive posterior-type stage 4A ROP with plus disease, documenting low anatomical success of LSV in progressive posterior stage 4A ROP, particularly associated with plus disease [143].

A consecutive, non-randomized, retrospective series comparing outcomes patients with stage 4 ROP treated with scleral buckle or lens-sparing vitrectomy found that LSV was associated with retinal reattachment in 72% of patients versus 31% of SB patients. At final follow-up, after further procedures, LSV and SB were found comparable in outcome as a first procedure. LSV was favoured in this study as more effective as a single procedure to stop stage 4 ROP [144].

The advent of anti-VEGF agents has led to widespread adjuvant use prior to vitrectomy in vasoproliferative disease to augment surgical outcome. Stage 4A ROP with plus disease has poorer surgical outcomes, and many reports have evaluated the benefit of bevacizumab prior to vitrectomy in these patients [145-148]. Several reports have documented the apparent pro-fibrotic effect of bevacizumab with contraction of fibrovascular membranes which may increased tractional retinal detachment [149] and require surgical treatment. Case reports document acute retinal fibrosis 1 day following bevacizumab despite acute resolution of the vascular component, with centripetal contraction of fibrovascular tissue and retinal detachment [150]. One series evaluated the efficacy of intravitreal bevacizumab 72 hour prior to vitrectomy or laser, finding improved visualisation in high risk ROP [151]. This finding has been demonstrated in other series [87,154], with no adverse effects attributable to bevacizumab in the short-term [152].

Author details

Vikas Tah[1], Walid Sharif[2], Imran Yusuf[5], Marcus Posner[4], Louise Ramskold[3], Farihah Tariq[1], Dev Mukhey[2] and Zuhair Sharif[2]

1 Stoke Mandeville Hospital, UK

2 UCL Institute of Ophthalmology, UK

3 East and North Hertfordshire NHS Trust, UK

4 Royal Free Hospital, UK

5 Oxford, UK

References

[1] Hartnett ME, Penn JS. Mechanisms and management of retinopathy of prematurity. *New England Journal of Medicine*. 2012; 367:2515-2526.

[2] Terry TL. Extreme prematurity and fibroblastic overgrowth of persistent vascular sheath behind each crystalline lens. *Am J Ophthalmol*. 1942;25:203-4

[3] Akkoyun I, Oto S, Yilmaz G, Gurakan B, Tarcan A, Anuk D, Akgun S, Akova YA. Risk factors in the development of mild and severe retinopathy of prematurity. *J AAPOS*. 2006 Oct; 10(5):449-53

[4] Kim TI, Sohn J, Pi SY, Yoon YH. Postnatal risk factors of retinopathy of prematurity. *Paediatr Perinat Epidemiol*. 2004 Mar; 18(2):130-4.

[5] Coats DK, Aaron MM, Mohamed AH. Involution of retinopathy of prematurity after laser treatment: Factors associated with development of retinal detachment. *Am J Ophthalmol.* 2005;140:214–22

[6] Fanaroff AA, Martin RJ, editors. Neonatal perinatal medicine. 7th ed. *Louis: Mosby;* 2002. pp. 676–74

[7] Saugstad OD. Is oxygen more toxic than currently believed? *Pediatrics.* 2001; 108:1203-1205

[8] Gilbert C. Retinopathy of prematurity ; a global perspective of the epidemics, population of babies at risk and implications for control. *Early Hum Dev.* 2008; 84;77-82

[9] Bouzas L, Bauer G, Novali L et al. Retinopathy of prematurity in the XXI century in a developing country; an emergency that should be resolved. *Annals de paediatrica.*2007; 66: 551-8

[10] Chen Y, Li X. Characteristics of severe retinopathy of prematurity patients in China: a repeat of the first epidemic? *Br J Ophthal.* 2006; 90: 268-271

[11] Palmer EA, Flynn JT, Hardy RJ et al. The cryotherapy for retinopathy cooperative study group. Incidence and early course of ROP. *Ophthalmology.* 1991; 98: 1628-1640

[12] Good VW, Hardy RJ, Dobson V et al. Early Treatment for Retinopathy of Prematurity Cooperative Study Group. The incidence and course of retinopathy of prematurity; findings from the early treatment for retinopathy of prematurity study. *Pediatrics.* 2005; 116: 15-23 (http://pediatrics.aappublications.org/cgi/content/full/116/1/15)

[13] Al-Amro SA, Al-Kharfi TM, Thabit AA et al. Retinopathy of prematurity at a university hospital in Riyadh, Saudi Arabia. *Saudi Medical Journal Online.* 2002. (http://www.smj.org.sa/DetailArticle.asp?ArticleId=862)

[14] Hussan N, Clive J, Bhandari V. Current incidence of retinopathy of prematurity 1989-97. *Pediatrics.* 1999 Sep;104(3):e26 (http://pediatrics.aappublications.org/cgi/content/full/104/e26)

[15] Fortes Filho JB, Eckert GU, Procianoy L. Incidence of retinopathy of prematurity in very low and in extremely low birthweight infants in a unit based approach in Brazil. *EYE(Lon).* Jan 2009; 23(1): 25-30 (http://nature.com/eye//journal/v23/n/full/6702924a.html)

[16] Good WV. Screening for retinopathy of prematurity; no ophthalmologist required? *Brit Ophthal.* 2000; 84: 124-7

[17] Shah VA, Yeo CL, LingYL et al. Incidence, risk factors of retinopathy of prematurity among very low birthweight infants in Singapore. *Annals Academy of Medicine.* 2005; 34: 169-178 (http://annals.edu.sg/pdf//34vol200501/V34N2p169.pdf)

[18] M Begué N, Perapoch Lopez J. Retinopathy of prematurity; incidence, severity and outcome. *Anales de Pediatria.* 2003: 58; 156-61

[19] Rekha S, Battu RR; Retinopathy of prematurity; incidence and risk factors. *Indian Pediatr.* 1996; 33(12): 999-1003 (http://indianpediatrics.net/dec1996/999.pdf)

[20] The International Committee for the Classification of Retinopathy of Prematurity. An International Classification of Retinopathy of Prematurity.. *Arch Ophthalmol.* 1984;102: 1130-1134

[21] An International Classification of Retinopathy of Prematurity. The International Committee for the Classification of Retinopathy of Prematurity. *Arch Ophthalol. 1987;* 105

[22] The International Classification of Retinopathy of Prematurity revisited. The International Committee for the Classification of Retinopathy of Prematurity. *Arch Ophthalmol.* 2005;123.

[23] Lucey JF, Dangman B. A re-examination of the role of oxygen in retrolental fibroplasia. *Pediatrics.*1984;73(1):82-96.

[24] Michaelson IC. The mode of development of the vascular system of the retina with some observations on its significance for certain retinal diseases. *Trans Ophthalmol Soc.* 1948; 68:137–180.

[25] Ashton N, Ward B, Serpell G. Effect of oxygen on developing retinal vessels with particular reference to the problem of retrolental fibroplasia. *Br J Ophthalmol.* 1954; 38:397–432.

[26] Patz A, Eastham A, Higginbotham DH, Kleh T. Oxygen studies in retrolental fibroplasia. *Am J Ophthalmol.* 1953;36:1511–1522.

[27] Kinsey VE, Arnold HJ, Kalina RE, et al. PaO2 levels and retrolental fibroplasia: a report of the cooperative study. *Pediatrics.* 1977;60(5):655–668.

[28] Flynn JT. Acute proliferative retrolental fibroplasia: multivariate risk analysis. *Trans Am Ophthalmol Soc.* 1983; 81:549–591.

[29] Smith LE. Pathogenesis of retinopathy of prematurity. *Semin Neonatol.* 2003;8(6):469–473.

[30] Tasman W, Patz A, McNamara JA, Kaiser RS, Trese MT, Smith BT. Retinopathy of prematurity: the life of a lifetime disease. *Am J Ophthalmol.* 2006;141(1):167–174.

[31] Lutty GA, Chan-Ling T, Phelps DL, et al. Proceedings of the Third International Symposium on Retinopathy of Prematurity: an update on ROP from the lab to the nursery (November 2003, Anaheim, California) *Mol Vis.* 2006;12:532–580.

[32] Silverman W. Retrolental fibroplasia: a modern parable. New York: *Grune and Stratton.*1980.

[33] Askie, LM. Optimal oxygen saturations in preterm infants: a moving target. *Current Opinion in Pediatrics.* 2013; 25: 2:188–192.

[34] Palmer EA, Hardy RJ, Dobson V, Phelps DL, Quinn GE, Summers CG et al. International Committee for the Classification of Retinopathy of Prematurity. The International Classification of Retinopathy of Prematurity Revisited. *Arch Ophthalmol.* 2005;123:991-999.

[35] Cryotherapy for Retinopathy of Prematurity Cooperative Group. Multicentre trial of cryotherapy for retinopathy of prematurity: Preliminary results. *Arch Ophthalmol.* 1988;106: 471-479.

[36] Cryotherapy for Retinopathy of Prematurity Cooperative group. Multicentric trial of cryotherapy for retinopathy of prematurity. Three-month outcome. *Arch Ophthalmol* 1990;108: 195-204.

[37] Cryotherapy for Retinopathy of Prematurity Cooperative Group. The natural ocular outcome of premature birth and retinopathy status at 1 year. *Arch Ophthalmol.* 1994; 112(7):903-912.

[38] Cryotherapy for Retinopathy of Prematurity Cooperative group. Multicentric trial of cryotherapy for retinopathy of prematurity: natural history ROP: ocular outcome at 5 ½ years in premature infants with birth weight less than 1251 g. *Arch Ophthalmol.* 2002;120: 595-599.

[39] Ellsbury, D, Ursprung, R. Comprehensive Oxygen Management for the Prevention of Retinopathy of Prematurity: The Pediatrix Experience. *Clinics in Perinatology.* 2010; 37:1: 203–215.

[40] Flynn JT, Chan-Ling T. Retinopathy of prematurity: two distinct mechanisms that underlie zone 1 and zone 2 disease. *Am J Ophthalmol.* 2006; 142(1):46-59.

[41] Stenson BJ, Tarnow-Mordi WO, Darlow Ba, et al. Oxygen Saturation and Outcomes in Pre-term Infants. *N Engl J Med.* 2013; 368:2094-2104.

[42] Mills, MD. Evaluating the Cryotherapy for Retinopathy of Prematurity Study (CRYO-ROP). *Arch Ophthalmol.* 2007;125 (9):1276-1281.

[43] The STOP-ROP Multi-center Study Group. Supplemental Therapeutic Oxygen for Pre-threshold Retinopathy of Prematurity (STOP-ROP), a randomized, controlled trial. I: primary outcomes. *Pediatrics.* 2000;105:295–310.

[44] Chow, LC. et al. Can Changes in Clinical Practice Decrease the Incidence of Severe Retinopathy of Prematurity in Very Low Birth Weight Infants? *Pediatrics.* 2003;111:1:339-345.

[45] Chen ML, Guo L, Smith LE, Dammann CE, Dammann O. High or low oxygen saturation and severe retinopathy of prematurity: a meta-analysis. *Pediatrics.* 2010;125:6: e1483-1492.

[46] Fleck BW, Stenson, BJ. Retinopathy of Prematurity and the Oxygen Conundrum: Lessons Learned from Recent Randomized Trials. *Clinics in Perinatology*. 2013; 40: 2229–2240.

[47] Wilson CM, Ells AL, Fielder AR. The Challenge of Screening for Retinopathy of Prematurity. *Royal College of Paediatrics and Child Health, Royal College of Ophthalmologists and British Association of Perinatal Medicine*. 2007.

[48] Blakeman, TC. Evidence for Oxygen Use in the Hospitalized Patient: Is More Really the Enemy of Good? *Respiratory Care*. 2013;58 :10: 1679-169.

[49] Guideline for the Screening and Treatment of Retinopathy of Prematurity. Royal College of Paediatrics and Child Health, Royal College of Ophthalmologists and British Association of Perinatal Medicine. 2008.

[50] Fielder AR, Haines L, Scrivener R, Wilkinson AR, Pollock JI on behalf of the Royal Colleges of Ophthalmologists and Paediatrics and Child Health and the British Association of Perinatal Medicine. Retinopathy of prematurity in the UK II: audit of national guidelines for screening and treatment. *Eye*. 2002; 16(3):285-291.

[51] Goble RR, Jones HS, Fielder AR. Are we screening too many babies for retinopathy of prematurity? *Eye*.1997; 11(Pt 4):509-514.

[52] Mathew MR, Fern AI, Hill R. Retinopathy of prematurity: are we screening too many babies? *Eye*. 2002; 16(5):538-542.

[53] Early Treatment for Retinopathy of Prematurity Cooperative Group. Revised indications for the treatment of retinopathy of prematurity: results of the early treatment for retinopathy of prematurity randomized trial. *Arch Ophthalmol*. 2003; 121(12): 1684-1694.

[54] AMERICAN ACADEMY OF OPHTHALMOLOGY, AMERICAN ASSOCIATION FOR PEDIATRIC OPHTHALMOLOGY AND STRABISMUS, AMERICAN ASSOCIATION OF CERTIFIED ORTHOPTISTS. Policy Statement: Screening Examination of Premature Infants for Retinopathy of Prematurity. *Pediatrics*. 2013;l: 131:89-195.

[55] Reynolds JD, Dobson V, Quinn GE, Fielder AR, Palmer EA, Saunders RA et al. Evidence-based screening criteria for retinopathy of prematurity: natural history data from the CRYO-ROP and LIGHT-ROP studies. *Arch Ophthalmol* 2002; 120(11): 1470-1476.

[56] Repka MX, Palmer EA, Tung B. Cryotherapy for Retinopathy of Prematurity Cooperative Group. Involution of retinopathy of prematurity. *Arch Ophthalmol* 2000; 118(5): 645-649.

[57] Kanski J. Clinical Ophthalmology; A Systematic Approach (7th Ed) Butterworth Heinemann 2011.

[58] Chen, J, Stahl, A, Hellstrom, A, Smith, LE. Current update on retinopathy of prematurity: screening and treatment. *Curr Opin Pediatr*. 2011; 23(2): 173–178.

[59] Löfqvist C, Hansen-Pupp I, Andersson E, et al. Validation of a new retinopathy of prematurity screening method monitoring longitudinal postnatal weight and insulin like growth factor I. *Arch Ophthalmol* 2009;127:622-627.

[60] Wu C, Löfqvist C, Smith LH, VanderVeen DK, Hellström A. Importance of early postnatal weight gain for normal retinal angiogenesis in very preterm infants: a multicenter study analyzing weight velocity deviations for the prediction of retinopathy of prematurity. *Arch Ophthalmol*. 2012;130:992–999.

[61] Zepeda-Romero LC, Hård AL, Gomez-Ruiz LM, et al. Prediction of retinopathy of prematurity using the screening algorithm WINROP in a Mexican population of preterm infants. *Arch Ophthalmol* 2012; 130:720-3.

[62] Mohamed, S, Murray, JC, Dagle, JM, Colaizy, T. Hyperglycemia as a risk factor for the development of retinopathy of prematurity. *BMC Pediatr*. 2013; 13

[63] Piyasena C, Dhaliwal C, et al. Prediction of severe retinopathy of prematurity using the WINROP algorithm in a birth cohort in South East Scotland. *Archives of Disease in Childhood Fetal and Neonatal Edition*. 2014; 99:1 29-33.

[64] Chiang MF, Keenan JD, Starren JB, Du YE, Schiff WM, Barile GR et al. Accuracy and reliability of remote retinopathy of prematurity diagnosis. *Arch Ophthalmol*. 2006; 124:322-327.

[65] Chiang MF, Starren JB, Du YE, Keenan JD, Schiff WM, Barile GR et al. Remote image based retinopathy of prematurity diagnosis: a receiver operating characteristic analysis of accuracy. *Br J Ophthalmol*. 2006; 90(10):1292-1296.

[66] Roth DB, Morales D, Feuer WJ, Hess D, Johnson RA, Flynn JT et al. Screening for retinopathy of prematurity employing the Retcam 120: sensitivity and specificity. *Arch Ophthalmol*. 2001; 119(2):268-272.

[67] Capone, A. The Photographic Screening for Retinopathy of Prematurity Study Group. The Photographic Screening for Retinopathy of Prematurity Study (Photo-ROP): Study design and baseline characteristics of enrolled patients. *Retina*. 2006; 26(7 Suppl):S4-S10.

[68] Aslam T, Fleck B, Patton N, Trucco M, Azegrouz H. Digital image analysis of plus disease in retinopathy of prematurity. *Acta Ophthalmologica*. 2009;87:4: 368–377.

[69] Wittenberg LA, Jonsson L, Chan RVP, Chiang, MF. Computer-Based Image Analysis for Plus Disease Diagnosis in Retinopathy of Prematurity. *Journal of Pediatric Ophthalmology and Strabismus*. 2012;49 :1: 11-19.

[70] Gelman R, Martinez-Perez M, Vanderveen D, Moskowitz A, Fulton A. Diagnosis of Plus Disease in Retinopathy of Prematurity using Retinal Image multiscale Analysis. *Invest Ophthalmol Vis Sci.* 2005;46(12):4734-4738

[71] Courtesy of Tygerberg Children's Hospital. From: http://www.tch-trust.org.za/improve-the-care-of-children-and-babies-by-acquiring-the-most-modern-technology/. (Accessed : 28/12/13)

[72] Courtesy of Hoag Levins. Clarity Medical Solutions. From: http://ldihealtheconomist.com/he000017.shtml. (Accessed:24/12/14)

[73] Courtesy of Minas Hambardzumyan.. From: https://picasaweb.google.com/lh/photo/47DVdk1Ed1eD6wmgEtcVyw (Accessed: 28/12/14)

[74] Courtesy of BIOPHOTONICS. From: http://photonics.com/Product.aspx?PRID=38590 (Accessed: 28/12/13)

[75] Kinsey VE. Retrolental fibroplasia; cooperative study of retrolental fibroplasia and the use of oxygen. *AMA Arch Ophthalmol* 1956;56:481-543.

[76] Higgins RD, Bancalari E, Willinger M, et al. Executive summary of the workshop on oxygen in neonatal therapies: controversies and opportunities for research. *Pediatrics* 2007;119:790-6.

[77] Kirchner L, Weninger M, Unterasinger L, et al. Is the use of early nasal CPAP associated with lower rates of chronic lung disease and retinopathy of prematurity? Nine years of experience with the Vermont Oxford Neonatal Network. *J Perinat Med* 2005;33:60-6.

[78] Flynn JT, Bancalari E, Bawol R, et al. Retinopathy of prematurity. A randomized, prospective trial of transcutaneous oxygen monitoring. *Ophthalmology* 1987;94:630-8.

[79] Berkowitz BA, Berlin ES, Zhang W. Variable supplemental oxygen during recovery does not reduce retinal neovascular severity in experimental ROP. *Curr Eye Res* 2001;22:401-4.

[80] Mills MD. STOP-ROP results suggest selective use of supplemental oxygen for prethreshold ROP. *Arch Ophthalmol* 2000;118:1121-2.

[81] Flynn JT, Bancalari E. Supplemental therapeutic oxygen for prethreshold retinopathy of prematurity (STOP-ROP), a randomized, controlled trial. I: Primary outcomes. *J Aapos* 2000;4:65-6.

[82] Hay WW, Jr., Bell EF. Oxygen therapy, oxygen toxicity, and the STOP-ROP trial. *Pediatrics* 2000;105:424-5.

[83] McGregor ML, Bremer DL, Cole C, et al. Retinopathy of prematurity outcome in infants with prethreshold retinopathy of prematurity and oxygen saturation >94% in room air: the high oxygen percentage in retinopathy of prematurity study. *Pediatrics* 2002;110:540-4.

[84] Askie LM, Henderson-Smart DJ, Irwig L, et al. Oxygen-saturation targets and outcomes in extremely preterm infants. *N Engl J Med* 2003;349:959-67.

[85] Askie LM, Brocklehurst P, Darlow BA, et al. NeOProM: Neonatal Oxygenation Prospective Meta-analysis Collaboration study protocol. *BMC Pediatr* 2011;11:6.

[86] Good WV. Final results of the Early Treatment for Retinopathy of Prematurity (ETROP) randomized trial. *Trans Am Ophthalmol Soc* 2004;102:233-48; discussion 248-50.

[87] Repka MX, Tung B, Good WV, et al. Outcome of eyes developing retinal detachment during the Early Treatment for Retinopathy of Prematurity Study (ETROP). *Arch Ophthalmol* 2006;124:24-30.

[88] Multicenter trial of cryotherapy for retinopathy of prematurity. One-year outcome--structure and function. Cryotherapy for Retinopathy of Prematurity Cooperative Group. *Arch Ophthalmol* 1990;108:1408-16.

[89] Palmer EA, Hardy RJ, Davis BR, et al. Operational aspects of terminating randomization in the Multicenter Trial of Cryotherapy for Retinopathy of Prematurity. Cryotherapy for Retinopathy of Prematurity Cooperative Group. *Control Clin Trials* 1991;12:277-92.

[90] Hardy RJ, Davis BR, Palmer EA, et al. Statistical considerations in terminating randomization in the Multicenter Trial of Cryotherapy for Retinopathy of Prematurity. Cryotherapy for Retinopathy of Prematurity Cooperative Group. *Control Clin Trials* 1991;12:293-303.

[91] Multicenter trial of cryotherapy for retinopathy of prematurity. 3 1/2-year outcome--structure and function. Cryotherapy for Retinopathy of Prematurity Cooperative Group. *Arch Ophthalmol* 1993;111:339-44.

[92] Multicenter Trial of Cryotherapy for Retinopathy of Prematurity: ophthalmological outcomes at 10 years. *Arch Ophthalmol* 2001;119:1110-8.

[93] Palmer EA, Hardy RJ, Dobson V, et al. 15-year outcomes following threshold retinopathy of prematurity: final results from the multicenter trial of cryotherapy for retinopathy of prematurity. *Arch Ophthalmol* 2005;123:311-8.

[94] Hardy RJ, Palmer EA, Dobson V, et al. Risk analysis of prethreshold retinopathy of prematurity. *Arch Ophthalmol* 2003;121:1697-701.

[95] Saunders RA, Donahue ML, Christmann LM, et al. Racial variation in retinopathy of prematurity. The Cryotherapy for Retinopathy of Prematurity Cooperative Group. *Arch Ophthalmol* 1997;115:604-8.

[96] Kivlin JD, Biglan AW, Gordon RA, et al. Early retinal vessel development and iris vessel dilatation as factors in retinopathy of prematurity. Cryotherapy for Retinop-

athy of Prematurity (CRYO-ROP) Cooperative Group. *Arch Ophthalmol* 1996;114:150-4.

[97] Schaffer DB, Palmer EA, Plotsky DF, et al. Prognostic factors in the natural course of retinopathy of prematurity. The Cryotherapy for Retinopathy of Prematurity Cooperative Group. *Ophthalmology* 1993;100:230-7.

[98] Quinn GE, Dobson V, Biglan A, et al. Correlation of retinopathy of prematurity in fellow eyes in the cryotherapy for retinopathy of prematurity study. The Cryotherapy for Retinopathy of Prematurity Cooperative Group. *Arch Ophthalmol* 1995;113:469-73.

[99] Dobson V, Quinn GE, Tung B, et al. Comparison of recognition and grating acuities in very-low-birth-weight children with and without retinal residua of retinopathy of prematurity. Cryotherapy for Retinopathy of Prematurity Cooperative Group. *Invest Ophthalmol Vis Sci* 1995;36:692-702.

[100] Dobson V, Quinn GE, Summers CG, et al. Effect of acute-phase retinopathy of prematurity on grating acuity development in the very low birth weight infant. The Cryotherapy for Retinopathy of Prematurity Cooperative Group. *Invest Ophthalmol Vis Sci* 1994;35:4236-44.

[101] Reynolds J, Dobson V, Quinn GE, et al. Prediction of visual function in eyes with mild to moderate posterior pole residua of retinopathy of prematurity. Cryotherapy for Retinopathy of Prematurity Cooperative Group. *Arch Ophthalmol* 1993;111:1050-6.

[102] Quinn GE, Dobson V, Repka MX, et al. Development of myopia in infants with birth weights less than 1251 grams. The Cryotherapy for Retinopathy of Prematurity Cooperative Group. *Ophthalmology* 1992;99:329-40.

[103] Bremer DL, Palmer EA, Fellows RR, et al. Strabismus in premature infants in the first year of life. Cryotherapy for Retinopathy of Prematurity Cooperative Group. *Arch Ophthalmol* 1998;116:329-33.

[104] Summers G, Phelps DL, Tung B, et al. Ocular cosmesis in retinopathy of prematurity. The Cryotherapy for Retinopathy of Prematurity Cooperative Group. *Arch Ophthalmol* 1992;110:1092-7.

[105] Gilbert WS, Quinn GE, Dobson V, et al. Partial retinal detachment at 3 months after threshold retinopathy of prematurity. Long-term structural and functional outcome. Multicenter Trial of Cryotherapy for Retinopathy of Prematurity Cooperative Group. *Arch Ophthalmol* 1996;114:1085-91.

[106] Quinn GE, Dobson V, Hardy RJ, et al. Visual fields measured with double-arc perimetry in eyes with threshold retinopathy of prematurity from the cryotherapy for retinopathy of prematurity trial. The CRYO-Retinopathy of Prematurity Cooperative Group. *Ophthalmology* 1996;103:1432-7.

[107] Quinn GE, Dobson V, Hardy RJ, et al. Effect of retinal ablative therapy for threshold retinopathy of prematurity: results of Goldmann perimetry at the age of 10 years. *Arch Ophthalmol* 2001;119:1120-5.

[108] Quinn GE, Dobson V, Siatkowski R, et al. Does cryotherapy affect refractive error? Results from treated versus control eyes in the cryotherapy for retinopathy of prematurity trial. *Ophthalmology* 2001;108:343-7.

[109] O'Keefe M, Burke J, Algawi K, et al. Diode laser photocoagulation to the vascular retina for progressively advancing retinopathy of prematurity. *Br J Ophthalmol* 1995;79:1012-4.

[110] Axer-Siegel R, Snir M, Cotlear D, et al. Diode laser treatment of posterior retinopathy of prematurity. *Br J Ophthalmol* 2000;84:1383-6.

[111] Rezai KA, Eliott D, Ferrone PJ, et al. Near confluent laser photocoagulation for the treatment of threshold retinopathy of prematurity. *Arch Ophthalmol* 2005;123:621-6.

[112] Gonzalez VH, Giuliari GP, Banda RM, et al. Confluent laser photocoagulation for the treatment of retinopathy of prematurity. *J Pediatr Ophthalmol Strabismus* 2010;47:81-5; quiz 86-7.

[113] Banach MJ, Ferrone PJ, Trese MT. A comparison of dense versus less dense diode laser photocoagulation patterns for threshold retinopathy of prematurity. *Ophthalmology* 2000;107:324-7; discussion 328.

[114] Uparkar M, Sen P, Rawal A, et al. Laser photocoagulation (810 nm diode) for threshold retinopathy of prematurity: a prospective randomized pilot study of treatment to ridge and avascular retina versus avascular retina alone. *Int Ophthalmol* 2011;31:3-8.

[115] Steinmetz RL, Brooks HL, Jr. Diode laser photocoagulation to the ridge and avascular retina in threshold retinopathy of prematurity. *Retina* 2002;22:48-52.

[116] Tasman W. To laser the ridge or not laser the ridge, that is the question. *Retina* 2002;22:4-5.

[117] Ells AL, Gole GA, Lloyd Hildebrand P, et al. Posterior to the ridge laser treatment for severe stage 3 retinopathy of prematurity. *Eye (Lond)* 2013;27:525-30.

[118] Mintz-Hittner HA, Kuffel RR, Jr. Intravitreal injection of bevacizumab (avastin) for treatment of stage 3 retinopathy of prematurity in zone I or posterior zone II. *Retina* 2008;28:831-8.

[119] Mintz-Hittner HA, Kennedy KA, Chuang AZ. Efficacy of intravitreal bevacizumab for stage 3+retinopathy of prematurity. *N Engl J Med* 2011;364:603-15.

[120] Kim J, Kim SJ, Chang YS, et al. Combined Intravitreal Bevacizumab Injection and Zone I Sparing Laser Photocoagulation in Patients with Zone I Retinopathy of Prematurity. *Retina* 2013.

[121] Sahin A, Sahin M, Cingu AK, et al. Intravitreal bevacizumab monotherapy for retinopathy of prematurity. *Pediatr Int.*

[122] Dani C, Frosini S, Fortunato P, et al. Intravitreal bevacizumab for retinopathy of prematurity as first line or rescue therapy with focal laser treatment. A case series. *J Matern Fetal Neonatal Med* 2012;25:2194-7.

[123] Spandau U. What is the optimal dosage for intravitreal bevacizumab for retinopathy of prematurity? *Acta Ophthalmol* 2013;91:e154.

[124] Mireskandari K, Adams GG, Tehrani NN. Recurrence of retinopathy of prematurity following bevacizumab monotherapy: is it only the tip of the iceberg? *JAMA Ophthalmol* 2013;131:544-5.

[125] Harder BC, Schlichtenbrede FC, von Baltz S, et al. Intravitreal bevacizumab for retinopathy of prematurity: refractive error results. *Am J Ophthalmol* 2013;155:1119-1124 e1.

[126] Karaca C, Oner AO, Mirza E, et al. Bilateral effect of unilateral bevacizumab injection in retinopathy of prematurity. *JAMA Ophthalmol* 2013;131:1099-101.

[127] Orozco-Gomez LP, Hernandez-Salazar L, Moguel-Ancheita S, et al. Laser-ranibizumab treatment for retinopathy of prematurity in umbral-preumbral disease. Three years of experience. *Cir Cir* 2011;79:207-214, 225-32.

[128] Mota A, Carneiro A, Breda J, et al. Combination of intravitreal ranibizumab and laser photocoagulation for aggressive posterior retinopathy of prematurity. *Case Rep Ophthalmol* 2011;3:136-41.

[129] Castellanos MA, Schwartz S, Garcia-Aguirre G, et al. Short-term outcome after intravitreal ranibizumab injections for the treatment of retinopathy of prematurity. *Br J Ophthalmol* 2013;97:816-9.

[130] Lin CJ, Chen SN, Hwang JF. Intravitreal ranibizumab as salvage therapy in an extremely low-birth-weight infant with rush type retinopathy of prematurity. *Oman J Ophthalmol*;5:184-6.

[131] Jang SY, Choi KS, Lee SJ. Delayed-onset retinal detachment after an intravitreal injection of ranibizumab for zone I plus retinopathy of prematurity. *J Aapos* 2010;14:457-9.

[132] Autrata R, Krejcirova I, Senkova K, et al. Intravitreal pegaptanib combined with diode laser therapy for stage 3+retinopathy of prematurity in zone I and posterior zone II. *Eur J Ophthalmol* 2012;22:687-94.

[133] Mintz-Hittner HA. Intravitreal pegaptanib as adjunctive treatment for stage 3+ROP shown to be effective in a prospective, randomized, controlled multicenter clinical trial. *Eur J Ophthalmol* 2012;22:685-6.

[134] Hartnett ME. Features associated with surgical outcome in patients with stages 4 and 5 retinopathy of prematurity. *Retina* 2003;23:322-9.

[135] Sears JE, Sonnie C. Anatomic success of lens-sparing vitrectomy with and without scleral buckle for stage 4 retinopathy of prematurity. *Am J Ophthalmol* 2007;143:810-3.

[136] Ratanasukon M, Visaetsilpanonta S, Tengtrisorn S, et al. Outcomes of scleral buckling for stage 4 retinopathy of prematurity in Thai children. *J Med Assoc Thai* 2006;89:1659-64.

[137] Hinz BJ, de Juan E, Jr., Repka MX. Scleral buckling surgery for active stage 4A retinopathy of prematurity. *Ophthalmology* 1998;105:1827-30.

[138] Chow DR, Ferrone PJ, Trese MT. Refractive changes associated with scleral buckling and division in retinopathy of prematurity. *Arch Ophthalmol* 1998;116:1446-8.

[139] Choi MY, Yu YS. Efficacy of removal of buckle after scleral buckling surgery for retinopathy of prematurity. *J Aapos* 2000;4:362-5.

[140] Ertzbischoff LM. A systematic review of anatomical and visual function outcomes in preterm infants after scleral buckle and vitrectomy for retinal detachment. *Adv Neonatal Care* 2004;4:10-9.

[141] Quinn GE, Dobson V, Barr CC, et al. Visual acuity of eyes after vitrectomy for retinopathy of prematurity: follow-up at 5 1/2 years. The Cryotherapy for Retinopathy of Prematurity Cooperative Group. *Ophthalmology* 1996;103:595-600.

[142] Singh R, Reddy DM, Barkmeier AJ, et al. Long-term visual outcomes following lens-sparing vitrectomy for retinopathy of prematurity. *Br J Ophthalmol* 2012;96:1395-8.

[143] Choi J, Kim JH, Kim SJ, et al. Long-term results of lens-sparing vitrectomy for progressive posterior-type stage 4A retinopathy of prematurity. *Korean J Ophthalmol* 2012;26:277-84.

[144] Hartnett ME, Maguluri S, Thompson HW, et al. Comparison of retinal outcomes after scleral buckle or lens-sparing vitrectomy for stage 4 retinopathy of prematurity. *Retina* 2004;24:753-7.

[145] Kychenthal A, Dorta P. Vitrectomy after intravitreal bevacizumab (Avastin) for retinal detachment in retinopathy of prematurity. *Retina*;30:S32-6.

[146] Xu Y, Zhang Q, Kang X, et al. Early vitreoretinal surgery on vascularly active stage 4 retinopathy of prematurity through the preoperative intravitreal bevacizumab injection. *Acta Ophthalmol*;91:e304-10.

[147] Axer-Siegel R, Snir M, Ron Y, et al. Intravitreal bevacizumab as supplemental treatment or monotherapy for severe retinopathy of prematurity. *Retina*;31:1239-47.

[148] Wu WC, Yeh PT, Chen SN, et al. Effects and complications of bevacizumab use in patients with retinopathy of prematurity: a multicenter study in taiwan. *Ophthalmology*;118:176-83.

[149] Sun HJ, Choi KS, Lee SJ. Adjunctive effect of intravitreal bevacizumab prior to lens-sparing vitrectomy in aggressive posterior retinopathy of prematurity: a case report. *Jpn J Ophthalmol* 2012;56:476-80.

[150] Honda S, Hirabayashi H, Tsukahara Y, et al. Acute contraction of the proliferative membrane after an intravitreal injection of bevacizumab for advanced retinopathy of prematurity. *Graefes Arch Clin Exp Ophthalmol* 2008;246:1061-3.

[151] Law JC, Recchia FM, Morrison DG, et al. Intravitreal bevacizumab as adjunctive treatment for retinopathy of prematurity. *J Aapos* 2010;14:6-10.

[152] Kychenthal A, Dorta P. Vitrectomy after intravitreal bevacizumab (Avastin) for retinal detachment in retinopathy of prematurity. *Retina* 2010;30:S32-6.

[153] Xu Y, Zhang Q, Kang X, et al. Early vitreoretinal surgery on vascularly active stage 4 retinopathy of prematurity through the preoperative intravitreal bevacizumab injection. *Acta Ophthalmol* 2013;91:e304-10.

[154] Ittiara S, Blair MP, Shapiro MJ, et al. Exudative retinopathy and detachment: a late reactivation of retinopathy of prematurity after intravitreal bevacizumab. *J Aapos* 2013;17:323-5

4

Fabry Disease – Ocular Manifestations and Visual Symptoms

Pinakin Gunvant Davey

1. Introduction

Fabry disease is a rare lysosomal disorder that has a prevalence of 1 in 40,000 males.[1] This disease follows x-linked inheritance and the individuals affected with the disease show multi system disorders that are present at birth and signs and symptoms worsen with time. The *GLA* gene mutation leads to the deficiency of an enzyme alpha galactidose A which leads to the progressive accumulation of globotriacylceramide (GB3) deposits in a variety of cells including those in kidneys, and the autonomic the cardiovascular systems.[2-4]

The ocular manifestations of Fabry disease includes a cornea verticillata which is a "vortex whorl" like corneal opacity. It is the most common finding and is seen in all hemizygotes and majority (up to 70%) of hetrozygotes.[5] The cornea verticillata is the outcome of the deposit of GB3 in the basal layer of the corneal epithelium. The cornea verticillata is visible using a slitlamp biomicroscope and in-vivo confocal microscopic studies have shown that even when the cornea verticillata may not be visible using a slitlamp there are intracellular inclusion bodies in the basal epithelial cells.[6] To a lesser degree and fewer Fabry disease patients have subtle lenticular deposits which is the Fabry cataract.[7] The Fabry cataract tends to be off axis dendritic or subcapsular opacities along the posterior suture lines. It is believed that patients with cornea verticillata will not have any visual symptoms due to the deposits. [7-9]

The role of the cornea and the crystalline lens is to provide the eye with necessary refractive power and unhindered path to the light rays that pass through them. To this accord the corneal physiology is finely tuned and causes the least amount of scatter of light rays in ocular healthy individuals. It can be hypothesized that individuals with Fabry disease could have problems with visual function given that both the cornea and the crystalline lens have deposits of GB3 and opacities. It can further be hypothesized that the vision problems would be present and will be worst at night time when compared to the day time, with patients with Fabry disease having additional problems of glare, blurry vision or dim vision (contrast sensitivity issues).

The patients with Fabry disease also experience anhydrosis or hypohydrosis as one of the symptom. This is due to the neurological manifestations of the disease. Prior reports have suggested that patients with Fabry disease may have deposits of GB3 in the ganglia or the lacrimal gland itself.[10-12] It can be hypothesized that patients with Fabry disease could also have symptoms of dry eyes.

The present study utilized an ocular symptom survey instrument to evaluate for the symptoms of general ocular problems like itching, tearing, dryness, burning sensation, sensation of foreign body or difficulty in vision or asthenopic symptoms in patients with Fabry disease and compared the findings to healthy controls.

2. Materials and methods

2.1. Study participants

A total of 95 individuals (75 patients with Fabry disease and 20 healthy controls) completed the survey. The mean age and standard deviation (SD) of the patients in the Fabry group and the control group was 32.5 and SD 19.1 years and 42.6 SD 14.7 years respectively. Ninety six percent of the participants completed all the survey questions, with 4 individuals not answering the question about "soreness and fatigue" of eyes.

The survey was administered live at the conferences for lysosomal disease storage which was conducted by the Fabry Support and Information Group in San Diego California, USA and the National Fabry Disease Foundation in Greensboro, North Carolina, USA. These events were attended by individuals that had a confirmed case of Fabry disease or by a family member who were tested and confirmed of being healthy and did not have Fabry disease or healthy spouse. The participants were instructed to answer the survey questions with regards to their self-perceived ocular and vision status when they were wearing optimal refractive correction. Data was collated and analyzed in a masked fashion with the data entry performed by a separate individual and the statistical analysis performed by the author.

2.2. Survey instrument

A modified survey instrument that was utilized by Lee et al [13] to investigate the ocular and visual symptoms in glaucoma patients was utilized in the present study. The survey instrument proposed by Lee et al[13] was called the Glaucoma Symptom Scale (GSS) and is a simple 10 question survey that was developed by modifying the survey used in the Ocular Hypertension Treatment Study. The GSS was tested and validated on a group of glaucoma patients in four tertiary care glaucoma centers. This survey instrument was administered to both patients with Fabry disease and their healthy family members (controls).

The survey administered in the present study is shown in Figure 1. The major difference between the GSS and the survey administered in the present study is the scale of the symptoms.

The GSS graded the symptoms in 4 point scale whereas the present study utilized a 6 point scale. The larger scale in the present survey allowed evaluating a wide range of symptom level as it was likely that the ocular symptoms in patients with the ocular manifestations of Fabry disease could be mild or minimal. The GSS survey instrument mainly evaluated for dryness and tear film and ocular surface issues in questions 1 to 4 and 7, whereas question 4 is designed to evaluate for general fatigue or asthenopic symptoms. The survey instruments question number 6, 8-10 were designed to evaluate vision related problems primarily the difficulty in contrast sensitivity issues, day time night time vision and glare respectively.

		Almost Never					Almost Always
1	Burning /stinging	1	2	3	4	5	6
2	Tearing	1	2	3	4	5	6
3	Dryness	1	2	3	4	5	6
4	Itching	1	2	3	4	5	6
5	Soreness/tiredness	1	2	3	4	5	6
6	Blurry/Dim vision	1	2	3	4	5	6
7	Feeling of something in your eyes	1	2	3	4	5	6
8	Hard to see in daylight; I need to wear sunglasses	1	2	3	4	5	6
9	Hard to see in dark places	1	2	3	4	5	6
10	Halos around light	1	2	3	4	5	6

Figure 1. Survey instrument administered to the study participants; Survey instrument used in the study was developed by Lee et al [13]. The only modification made to the survey was the scale. The present study used a 6 point scale where as the survey instrument used by Lee et al had a 4 point scale.

2.3. Statistical analysis

The difference in the mean age between the groups was analyzed using a one–way analysis of variance (ANOVA). The severity for each variable was graded in an ordinal scale with 1 being "almost never" and 6 as "almost always". A Mann-Whitney test was performed to evaluate the median difference between the Fabry group and the healthy control for each symptom survey question. A p-value of <0.05 was considered to be significant.

3. Results

The mean age of the control group was greater than the mean age of the Fabry group (ANOVA $F=4.75$; $p=0.03$). The table-1 provides the mean symptom severity score for the Fabry group and the control group and the p-value obtained using the Mann-Whitney test.

	Symptom	Mean Severity Score		p-value
		Fabry group	Control group	
1	Burning /stinging	1.9	1.5	0.06
2	Tearing	2.0	1.9	0.2
3	Dryness	2.3	1.5	**0.02**
4	Itching	2.0	1.8	0.3
5	Soreness/tiredness	2.4	1.7	***0.009***
6	Blurry/Dim vision	2.2	1.6	**0.02**
7	Feeling of something in your eyes	2.0	1.5	0.07
8	Hard to see in daylight; I need to wear sunglasses	2.4	1.7	0.15
9	Hard to see in dark places	2.6	1.6	**0.01**
10	Halos around light	2.4	1.7	**0.01**

p-value in bold are significant at $p<0.05$ and in bold and italics are significant $p<0.01$

Table 1. Symptoms surveys and the median severity of groups and statistical significance

Of the survey instruments items, it was found that patients in the Fabry group had more complaints of "dryness" of eyes (p=0.02). The Fabry group also showed significantly greater symptom severity score and complained of "Blurry/Dim vision", "hard to see in dark places" and "halos around light" (p=0,02, 0.01 and 0.01 respectively). The Fabry group also had a mean severity score for "soreness/tiredness" significantly higher than the control group (p=0.009). The tally of number of participants with symptoms and without symptoms is given in Table 2

4. Discussion

The survey instrument (GSS) utilized in this study was designed by Lee et al [13] to study the ocular and vision issues in glaucoma patients with the purpose of surveying daytime and night time vision, contrast sensitivity, glare, dryness and tear film related problems. The present study utilized the GSS survey instrument to identify ocular and visual symptoms in the Fabry disease and ocular healthy controls. The study results indicate that compared to healthy controls, the patients with Fabry disease had greater ocular symptom severity score in particularly areas related to night vision, contrast sensitivity and glare. Further they also have greater symptom severity score and complaint of soreness/tiredness and dry eyes.

Prior reports have indicated that patients with Fabry disease do not have any visual problems due to the cornea verticillata. [7-9] This is perhaps true to the point that the cornea verticillata may not cause a decline in Snellen visual acuity charts that uses 100% contrast optotypes (black letters on white background) as long as the patients wear appropriate refractive error correction. The findings of this study indicate that the symptoms of "dim vision", "hard to see in dark places" perhaps indicates decrease in contrast sensitivity or difficulty in identifying targets in day to day life that are in shades of grey not of 100% contrast.. The Fabry group also had a symptom severity score significantly higher for the survey item seeing "Halo around lights" which is perhaps a result due to the scatter or glare problems that patients experience. This problem may perhaps be further exaggerated at night time.

Symptoms		Problem	No Problem
Burning and stinging	Disease	38	37
	No disease	5	15
Tearing	Disease	44	31
	No disease	11	9
Dryness*	Disease	44	31
	No disease	7	13
Itching	Disease	44	31
	No disease	9	11
Soreness tiredness*	Disease	52	23
	No disease	6	14
Blurry, Dim vision*	Disease	48	27
	No disease	7	13
Feeling something in your eyes	Disease	40	35
	No disease	6	14
Hard to see in daylight, I need sunglasses	Disease	39	36
	No disease	7	13
Hard to see in dark places*	Disease	45	30
	No disease	7	13
Halos around light*	Disease	44	31
	No disease	6	14

* indicates symptoms that was statistically significant greater severity score between the groups

Table 2. The tally of study participants that reported experiencing symptoms in the Fabry group and the control group

The vision problems related to scotopic (night) vision, contrast sensitivity and glare are most likely due to the deposits of GB3 in corneal epithelium and lens which causes increased scatter of light rays and decreased transmittance of light (See figures 2 A-C). The confocal microscopic studies have revealed that even when there is no clinically visible cornea verticillata the basal layer of the epithelium show hyper reflectivity due to the intracellular inclusion bodies. Thus although one can expect the symptom severity score to be related to the amount of corneal deposits visible, the patients that do not have visible deposits or cornea verticillata may still have some visual problems given that have the intracellular inclusion bodies in the corneal epithelial cells.

The Fabry group also had greater complaints of "dryness" compared to the control group. This could be due to the fact that GB3 gets deposited both in the ganglia and the lacrimal gland. [10-12] Prior researchers have also suggested that patients with Fabry disease can have a dry

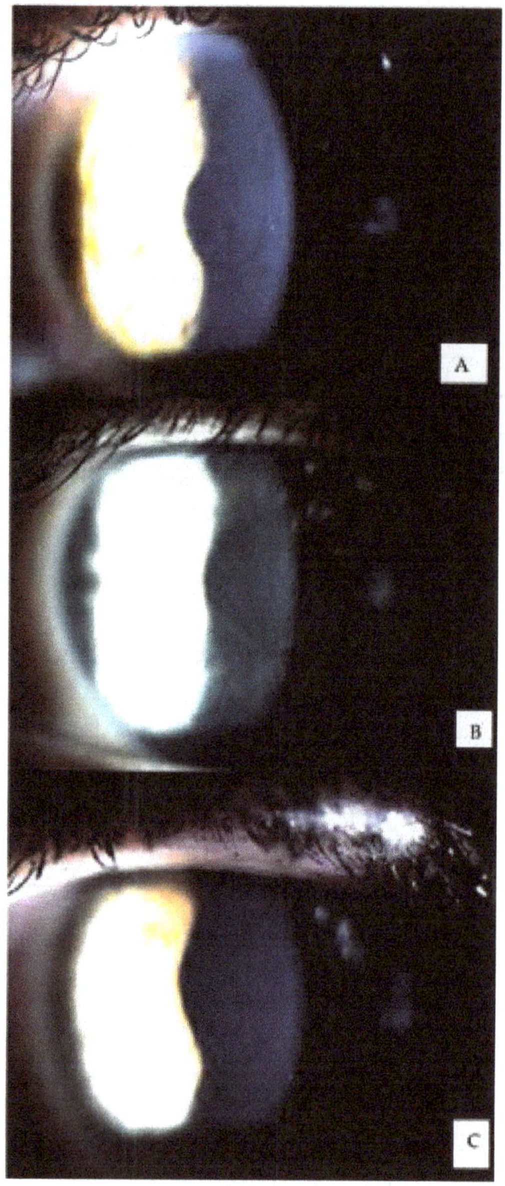

Figure 2. Cornea verticillata in patients with Fabry disease A: Top panel: Cornea verticillata giving a even spread of smear of deposits throughout the cornea. B: Middle panel: A vortex like deposits. C: Bottom panel: A subtle verticillata in a patient with Fabry disease

eye syndrome.[9] The report of this survey quantifies that patients may have a subtle yet clinically significant dry eye.

The patients with Fabry disease also complain of lack of energy or chronic fatigue. [14] It is intriguing to note that symptom survey score for "soreness/tiredness of eyes was significantly greater than the control group. This could have multiple reasons. The simplest explanation is they experience chronic fatigue of their body and thus also experience "soreness/tiredness" with eyes. Although it is possible that dry eye, dim vision may contribute to some of these asthenopic problems. It will be interesting to see if this symptom severity score would decrease if appropriate therapy using glare filters, contrast enhancing filters or treatment for dry eyes was administered.

The cornea verticillata in patients with Fabry disease can vary significantly; they can be absent, subtle, or dramatic in appearance. The figures 2 A-C provide slit lamp photographs of cornea verticillata in patients with known Fabry disease. The figures 3 A B provide images of of conjunctival vascular findings in patients with Fabry disease. It should be noted that the cornea verticillata is not limited to Fabry disease and patients on medication like amiodorone or aminoquinolones on chronic use can have similar corneal appearance.[7] It can be postulated that any person with cornea verticillata can have vision problems pertaining to night time, contrast discrimination and glare.

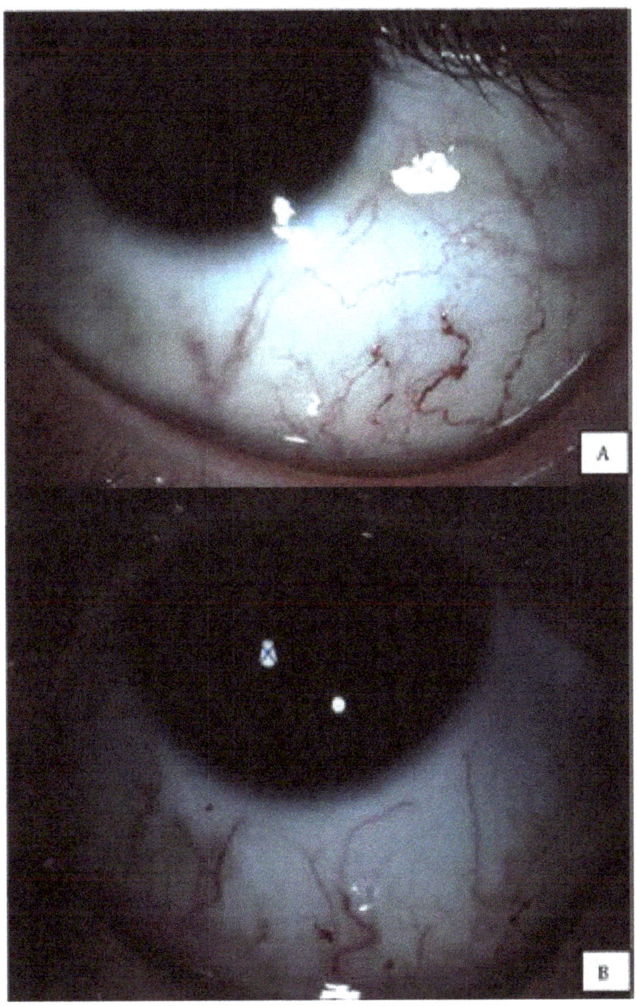

Figure 3. Conjunctival tortousity with aneurysms like out pouching (A: Top and B: Bottom panel)

This is first report to my knowledge that has evaluated the ocular symptom severity survey in patients with Fabry disease. Future studies are needed and should look at quantifying the problems and symptoms with contrast sensitivity function testing, glare testing and investigate tear function tests to evaluate the vision related difficulty and dry eye problems.

Acknowledgements

I would like to thank Mr. Jerry Walter Founder and President National Fabry Disease Foundation (NFDF) and Mr. Jack Johnson Executive Director Fabry Support & Information Group for their kind help in administering the survey to Fabry patients I would like to thank Mr. Nate Klingensmith of Haag Striet USA for his assistance in ocular imaging of Fabry group and Mr. Jack Greenan for the data entry related to the study. A special thank you to Dr. Rebecca Kammer for interesting discussion on ocular survey instruments and all the study participants for their time and efforts in completing the survey.

Author details

Pinakin Gunvant Davey

Western University of Health Sciences, College of Optometry, Pomona CA, USA

References

[1] Meikle PJ, Hopwood JJ, Clague AE, et al. Prevalence of lysosomal storage disorders. JAMA 1999;281:249-54.

[2] MacDermot KD, Holmes A, Miners AH. AndersoneFabry disease: clinical manifestations and impact of disease in a cohort of 98 hemizygous males. J Med Genet 2001;38:750-60.

[3] MacDermot KD, Holmes A, Miners AH. AndersoneFabry disease: clinical manifestations and impact of disease in a cohort of 60 obligate carrier females. J Med Genet 2001;38:769-75

[4] Branton MH, Schiffmann R, Sabnis SG, et al. Natural history of Fabry renal disease: influence of a-galactosidase A activity and genetic mutations on clinical course. Medicine 2002;81:122-38

[5] Desnick RJ, Brady RO. Fabry disease in childhood. J Pediatr 2004;144:20-26.

[6] Wasielica-Poslednik J, Pfeiffer N, Reinke J, Pitz S Confocal laser-scanning microscopy allows differentiation between Fabry disease and amiodarone-induced keratopathy Graefes Arch Clin Exp Ophthalmol (2011) 249:1689–1696

[7] Samiy N: Ocular Features of Fabry Disease: Diagnosis of a Treatable Life-threatening Disorder Surv Ophthalmol 53:416--423, 2008.

[8] Sodi A, Ioannidis A, Pitz S. Ophthalmological manifestations of Fabry disease. In: Metha A, Beck M, Sunder-Plassmann G, eds. Fabry disease. Perspectives from 5 years of FOS. Oxford, UK: Oxford Pharmagenesis Ltd, 2006:249-61.

[9] Sivley MD Fabry Disease: A Review of Ophthalmic and Systemic Manifestations Optom Vis Sci 2013;90:e63-e78

[10] Cable WJ, Kolodny EH, Adams RD. Fabry disease: impaired autonomicfunction. Neurology 1982;32:498-502.

[11] Hilz MJ. Evaluation of peripheral and autonomic nerve function in Fabry disease. Acta Paediatr Suppl 2002;91:38-42.

[12] Kolodny EH, Pastores GM. Anderson-Fabry disease: extrarenal, neurologic manifestations. J Am Soc Nephrol 2002;13(Suppl. 2):S150-3.

[13] Lee BL, Gutierrez P, Gordon M, Wilson MR, Cioffi GA, Ritch R, Sherwood M, MangioneCM The Glaucoma Symptom Scale. A brief index of glaucoma-specific symptoms. Arch Ophthalmol. 1998 Jul;116(7):861-6

[14] Zarate YA, Hopkin RJ Fabry's disease. Lancet. 2008 Oct 18;372(9647):1427-35

5

Excitotoxicity and Glaucoma

Makoto Ishikawa, Takeshi Yoshitomi and
Yukitoshi Izumi

1. Introduction

Glutamate is a major excitatory neurotransmitter in the visual perception pathway. In the retina, rod and cone photoreceptor cells continuously release glutamate and partially depolarized in darkness, and light decreases the glutamate release in a graded manner. The photoreceptor signals are transmitted to bipolar cells and horizontal cells. The two-types of bipolar cells, ON-and OFF-bipolar cells, continuously release glutamate in lightness and in darkness, respectively [1,2]. Bipolar cells respond to light with sustained and graded potential as photoreceptor cells do. Bipolar cell signals are then transmitted to ganglion cells, which produce action potentials as a signal transduction to the brain via the axon of the ganglion cell.

Glutamate released from the presynaptic terminals diffuse to bind to the glutamate receptors on the postsynaptic membrane via the synaptic cleft. Retinal glutamate receptors are mainly located in the outer plexiform layer where glutamatergic synapses connect photoreceptors to bipolar and horizontal cells; and also in the inner plexiform layer which contains the bulk of glutamatergic synapses from bipolar cells to ganglion cells and amacrine cells [3-6].

Multiple glutamate receptor types have been identified. Though glutamate will bind onto all glutamate receptors, each receptor is characterized by its sensitivity to specific glutamate analogues and by the features of the glutamate-elicited current. Glutamate receptors are divided into three groups, N-methyl-D-aspartate (NMDA) receptors, AMPA (α-amino-3-hydroxyl-5-methyl-4-isoxazole-propionate)/kainic acid receptors (non-NMDA receptors), and metabotropic receptors. NMDA and non-NMDA receptors are called ionotropic glutamate receptors, and form ion channel pores for ion influx and efflux, when glutamate binds to the receptor [7-9].

When glutamate is in excess, glutamate binds to cell surface ionotropic glutamate receptors, triggering massive Ca^{2+}influx and activation of pro-apoptotic signaling cascades. It can become toxic to the retinal neurons [10-13]. Olney (1969)coined the term excitotoxicity to describe the process of neuronal death caused by excessive or prolonged activation of receptors for excitatory amino acid neurotransmitters [14]. Like excitotoxicity has been considered as an important contributor to the retinal ganglion cell death in ischemic retinal diseases such as vascular occlusions [15] or diabetic retinopathy [16-18] excitotoxicity may be involved in ganglion cell death in glaucoma [19].

Although massive glutamate release is characteristic for the ischemic retinal diseases [20-22], this is not necessarily required for pathogenesis of glaucoma. In fact, several studies were unable to detect the elevation of extracellular concentration of glutamate in vitreous humor samples from experimental animals with ocular hypertension, and in human glaucoma [23-27]. Correspondingly, it has been revealed that retinal glial cells play critical roles in the prevention of excitotoxocity. For example, Müller cells are responsible for the uptake of excess glutamate via GLAST (Glutamate Aspartate Transporter) [28.29], which is essential to maintain physiological concentrations of glutamate. Glutamate at physiological levels can be neurotoxic, if glutamate metabolism is impaired. Therefore, it is considered that impaired metabolism of glutamate more likely contributes to the excitotoxic injury even if glutamate is not in excess.

This review summarizes the present knowledge regarding the glutamate metabolism in glaucoma and the possible neuroprotective therapy of glaucoma.

2. Glutamate uptake and glaucoma

Glutamate released from the presynaptic terminals reaches the receptor molecules of the postsynaptic plasma membrane; but majority of glutamate are taken up by Müller glia or by retinal neurons via glutamate transporters. Glutamate transported into Müller glia is amidated to glutamine by a glutamate degrading enzyme, glutamine synthetase [30-33] (Figure 1).

2.1. Physiology of glutamate transporters

Glutamate uptake is mediated by five distinct glutamate transporters (EAAT1-5): GLAST (EAAT1) [34], GLT-1 (EAAT2) [35], EAAC1 (EAAT3) [36], EAAT4 [37] and EAAT5 [38]. In five EAATs, GLAST (EAAT1) and GLT-1 (EAAT2) are the major glutamate transporters in the retina. GLAST is mainly expressed in the Müller cells, whereas GLT1 and EAAC1 are in retinal neurons. We describe the physiological roles of GLAST and GLT-1, respectively.

a. GLAST

GLAST is the prominent glutamate transporter in the retina, and mainly expressed in the Müller cells [10, 31-33, 39, 40]. Müller cells remove the majority of glutamate from extracellular sites [41-47]. When Müller glial uptake is pharmacologically blocked, extracellular glutamate concentration increase [48], and severe excitotoxicity is induced [48, 49]. In GLAST KO mice, the Vmax for Müller glial glutamate transport is suppressed by 50%, suggesting that approximately 50% of glutamate is taken up via GLAST, another 40% through electroneutral, sodium-dependent (presently undefined) glutamate transporters, and 10% via sodium-independent

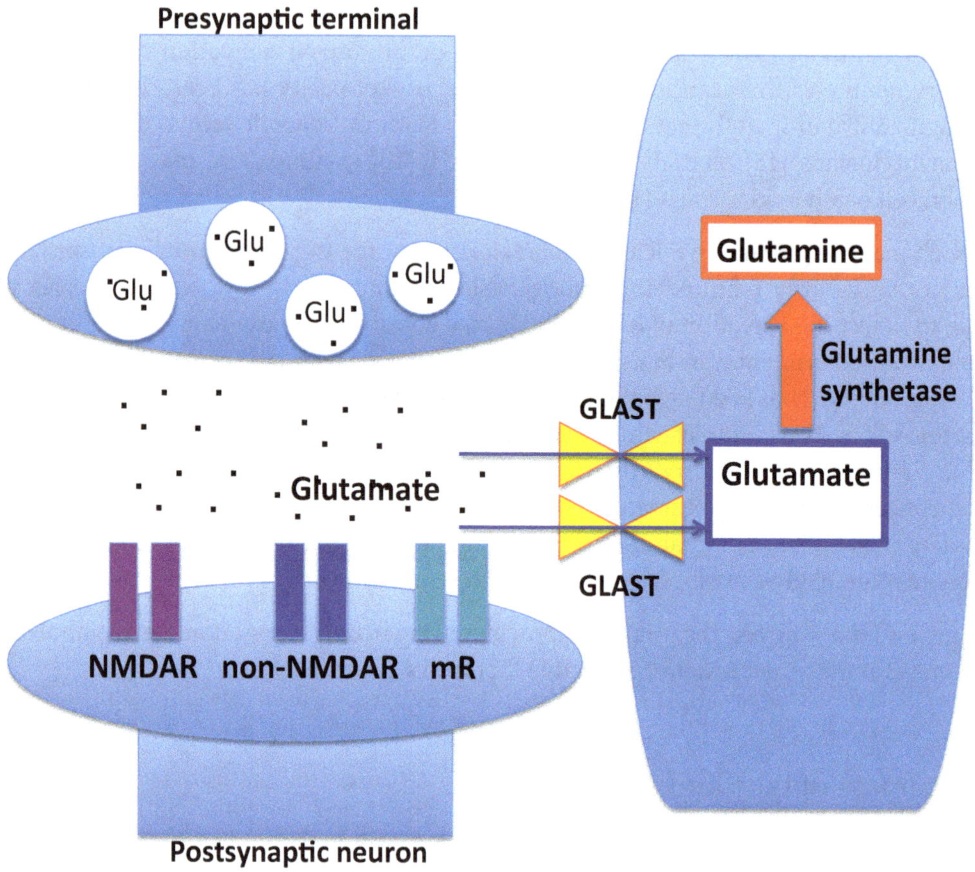

Figure 1. After release from the presynaptic terminal, glutamate binds to the post-synaptic glutamate receptors.Then, excess of glutamate is transported into the Mulller glia via glial glutamate transporter, GLAST, and catalyzed by glutamine synthetase to the nontoxic amino acid glutamine. Glutamate is also transported into retinal neurons via neuronal glutamate transporter, GLT-1.

transporters or exchangers [50]. Although antisense GLAST fails to induce apparent excitotoxicity [51], antisense suppresses the b-wave and oscillatory potentials of electrocardiogram [46, 51], and doubles total glutamate levels in the retina [50]. These results indicate that GLAST is essential to maintain the homeostasis of glutamate metabolism and physiological neural functions. In support of this, it has been shown that retinas from mice with targeted deletions of GLAST are extremely sensitive to ischemic insults [46].

b. GLT-1

GLT-1 (EAAT2) is the neuronal glutamate transporter, and exists in several distinct forms, including the originally described form (GLT-1, also referred as GLT-1a), along with GLT-1b (also called GLT1v) and GLT1c [48]. GLT-1a appears to be associated mainly with a population of amacrine cells and bipolor cells, whereas GLT-1b is associated with cone photoreceptors and subpopulations of bipolar cells [52,53]. GLT-1c is normally only expressed by the photoreceptors in the mammalian retina [54]. GLT1 knockout mice appear to exhibit minimal compromise of retinal function, suggesting that GLAST is essential for the maintenance of normal synaptic transmission [46, 49]. However, it is still controversial because other researchers reported that treatment with antisense oligonucleotides against GLT-1 induced the excitotoxic ganglion cell death in the rat retina [42].

2.2. Impairment of glutamate removal in glaucoma

a. GLAST

Some studies have shown that GLAST expression diminishes [55-57] or remains stable [58] in experimental glaucoma, whereas others have reported increased expression [59]. Thus, it remains unclear whether elevated intraocular pressure (IOP) alters glutamate uptake by modulating GLAST. After experimental IOP elevation in rats, Holcombe et al. (2008) [47] immunohistochemically determined the glutamate transport activity as aspartate uptake into Müller glia, and found that Müller glial uptake is normal even IOP is as high as 70 mmHg but compromised at 80 mmHg or higher. These results suggest that GLAST is functional as long as retinal perfusion is maintained.

We [60] used a rat *ex vivo* model incubating rat eye cups under hydrostatic pressure at the bottom of a deep cylinder. Such acute high pressures can induce retinal ischemia clinically and in *in vivo* glaucoma models [61-63] but not in this *ex vivo* model. The advantages of *ex vivo* hydrostatic pressure model include better preservation of eyecup samples without ischemia, making it possible to investigate direct effects of pressure-induced retinal injury on glutamate metabolism. In this acute *ex vivo* model, axonal damage of the retinal ganglion cells were prominent, and Western blot and real-time RT-PCR analyses revealed that 75 mm Hg pressure depressed GLAST expression [64]. Administration of glutamate receptor blockers prevented axonal damages, indicating that IOP elevation induces excitotoxicity via depression of GLAST. It should be also noticed that IOP elevation can depress GLAST activity even if retinal perfusion is preserved.

Harada et al. (2007) [65] show that GLAST-deficient mice demonstrate spontaneous RGC loss and optic nerve degeneration in spite of normal IOP. In GLAST-deficient mice, administration of glutamate receptor blockers prevented RGC loss.

These findings suggest that glutamate transporters are necessary to prevent glaucomatous excitotoxic retinal damages.

b. GLT-1

GLT-1, the main neuronal glutamate transporter in the retinal neurons, is reported to be down-regulated in glaucomatous eyes in rats [58, 66] and mice [57]. By contrast, Park et al. [58] reported that the expression of GLT-1 was expressed in cone photoreceptors and the level of expression in some cone bipolar cells was significantly increased in *in vivo* glaucoma model. They also demonstrated that GLAST expression in Müller cells remained stable during the experimental period. These results suggest that integrity of GLT-1 may be a prerequisite for the maintenance of glutamate homeostasis in the retina undergoing glaucoma [67].

Sullivan et al. (2006) [68] reported the expressional changes of the splice variant of GLT-1 (GLT-1c) in the glaucoma eyes. In normal eyes of humans and rats, GLT-1c is expressed only in photoreceptors. In glaucoma, additional robust expression of GLT-1c is detected in retinal ganglion cells, including occasional displaced ganglion cells [106]. The new induction of GLT-1c expression by retinal ganglion cells may imply abnormalities in glutamate homeostasis in glaucomatous RGCs. The same authors said that GLT-1c may be a useful indicator of the extent of stress of the RGCs and thus a tool for examining outcomes of potential therapeutic and experimental interventions.

2.3. Neuroprotection by upregulation of glutamate transporters

Several studies [56, 64] revealed that the expression of the major glutamate transporter, GLAST, decreases after pressure loading. Therefore, agents that effectively enhance glutamate transporter function may serve as potential therapeutics against the pressure-induced injury. Enhancement of glutamate transport is developing into a new strategy for reducing excitotoxicity also in brain injury and neurodegenerative disease [69-71]. Lee et al. (2009) [72] reported that tamoxifen, estrogen modulator, possessed neuroprotective properties against excitotoxicity by the up-regulation of GLAST at protein and mRNA levels in the mannganese-induced excitotoxicity. Estradiol and its derivative also reported to increase GLAST expression, though these drugs have not been applied to glaucoma patients.

Recently, the daily treatment with 17β-estradiol (E2) eye drops resulted in significant E2 concentration in the retina with concomitant profound neuroprotective therapeutic benefits, even in the presence of continually elevated IOP [73]. However, E2 eye drop induces the adverse effect to other organs induced by stimulation of estrogen receptors. It seems safe to apply E2 eye drops to postmenopausal women. Taking all above into consideration, there is a long way to go before topical estrogen drops becomes a new therapeutics of glaucoma.

3. Enzymatic degradation of glutamate and glaucoma

In the Müller cells, glutamate is rapidly converted into glutamine by the glia-specific enzyme, glutamine synthetase [33]. Glutamine synthetase is specifically localized in the cytosol of Müller cells [74].Glutamine synthetase catalyzes the following reaction,

$$\text{Glutamate} + NH^{4+} + ATP \rightarrow \text{glutamine} + ADP + P_i + H^+,$$

in the presence of Mn^{2+}or Mg^{2+}.

The activity of the glutamine synthetase influences the rate of the glutamate uptake by the Müller cells [41]. The rapid metabolization of glutamate to glutamine causes a stronger driving force for the glutamate uptake in the Müller cells than in neurons, which have intracellular free glutamate concentrations two orders of magnitude higher than the Müller cells [75]. A prerequisite for an effective glutamate-glutamine cycle in Müller cells would be the regulated coordination between glutamate uptake and glutamate degradation [39].

The activity of glutamine synthetase is stimulated by glucocorticoids [76,77]. In chick embryo retinas the stimulated glutamine synthetase by glucocorticoids is correlated with amounts of released glutamine from Müller glia, suggesting that the activity of glutamine synthetase influences glutamate uptake [78]. Conversely, it is also reported that basic fibrogrowth factor (bFGF) suppresses the activity of glutamine synthetase presumably through inhibition of glucocorticoid actions [79].

Glutamine, synthesized from glutamate in Müller glia, is the major source of glutamate found in retinal neurons. MSO, an inhibitor of glutamine synthetase, rapidly abolish free glutamate from bipolar cells and retinal ganglion cells [80]. Therefore, glutamine synthetase is a key enzyme in glutamate-glutamine cycle.

3.1. Impairment of glutamate metabolism and glaucoma

Several studies have shown increases in the expression of glutamine synthetase [78] after pressure elevation [81,82], whereas others have reported decreases. Thus, it remains controversial whether elevated IOP alters glial cell glutamate metabolism as a potential mechanism of retinal excitotoxicity [83].

In primary glaucoma in dogs [84], decreases in immunoreactivity of glutamine synthetase were associated with glutamate redistribution. These decreases in glutamine synthetase occurred even in mildly damaged regions of retina before retinal thinning. Reactive Müller cells were seen primarily in chronic primary glaucoma in severely damaged regions. Decreases in glutamine synthetase may potentiate ischemia-induced early glutamate redistribution and neuronal damage in canine primary glaucoma.

We (2010) [60] reported that pressure elevation induced reduction of glutamine synthetase activity compared with control pressure in an acute*ex vivo* model. The result suggests that the neural degeneration observed during pressure elevation is caused by impaired glial glutamate metabolism.

Although GLAST and the activities of glutamine synthetase are intimately intertwined [85], both are simultaneously suppressed by high pressure-loading. Thus, it is also possible that suppression of GLAST and the activities of glutamine synthetase occur separately during pressure-loading [86]. However, a series of observations using acute *ex vivo* model suggest that during pressure-loading, the impairment of GLAST expression precedes the depression of glutamine synthetase activity. Pharmacologic inhibition of glutamine synthetase activity with MSO fails to modulate GLAST expression, whereas inhibition of GLAST with TFB-TBOA substantially suppresses glutamine synthetase activity. Based on these findings, it is hypothesize that during pressure-loading, impairment of GLAST takes place first and results in downregulation of activities of glutamine synthetase as a secondary effect [62], though it is also possible that changes in the activities of glutamine synthetase influence GLAST activities [78].

3.2. Neuroprotection by upregulation of glutamine synthetase

Hydrocortisone, which is shown to increase the expression of glutamine synthetase in the Müller cells, is considered as neuroprotectve against excitotoxicity [87-89]. Upregulation of glutamine synthetase by hydrocortisone may be related to the fact that the upstream region of the glutamine synthetase gene contains a glucocorticoid response element that can bind the glucocorticoid receptor protein [53]. Glutamine synthtase was also reported upregulated by taurine supplementation in the diabetic retina [90]. These agents that effectively enhance glutamine synthetase function and expression may serve as potential therapeutics against the pressure-induced injury.

4. Glutamate receptors

The excitotoxicity is predominantly mediated by the overstimulation of NMDA receptors due to their extreme permeability to calcium ions [94]. Many researchers have concluded, therefore, that excitotoxicity occurs, in part, via NMDA receptors activation [99,100]. There is still remained a possibility that glutamate acts via non-NMDA receptors to initiate neurotoxicity [101-105]. However, the role of non-NMDA receptorsin pathogenesis of glaucoma has not been elucidated.

We describe the present knowledge concerning the molecular function of NMDA receptors and its relation to excitotoxicity.

a. NMDA receptors

Retinal ganglion cells express abundant NMDA receptors [106-109]. A number of studies demonstrated that ganglion cells are extremely vulnerable to exogenously applied NMDA, which inducesganglion cell degeneration.It has been also shown that NMDA receptor antagonists are neuroprotective in experimental glaucoma models [110-117]. NMDA receptors permit the influx of sodium ions (Na^+) and calcium ions (Ca^{2+}) and the efflux of potassium ions (K^+).

Although all NMDA receptors express the NR1 subunit [122,123,124], NR2 subunits are major determinants of the functional properties of NMDA receptor [125]. Recently, Bai et al. (2013) [126] reported the roles of the four different NR2 subtypes (NR2a, NR2b, NR2c, NR2d) in NMDA-induced retinal cell death using mice lacking specific NR2 subunits. They also evaluated the neuroprotective effect of 7-hydroxy-6-methoxy-2-methyl-1-(2-(4-(trifluoromethyl)phenyl)ethyl)-1,2,3,4-tetra-hydro-isoquinoline hydrochloride (HON0001) [127], an specific NR2b antagonist, on ganglion cell degeneration due to glutamate excitotoxicity in GLAST-deficient mice. As the results, NR2b-and NR2d-deficiency protected ganglion cells from NMDA-induced excitotoxicity. Pharmacological inhibition of the NR2b subunit by HON0001 attenuated ganglion cell loss in GLAST deficient mice. These findings suggest that NR2b-and NR2d-containing NMDA receptors play a critical role in NMDA receptor-mediated excitotoxicity in the retina. Based on these findings,inhibition of NR2b and NR2d activity is a potential therapeutic strategy for the treatment of retinal neurodegeneration induced by excitotoxicity.

The same authors demonstrate that NR2d deficiency attenuates ganglion cell loss in GLAST-deficient mice [126]. Furthermore, Dock3, a guanine nucleotide exchange factor, binds to the NR2d C-terminal domain and reduces the expression of NR2d, thereby protects ganglion cells from excitotoxicity. These results suggest that NR2d is involved in the excitotoxic ganglion cell death, and that the interaction between NR2d and Dock3 may have a neuroprotective effect. These findings indicate the possibility that NR2d and Dock3 might be therapeutic targets for glaucoma.

b. Neuroprotection by NMDA receptor antagonists

Classical pharmacological approaches for reducing excitotoxicity have focused on antagonism of glutamate receptors. Memantine is an uncompetitive NMDA antagonist, binding near the Mg^{2+}site within the ion channel [128]. The degree of blockade of the NMDA receptors is changed according to the concentration of memantine [128]. Memantine is a neuroprotective agent that has completed phase III clinical trial in patients with glaucoma [129, 130]. The trial showed that memantine was ineffective by the primary end point, with the variable mechanisms of retinal ganglion apoptosis being offered as an explanation [131].

A recent study demonstrated that NR2c-and NR2d-containing NMDA receptors are the primary targets of memantine [132]. It has been reported that memantine prevents the loss of retinal ganglion cells in GLAST knockout mice, a model of normal tension glaucoma (NTG), suggesting that NR2d-containing receptors may be involved in ganglion cell loss in glaucoma [125, 126]. It was also demonstrated that Mg^{2+}regulates the sensitivity of NMDA receptors to memantine [133]. In a physiological concentration (1 mM) of extracellular Mg^{2+}, memantine exerts a more potent blocking effect at NR2c and NR2d subunits than at NR2a and NR2b subunits. These findings suggest that NR2c-and NR2d-containing NMDA receptors are likely to be the main targets of memantine.

5. Concluding comments

Glutamate accumulation in extracellular spaces can be potentially neurotoxic if glutamate is not removed in an appropriate manner. It should be noticed that excitotoxicity does not always due to excess of glutamate. Extracellular glutamate level duringretinal ischemia may not be sufficient to induceneuronal damage under normal conditions. This suggeststhat clearance of glutamate is essential in preventingretinal excitotoxicity. In glaucomatous models, glutamate metabolism can be impaired by inhibition of glutamate transporter and glutamine synthetase, resulting in excitotoxic glaucomatous damages of retinal ganglion cells. A series of observations using ex vivo glaucomatous model suggest that during pressure-loading, the impairment of glutamate transporter expression precedes the depression of glutamine synthetase activity. Therefore, it is also possible that changes in the activities of glutamine synthetase influence GLAST activities.Agents that effectively enhance glutamate transporter function may serve as potential therapeutics against the pressure-induced injury. Enhancement of glutamine synthetase may be a therapeutic strategy for reducing excitotoxicity.

Acknowledgements

I thank Yoko Hayami, and Sanae Takaseki (Department of Ophthalmology Akita Graduate University School of Medicine) for instructions and suggestions. This work was supported by JSPS KAKENHI Grant Numbers 24592666 to M.I.

Author details

Makoto Ishikawa[1*], Takeshi Yoshitomi[1] and Yukitoshi Izumi[2]

*Address all correspondence to: mako@med.akita-u.ac.jp

1 Department of Ophthalmology, Akita Graduate University Faculty of Medicine, Akita, Japan

2 Department of Psychiatry, Washington University School of Medicine, St. Louis, M.O., USA

References

[1] Crevetto, L, & Piccolino, M. Synaptic trans-mission between photoreceptors and horizontal cells in the turtle retina. Science (1974)., 183, 417-419.

[2] Dowling, J. E, & Ripps, H. Effect of magnesium on horizontal cell activity in the skate retina. Nature London(1973)., 242, 101-103.

[3] Gruender, T, Kohler, K, Kaletta, A, & Guenther, E. The distribution and developmental regulation of NMDA receptor subunit proteins in the outer and inner retina of the rat. J. Neurobiol (2000)., 44, 333-342.

[4] Lagrèze, W. A, Darstein, M, Feuerstein, T. J, Otto, T, & Landwehrmeyer, G.B. NMDA receptor subunit mRNA expression in human retinal ganglion cells.Graefe's Archives of Clinical & Experimental Ophthalmology (2000)., 238, 486-490.

[5] Lukasiewicz, P. Synaptic mechanisms that shape visual signaling at the inner retina. Progress in Brain Research (2005).. 147, 205-218.

[6] Peng, Y. W, Blackstone, C. D, Huganir, R. L, &Yau, K. W, Distribution of glutamate receptor subtypes in the vertebrate retina. Neuroscience (1995)., 66, 483-497.

[7] Thoreson, W. B, & Witkovsky, P. Glutamate receptors and circuits in the vertebrate retina. Progress in Retinal and Eye Research(1999)., 18, 765-810.

[8] Massey, S. C, & Miller, R. F. Excitatory amino acid receptors of rod-and cone-driven horizontal cells in the rabbit retina. Journal of Neurophysiology (1987)., 57, 645-59.

[9] Massey, S. C, & Miller, R. F. N-methyl-D-aspartate receptors of ganglion cells in rabbit retina. Journal of Neurophysiology (1990)., 63, 16-30.

[10] Lucas, D. R, & Newhouse, J. P. The toxic effect of sodium l-glutamate on the inner layers of the retina. Archives of Ophthalmology (1957)., 58, 193–201.

[11] Sisk, D. R, & Kuwabara, T. Histologic changes in the inner retina of albino rats following intravitreal injection of monosodium l-glutamate. Graefe's Archives of Clinical&Experimental Ophthalmology (1985)., 223, 250–258.

[12] Olney, J. W. The toxic effects of glutamate and related compounds in the retina and the brain, Retina(1982)., 2, 341–359.

[13] Vorwerk, C. K, Lipton, S. A, Zurakowski, D, Hyman, B. T, Sabel, B. A, &Dreyer, E. B. Chronic low-dose glutamate is toxic to retinal ganglion cells. Toxicity blocked by memantine. Invest igative Ophthalmology & Visual Science (1996)., 37, 1618–1624.

[14] Olney J. W. Glutaate-induced retinal degeneration in neonatal mice. Electron microscopy of the acutely evolving lesion. Journal of Neuropatholgy & Experimental Neurology(1969)., 28(3):455-74.

[15] Ju, W. K, &Kim, K. Y. Measuring glutamate receptor activation-induced apoptotic cell death in ischemic rat retina using the TUNEL assay. Methods in Molecular Biology(2011)., 740:149-56.

[16] Casson, R. J. Possible role of excitotoxicity in the pathogenesis of glaucoma. Clinical & Experimental Ophthalmology (2006)., 34, 54-63.

[17] Kaur, C, Foulds, W. S, & Ling, E. A. Hypoxia-ischemia and retinal ganglion cell damage.
Clinical Ophthalmology(2008)., 2, 879-889.

[18] Hernández, C, & Simó, R. Neuroprotection in diabetic retinopathy.
Current Diabtes Report (2012).,12, 329-337.

[19] Vorwerk C. K, Gorla M. S, &Dreyer, E. B. An experimental basis for implicating excitotoxicity in glaucomatous optic neuropathy. Survey of Ophthalmology(1999)., 43 Suppl 1, S142-150.

[20] Choi, D. W, &Rothman, S. M. The role of glutamate neurotoxicity in hypoxicischemic neuronal death. Annual Review of Neuroscience (1990)., 13, 171-182.

[21] Bertram, K. M, Bula, D. V, Pulido, J. S, Shippy, S. A, Gautam, S, Lu, M. J, Hatfield, R. M, Kim, J. H, Quirk, M. T, &Arroyo, J. G. Amino-acid levels in subretinal and vitreous fluid of patients with retinal detachment. Eye(2008).,22, 582-589.

[22] Diederen, R.M. H, La Heij, E. C, Deutz, N.E. P, Kijlstra, A, Kessels, A.G. H, van Eijk, H.M. H, Liem, A.T. A, Dieudonné, S, & Hendrikse, F. Increased glutamatelevels in the vitreous of patients with retinal detachment. Experimantal Eye Research (2006)., 83, 45-50.

[23] Carter-Dawson, L, Crawford, M.L. J, Harwerth, R. S, Smith, E. L, Feldman, R, Shen, F. F, Mitchell, C. K, & Whitetree, A. Vitreal glutamate concentration in monkeys with experimental glaucoma. Investigative Ophthalmology & Visual Science(2002)., 43, 2633e2637.

[24] Honkanen, R. A, Baruah, S, Zimmerman, M. B, Khanna, C. L, Weaver, Y. K, Narkiewicz, J, Waziri, R, Gehrs, K. M, Weingeist, T. A, Boldt, H. C, Folk, J.C., Russell, S. R, &Kwon, Y. H. Vitreous amino acid concentrations in patients with glaucoma undergoing vitrectomy. Archives of Ophthalmology (2003)., 121, 183-188.

[25] Kwon, Y. H, Rickman, D. W, Baruah, S, Zimmerman, M. B, Kim, C.S., Boldt, H. C, Russell, S. R, &Hayreh, S. S. Vitreous and retinal amino acid concentrations in experimental central retinal artery occlusion in the primate. Eye (2004)., 19, 455-463.

[26] Levkovitch-Verbin, H, Martin, K. R, Quigley, H. A, Baumrind, L. A, Pease, M. E, & Valenta, D. Measurement of amino acid levels in the vitreous humor of rats after chronic intraocular pressure elevation or optic nerve transection. Journal of Glaucoma (2002)., 11, 396-405.

[27] Wamsley, S, Gabelt, B. T. Dahl, D. B, Case, G. L, Sherwood, R. W. May, C.A., Hernandez, M. R,& Kaufman, P.L. Vitreous glutamate concentration and axon loss in monkeys with experimental glaucoma. Archives of Ophthalmology(2005)., 123, 64-70.

[28] Barnett, N. L Pow, D. V, &Bull, N. D. Differential perturbation of neuronal and glial glutamate transport systems in retinal ischemia. Neurochemistry International(2001)., 39(4), 291-299.

[29] Otori, Y, Shimada, S, Tanaka, K, Ishimoto, I. Tano, Y, & Tohyama, M. Marked increase in glutamate-aspartate transporter (GLAST/GluT-1) mRNA following transient retinal ischemia. Molecular Brain Research (1994)., 27, 310–314.

[30] Derouiche, A, & Rauen, T. Coincidence of L-glutamate/L-aspartate transporter (GLAST) and glutamine synthetase (GS) immunoreactions in retinal glia: evidence for coupling of GLAST and GS in transmitter clearance. Journal of Neuroscience Research (1995)., 42, 131-143.

[31] Higgs, M. H, & Lukasiewicz, P. D. Glutamate uptake limits synaptic excitation of retinal ganglion cells. Journal of Neuroscience (2002)., 19, 3691–3700.

[32] Matsui, K, Hosoi, N, & Tachibana, M. Active role of glutamate uptake in the synaptic transmission from retinal nonspiking neurons. Journal of Neuroscience (1999)., 19, 6755–6766.

[33] Bringmann, A, Pannicke, T, Biedermann, B, Francke, M, Iandiev, I, Grosche, J, Wiedemann, P, Albrecht, J, & Reichenbach, A. Role of retinal glial cells in neurotransmitter uptake and metabolism. Neurochemistry International (2009)., 54, 143-160.

[34] Storck, T, Schulte, S, Hofmann, K, &Stoffel, W. Structure, expression, and functional analysis of a Na(+)-dependent glutamate/aspartate transporter from rat brain. Proceedings ofthe National Acaddemy of Sciences of the United States of America(1992)., 89:10955–10959.

[35] Pines, G, Zhang, Y, & Kanner, B. I. Glutamate 404 is involved in the substrate discrimination of GLT-1, a (Na++K+)-coupled glutamate transporter from rat brain. Journal of Biological Chemistry (1995)., 270,17093-17097.

[36] Kanai, Y, & Hediger, M. A. Primary structure and functional characterization of a high-affinity glutamate transporter. Nature(1992)., 360, 467-471.

[37] Fairman, W. A, Vandenberg, R. J, Arriza, J. L, Kavanaugh, M. P, & Amara, S. G. An excitatory amino-acid transporter with properties of a ligand-gated chloride channel. Nature(1995)., 375, 599-603.

[38] Arriza, I. L, Eliasof, S, Kavanaugh, M. P, & Amara, S. G. Excitatory amino acid transporter 5, a retinal glutamate transporter coupled to a chloride conductance. Proceedings ofthe National Acaddemy of Sciences of the United States of America(1997)., 94, 4155-4160.

[39] Rauen, T, & Wiessner, M. Fine tuning of glutamate uptake and degradation in glial cells: common transcriptional regulation of GLAST1 and GS. Neurochemistry International (2000)., 37, 179–189.

[40] Kanai, Y, & Hediger, M. A. The glutamate/neutral amino acid transporter family SLC1: molecular, physiological and pharmacological aspects. Pflugers Archiv(2004)., 447, 469–479.

[41] Rauen, T, Taylor, W. R, Kuhlbrodt, K, & Wiessner, M. High-affinity glutamate transporters in the rat retina: a major role of the glial glutamate transporter GLAST-1 in transmitter clearance. Cell &Tissue Research (1998)., 291, 19–31.

[42] Rauen, T. Diversity of glutamate transporter expression and function in the mammalian retina. Amino Acids(2000)., 19, 53–62.

[43] Pow, D. V, Barnett, N. L, & Penfold, P. Are neuronal transporters relevant in retinal glutamate homeostasis? Neurochemistry International (2000)., 37, 191–198.

[44] White, R. D, & Neal, M. J. The uptake of L-glutamate by the retina. Brain Research (1976)., 111, 79–93.

[45] Ladanyi, M, & Beaudet, A. In-vivo labeling of (3H)D-aspartate uptake sites in monkey retina. Cell & Tissue Research (1986)., 243, 59–63.

[46] Harada, T, Harada, C, Watanabe, M, Inoue, Y, Sakagawa, T, Nakayama, N, Sasaki, S, Okuyama, S, Watase, K, Wada, K, & Tanaka, K. Functions of the two glutamate transporters GLAST and GLT-1 in the retina. Proceedings ofthe National Acaddemy of Sciences of the United States of America(1998).,95, 4663–4666.

[47] Holcombe, D. J, Lengefeld, N, Gole, G. A, &Barnett, N. L. (The effects of acute intraocular pressure elevation on rat retinal glutamate transport. Acta Ophthalmologica Scandinavia, (2008)., 86, 408–414.

[48] Sarthy, V. P, Pignataro, L, Pannicke, T. Weick, M, Reichenbach, A, Harada, T, Tanaka, K, &Marc, R. Glutamate transport by retinal Mülle cells in glutamate/aspartate transporter-knockout mice. Glia(2005)., 49, 184–196.

[49] Barnett, N. L, & Pow, D. V. Antisense knockdown of GLAST, a glial glutamate transporter, compromises retinal function. Investigative Ophthalmology & Visual Science (2000)., 41, 585–591.

[50] Izumi, Y, Shimamoto, K, Benz, A. M, Hammerman, S. B, Olney, J. W, &Zorumski, C. F. Glutamate transporters and retinal excitotoxicity. Glia (2002). 39, 58–68.

[51] Reye, P, Sullivan, R, Fletcher, E. L, & Pow, D. W. Distribution of two splice variants of the glutamate transporter GLT1 in the retinas of humans, monkeys, rabbits, rats, cats, and chickens. Journal of Comparative Neurology (2002)., 445, 1–12.

[52] Reye, P, Sullivan, R, &Pow, D. V. Distribution of two splice variants of the glutamate transporter GLT-1 in the developing rat retina. Journal of Comparative Neurology (2002)., 447, 323–330.

[53] Rauen, T, Wiessner, M, Sullivan, R, Lee, A, & Pow, D. V. A new GLT1 splice variant: cloning and immunolocalization of GLT1c in the mammalian retina and brain,. Neurochemistry International (2004)., 45, 1095–1106.

[54] Naskar, R, Vorwerk, C. K, &Dreyer, E. B. Concurrent downregulation of a glutamate transporter and receptor in glaucoma. Investigative Ophthalmology & Visual Science (2000)., 41, 1940–1944.

[55] Martin, K. R, Levkovitch-Verbin, H, Valenta, D., L, Baumrind, L, Pease, M. E, &Quigley, H. A. Retinal glutamate transporter changes in experimental glaucoma and after optic nerve transection in the rat. Investigative Ophthalmology & Visual Science (2002)., 43, 2236–2243.

[56] Schuettauf, F, Thaler, S. Bolz, S, Kalbacher, S. H, Mankowska, A, Zurakowski, D, Zrenner, E, & Rejdak, R. Alterations of amino acids and glutamate transport in the DBA/2J mouse retina; possible clues to degeneration. Graefe's Archives of Clinical&Experimental Ophthalmology (2007)., 245, 1157–1168.

[57] Park, C. K, Cha, J, Park, S. C, Lee, P. Y, Kim, J. H, Kim, H. S, Kim, S. A, Kim, I. B, & Chun, M. H. "Differential expression of two glutamate transporters, GLAST and GLT-1, in an experimental rat model of glaucoma. Experimental Brain Research (2009).. 197, 101–109.

[58] Ishikawa, M, Yoshitomi, T, Zorumski, C. F, & Izumi, Y. Effects of acutely elevated hydrostatic pressure in a rat ex vivo retinal preparation, Investigative Ophthalmology & Visual Science (2010)., 51,6414-6423.

[59] Park, S. W., Kim, K. Y, Lindsey, J. D, Dai, Y, Heo, H. Nguyen, D. H, Ellisman, M. H, Weinreb, R. N, & Ju, W. K. A selective inhibitor of drp1, mdivi-1, increases retinal ganglion cell survival in acute ischemic mouse retina. Investigative Ophthalmology & Visual Science (2011)., 52, 2837-2843.

[60] Yoneda, S, Tanaka, E, Goto, W, Ota, T, & Hara, H. Topiramate reduces excitotoxic and ischemic injury in the rat retina. Brain Research (2003)., 967, 257-266.

[61] Whitlock, N. A, Agarwal, N. Ma, J. X, & Crosson, C. E. Hsp27 upregulation by HIF-1 signaling offers protection against retinal ischemia in rats. Investigative Ophthalmology & Visual Science (2005)., 46, 1092-1098.

[62] shikawa, M, Yoshitomi, T, Zorumski, C. F., & Izumi, Y. Downregulation of glutamine synthetase via GLAST suppression induces retinal axonal swelling in a rat ex vivo hydrostatic pressure model. Investigative Ophthalmology & Visual Science (2011).. 52, 6604-6616.

[63] Harada T, Harada, C, Nakamura, K, Quah, H. M, Okumura, A, Namekata, Saeki, K, Aihara, M, Yoshida, H, Mitani, A, &Tanaka, K. The potential role of glutamate transporters in the pathogenesis of normal tension glaucoma. Journal of Clinical Investigation (2007)., 117, 1763–1770.

[64] Russo, R, Cavaliere, F, Varanom G. P, Milanese, M, Adornetto, A, Nucci, C, Bonanno, G, Morrone, L. A, Corasaniti, M. T, & Bagetta, G. Impairment of Neuronal Glutamate Uptake and Modulation of the Glutamate Transporter GLT-1 Induced by Retinal Ischemia. PLoS One(2013)., 8, e69250.

[65] Persson, M, & Rönnbäck, L. Microglial self-defence mediated through GLT-1 and glutathione. Amino Acids(2012)., 42, 207-219.

[66] Sullivan, R. K, Woldemussie, E, Macnab, L, Ruiz, G, Pow, DV. Evoked expression of the glutamate transporter GLT-1c in retinal ganglion cells in human glaucoma and in a rat model. Investigative Ophthalmology & Visual Science(2006)., 47(9):3853-3859.

[67] Shi, J, Zhang, Y. Q, & Simpkins, J. W. Effects of 17beta-estradiol on glucose transporter 1 expression and endothelial cell survival following focal ischemia in the rats. Experimantal Brain Research (1997)., 117, 200–206.

[68] Namekata, K, Harada, C, Guo, X, Kikushima, K, Kimura, A, Fuse, N, Mitamura, Y, Kohyama, K, Matsumoto, Y, Tanaka, K, & Harada, T. Interleukin-1 attenuates normal

tension glaucoma-like retinal degeneration in EAAC1-deficient mice. Neuroscience Letter (2009)., 465, 160-164.

[69] Dhandapani, K. M, & Brann, D. W. Protective effects of estrogen and selective estrogen receptor modulators in the brain. Biology of Reproduction (2002)., 67, 1379–1385.

[70] Lee, E. S, Sidoryk, M, Jiang, H, Yin, Z, & Aschner, M. Estrogen and tamoxifen reverse manganese-induced glutamate transporter impairment in astrocytes. Journal of Neurochemistry (2009)., 110, 530-544.

[71] Prokai-Tatrai, K, Xin, H, Nguyen, V, Szarka, S, Blazics, B, Prokai, L, & Koulen, P. 17β-estradiol eye drops protect the retinal ganglion cell layer and preserve visual function in an in vivo model of glaucoma. Molecular Pharmacology (2013)., 10, 3253-3261.

[72] Riepe, R. E, &Norenburg, M. D. Müller cell localisation of glutamine synthetase in rat retina. Nature(1977)., 268(5621):654-655.

[73] Marc, R. E, Murry, R. F, & Basinger, S. F. Pattern recognition of amino acid signatures in retinal neurons. Journal of Neuroscience (1995)., 15, 5106–5129.

[74] Gorovits, R, Yakir, A, Fox, L. E, & Vardimon, L. Hormonal and non-hormonal regulation of glutamine synthetase in the developing neural retina. Brain Research & Molecular Brain Research (1996)., 43, 321–329,

[75] Vardimon L. Neuroprotection by glutamine synthetase. Israel Medical Association Journal(2000)., Suppl:46-51

[76] Shaked, I, Ben-Dror, I, &Vardimon, L. Glutamine synthetase enhances the clearance of extracellular glutamate by the neural retina. Journal of Neurochemistry(2002)., 83(3):574-580.

[77] Kruchkova, Y, Ben-Dror, I, Herschkovitz, A, David, M, Yayon, A, &Vardimon, L. Basic fibroblast growth factor: a potential inhibitor of glutamine synthetase expression in injured neural tissue. Journal of Neurochemistry (2001).,77(6), 1641-1649.

[78] Pow, D. V, &Robinson, S. R. Glutamate in some retinal neurons is derived solely from glia. Neuroscience. (1994).,60(2), 355-366

[79] Izumi, Y., Hammerman, S. B., Kirby, C. O., Benz, A. M, Olney, J. W, & Zorumski, C. F. Involvement of glutamate in ischemic neurodegeneration in isolated retina. Visual Neuroscience (2003)., 20, 97-107.

[80] Shen, F, Chen, B, J., Danias, J, Lee, K. C, Lee, K. H, Su, Y, Podos, S. M, &Mittag, T. W. Glutamate-induced glutamine synthetase expression in retinal Müller cells after short-term ocular hypertension in the rat. Investigative Ophthalmology & Visual Science (2004)., 45, 3107–3111.

[81] Zeevalk, G. D, &Nicklas, W. J. Evidence that the loss of the voltage-dependent Mg2+block at the N-methyl-D-aspartate receptor underlies receptor activation dur-

ing inhibition of neuronal metabolism. Journal of Neurochemistry (1992).. 59, 1211–1220.

[82] Chen, C-H, Alyahya, K, Gionfriddo, J. R, Dubielzig, R. R, &Madl, J. E. Loss of glutamate synthetase immunoreactivity from the retina in canine primary glaucoma, Veterinary Ophthalmology (2008)., 11, 150–157.

[83] Derouiche, A, & Rauen, T. Coincidence of L-glutamate/L-aspartate transporter (GLAST) and glutamine synthetase (GS) immunoreactions in retinal glia: evidence for coupling of GLAST and GS in transmitter clearance. Journal of Neuroscience Research (1995)., 42:131–143.

[84] Jablonski, M. M, Freeman, N. E, Orr, W. E, Templeton, J. P, Lu, L, Williams, R. W, & Geisert, E. E. Genetic pathways regulating glutamate levels in retinal Mülle cells. Neurochemical Research (2011)., 36, 594–603.

[85] Carter-Dawson, L, Crawford, M. L, Harwerth, R. S, Smith, E. L, Feldman, R, Shen, F. F, Mitchell, C. K, & Whitetree, A. Vitreal glutamate concentration in monkeys with experimental glaucoma.
Investigative Ophthalmology & Visual Science (2002).., 43:2633-2637.

[86] Louzada-Junior, P, Dias, J. J, Santos, W. F, Lachat, J. J, Bradford, H. F, & J. Coutinho-Netto. Glutamate release in experimental ischaemia of the retina: an approach using microdialysis. Journal of Neurochemistry (1992).,59, 358–363.

[87] Neal, M. J, Cunningham, J. R, Hutson, P. H, & Hogg,, J. Effects of ischemia on neurotransmitter release from the isolated retina. Journal of Neurochemistry(1994)., 62, 1025–1033.

[88] Zeng, K, Xu, H, Mi, M, Zhang, Q, Zhang, Y, Chen, K, Chen, F, Zhu, J, Yu, X. Dietary taurine supplementation prevents glial alterations in retina of diabetic rats. Neurochemical Research(2009)., 34(2), 244-54.

[89] Zuo, ZF, Zhang, Q, Liu, XZ. Protective effects of curcumin on retinal Müller cell in early diabetic rats. International Journal of Ophthalmology(2013)., 6(4):422-424.

[90] El-Remessy, A. B, Khalifa, Y, Ola, S, Ibrahim, A. S, &Liou, GI. Cannabidiol protects retinal neurons by preserving glutamine synthetase activity in diabetes. Molecular Vision(2010)., 16:1487-95

[91] Shen, X, Xie, B, Cheng, Y, Jiao, Q, &Zhong Y. Effect of pigment epithelium derived factor on the expression of glutamine synthetase in early phase of experimental diabetic retinopathy. Ocular Immunology & Inflammation(2011).,19(4), 246-254.

[92] Ferreira, I. L, Duarte, C. B, &Carvalho, A. P. Ca2+influx through glutamate receptor-associated channels in retina cells correlates with neuronal cell death.Europian Journal of Pharmacology(1996)., 302:153-162.

[93] Osborne, N.N, DeSantis, L, Bae, J. H, Ugarte, M, Wood, J.P. M. Nash, M. S, & Chidlow, G. Topically applied betaxolol attenuates NMDA-induced toxicity to ganglion

cells and the effects of ischaemia to the retina. Experimental Eye Research(1999)., 69, 331–342.

[94] Osborne, N.N, Safa, R, &Nash, M.S. Photoreceptors are preferentially affected in the rat retina following permanent occlusion of the carotid arteries. Vision Research (1999).. 39, 3995–4002.

[95] Osborne, N. N, Ugarte, M, Chao, M, Chidlow, G, Bae, J. H, Wood, J.P.M., &Nash, M. S. Neuroprotection in relation to retinal ischemia and relevance to glaucoma. Survey of Ophthalmology (1999).. 43 (Suppl. 1), 102–128.

[96] Osborne, N. N, Wood, J.P. M, Chidlow, G, Bae, J. H, Melena, J, &Nash, M. S., Ganglion cell death in glaucoma: what do we really know? British Journal of Ophthalmology(1999).83, 980–986.

[97] Olney, J. W, Price, M. T, Salles, K. S, Labruyere, J, Ryerson, R, Mahan, K, Frierdich, G, & Samson, L. L-homocysteic acid: an endogenous excitotoxic ligand of the NMDA receptor. Brain Research Bulletin (1987)., 19, 597–602.

[98] el-Asrar A. M, Morse P. H, Maimone, D, Torczynski, E, &Reder, A. T. MK-801 protects retinal neurons from hypoxia and the toxicity of glutamate and aspartate. Investigative Ophthalmology &Visual Science(1992)., 33(12):3463-3468.

[99] Izumi, Y, Hammerman, S. B, Kirby, C. O, Benz, A. M, Olney, J. W, &Zorumski, C. F. Involvement of glutamate in ischemic neurodegeneration in isolated retina. Visual Neuroscience (2003)., 20, 97-107.

[100] Romano, C, Price, M. T, Almli, T, Olney, J. W. Excitotoxic neurodegeneration induced by deprivation of oxygen and glucose in isolated retina. Investigative Ophthalmology & Visual Science(1998)., 39(2), 416-23.

[101] Lees, G. J, & Leong, W. Differential effects of NBQX on the distal and local toxicity of glutamate agonists administered intrahippocampally. Brain Research (1993).. 628, 1–7.

[102] Osborne, N. N,&Herrera, A. J. The effect of experimental ischaemia and excitatory amino acid agonists on the GABA and serotonin immunoreactivities in the rabbit retina. Neuroscience (1994).59,1071–1081.

[103] Weber, M, Bonaventure, N, &Sahel, J. A. Protective role of excitatory amino acid antagonists in experimental retinal ischemia. Graefes Archives of Clinical & Experimental Ophthalmology (1995)., 233, 360–365.

[104] Massey, S. C. Cell types using glutamate as a neurotransmitter in the vertebrate retina. In: Osborne, N.N., Chader, G.J. (Eds.), Progress in Retinal Research. Pergamon Press, Oxford, (1990)., pp. 399–425.

[105] Dixon D. B, &Copenhagen, D. R. Two types of glutamate receptors differentially excite amacrine cells in the tiger salamander retina. Journal of Physiology(1992)., 449, 589-606

[106] Diamond, J. S, &Copenhagen, D. R. The contribution of NMDA and non-NMDA receptors to the light-evoked input-output characteristics of retinal ganglion cells. Neuron(1993).,11(4), 725-38.

[107] Cohen, E. D, &Miller, R. F. The role of NMDA and non-NMDA excitatory amino acid receptors in the functional organization of primate retinal ganglion cells.Visual Neuroscience(1994).,11(2), 317-32.

[108] Dong, C-J, Guo, Y, Agey, P, Wheeler, L, & Hare, W.A, Alpha-2 adrenergic modulation of NMDA receptor function as a major mechanism of RGC protection in experimental glaucoma and retinal excitotoxicity. Investigative Ophthalmology & Visual Science(2008)., 49, 4515-4522.

[109] Hare, W. A, WoldeMussie, E, Lai, R. K, Ton, H, Ruiz, G, Chun, T, & Wheeler, L. Efficacy and safety of memantine treatment for reduction of changes associatedwith experimental glaucoma in monkey, I: functional Measures. Investigative Ophthalmology & Visual Science (2004)., 45, 2625-2639.

[110] Lam, T. T, Abler, A.S., Kwong, J.M. K, Tso, M.O. M. N-methyl-D-aspartate (NMDA)-induced apoptosis in rat retina. Investigative Ophthalmology & Visual Science(1999)., 40, 2391-2397.

[111] Manabe, S, &Lipton, S. Divergent NMDA signals leading to proapoptotic and antiapoptotic pathways in the rat retina. Investigative Ophthalmology & Visual Science (2003).. 44, 385-392.

[112] Reichstein, D, Ren, L, Filippopoulos, T, Mittag, T, & Danias, J., Apoptotic retinal ganglion cell death in the DBA/2 mouse model of glaucoma. Experimental Eye Research (2007)., 84, 13-21.

[113] Russo, R, Cavaliere, F, Berliocchi, L, Nucci, C, Gliozzi, M, Mazzei, C., Tassorelli, C, Corasaniti, M. T, Rotiroti, D, Bagetta, G, &Morrone, L. A. Modulation of prosurvival and death-associated pathways under retinal ischemia/reperfusion: effects of NMDA receptor blockade. J.ournal of Neurochemistry (2008)., 107, 1347-1357.

[114] Schuettauf, F, Stein, T, Choragiewicz, T, Rejdak, R, Bolz, S, Zurakowski, D. Varde, M, Laties, A, & Thaler, S. Caspase inhibitors protect against NMDAmediated retinal ganglion cell death. Clinical & Experimental Ophthalmology (2010)., 39, 545-554.

[115] Shimazawa, M, Yamashima, T, Agarwal, N, & Hara, H. Neuroprotective effects of minocycline against in vitro and in vivo retinal ganglion cell damage. BrainResearch (2005)., 1053, 185-194

[116] Kutsuwada, T, Kashiwabuchi, N, Mori, H, Sakimura, K, Kushiya, E, Araki, K, Meguro, H, Masaki, H, Kumanishi, T, Arakawa, M, &Mishina, M. Molecular diversity of the NMDA receptor channel. Nature (1992)., 358, 36–41.

[117] Moriyoshi, K, Masu, M, Ishii, T, Shigemoto, R, Mizuno, N, &Nakanishi, S. Molecular cloning and characterization of the rat NMDA receptor. Nature(1991).,354(6348), 31-37.

[118] Ikeda, K, Nagasawa, M, Mori, H, Araki, K, Sakimura, K, Watanabe, M, Inoue, Y, &Mishina, M. Cloning and expression of the epsilon 4 subunit of the NMDA receptor channel. FEBS Letter (1992)., 313(1), 34-38.

[119] Meguro, H, Mori, H, Araki, K, Kushiya, E, Kutsuwada, T, Yamazaki, M, Kumanishi, T, Arakawa, M, Sakimura, K, &Mishina, M. Functional characterization of a heteromeric NMDA receptor channel expressed from cloned cDNAs. Nature(1992) 357 (6373), 70-4.

[120] Ishii, T, Moriyoshi, K, Sugihara, H, Sakurada, K, Kadotani, H, Yokoi, M, Akazawa, C, Shigemoto, R, Mizuno, N, Masu, M, &Shigetada N. Molecular characterization of the family of the N-methyl-D-aspartate receptor subunits. Journal of Biological Chemistry(1993).,268(4), 2836-43

[121] Monyer, H, Sprengel, R, Schoepfe,r R, Herb, A, Higuchi, M, Lomeli, H, Burnashev, N, Sakmann, B, &Seeburg, P. H. Heteromeric NMDA receptors: molecular and functional distinction of subtypes. Science (1992).,256(5060), 1217-21

[122] Nakanishi, S. Molecular diversity of glutamate receptors and implications for brain function. Science(1992).,258(5082), 597-603.

[123] Bai, N, Aida, T, Yanagisawa, M, Katou, S, Sakimura, K, Mishina, M, & Tanaka, K. NMDA receptor subunits have different roles in NMDA-induced neurotoxicity in the retina. Molecular Brain(2013)., 6:34e

[124] Bai, N, Hayashi, H, Aida, T, Namekata, K, Harada, T, Mishina, M, &Tanaka, K. Dock3 interaction with a glutamate-receptor NR2D subunit protects neurons from excitotoxicity. Molecular Brain (2013)., 6:22e.

[125] Suetake-Koga, S, Shimazaki, T, Takamori, K, Chaki, S, Kanuma, K, Sekiguchi, Y, Suzuki, T., Kikuchi, T, Matsui, Y, & Honda, T. In vitro and antinociceptive profile of HON0001, an orally active NMDA receptor NR2B subunit antagonist. Pharmacology Biochemistry and Behavior (2006)., 84:134-141.

[126] Lipton, S. A. Possible role for memantine in protecting retinal ganglion cells from glaucomatous damage. Survey of Ophthalmology(2003)., (Suppl 1), S38-S46.

[127] Reisberg, B, Doody, R, Stoffler, A, Schmitt, F, Ferris, S, & Mobius, H. J. Memantine in moderate-to-severe Alzheimer's disease. New England Journal of Medicine (2003)., 348, 1333–1341.

[128] Baltmr, A, Duggan, J, Nizari, S, Salt, T. E & Cordeiro, M. F. Neuroprotection in glaucoma-Is there a future role? Experimental Eye Research (2010)., 91, 554-566.

[129] Osborne, N. N. Pathogenesis of ganglion "cell death" in glaucoma and neuroprotection: focus on ganglion cell axonal mitochondria. Progress in Brain Research(2008)., 173, 339–352

[130] Roberts, P. D, Spiros, A, &Geerts, H. Simulations of symptomatic treatments for Alzheimer's disease: computational analysis of pathology and mechanisms of drug action. Alzheimer's Research & Therapy(2012).,4(6), 50.

[131] Wrighton, D. C, Baker, E. J, Chen, P. E, &Wyllie, D. J. Mg2+and memantine block of rat recombinant NMDA receptors containing chimeric NR2A/2D subunits expressed in Xenopus laevis oocytes. Journal of Physiology(2008).,586(1), 211-225.

6

Utilization of Portable Digital Camera for Detecting Cataract

Retno Supriyanti, Hitoshi Habe and Masatsugu Kidode

1. Introduction

Cataract is a kind of eye disease [1]; that is a clouding in the lens of the eye that affects vision. Cataract exhibits a lot of whitish color inside a pupil. The three classes of cataracts are immature, mature and hypermature, which differ in seriousness. In an immature cataract, a whitish color appears inside the pupil but less so than in mature or hypermature cataracts. Usually, the condition is not yet serious. A Hypermature cataract exhibits much whitish color inside the pupil and can cause the lens of the eye to break if surgery is not carried out. This condition is very dangerous. Figure 1 shows examples of the range of serious and non-serious conditions.

The World Health Report published in 2001 estimated that there were 20 million people who are bilaterally blind (i.e., with eyesight of less than 3/60 in the better eye) whose blindness was caused by age related cataracts [2]. That number will have increased to 40 million by the year 2020. Increasing age is associated with an increasing prevalence of cataracts, but in most developing countries, cataracts often occur earlier in life. One of the developing countries that have the highest number of people with cataracts is Indonesia. There are about 6 million people in Indonesia who suffer from cataracts, but Indonesia only has about 1160 ophthalmologists for a population of more than 200 million people (one for every 350.000 people). In addition, ophthalmologists are not evenly distributed. Many ophthalmologists are located in the capital city, yet many people have no access to ophthalmologists because of geographic conditions.

Usually ophthalmologists will use various equipment like slit lamp or ophthalmoscope to determine the type, opacities and the location of the cataract, and to distinguish it from other eye diseases that have symptoms similar to cataracts. Basically, both equipments use a light source to determine the condition of the patient's eye lens. By using these kinds of equipment, lens opacities can be assessed by observing the width of the edge of the iris in a cloudy lens. If the remote location and the large shadow means immature cataracts, if it is a small shadow and close to the pupil occurs in mature cataracts. It is expected with early diagnosis, the cataract can be monitored whether to continue or will cause complications that must be treated to prevent blindness; However, using this equipment have some limitations including expensive price and special training needed. It will be a problem for some developing countries which has a limited number of both ophthalmologists and health facilities like Indonesia, Nepal, and Vietnam, for example. To solve this problem, we developed a method for detecting cataract based on digital image processing techniques. These techniques support the use of low-cost and easy-to-use equipment such as digital camera. We choose to use a digital camera as the main equipment with reference to the working principle of the slit-lamp camera and ophthalmoscope in which this equipment using the light to check the condition of the eye lens, so we adopted the use of the slit-lamp camera or ophthalmoscope light with a flash light on digital camera lenses to represent the condition. The two types of equipment are shown in Figure 2.

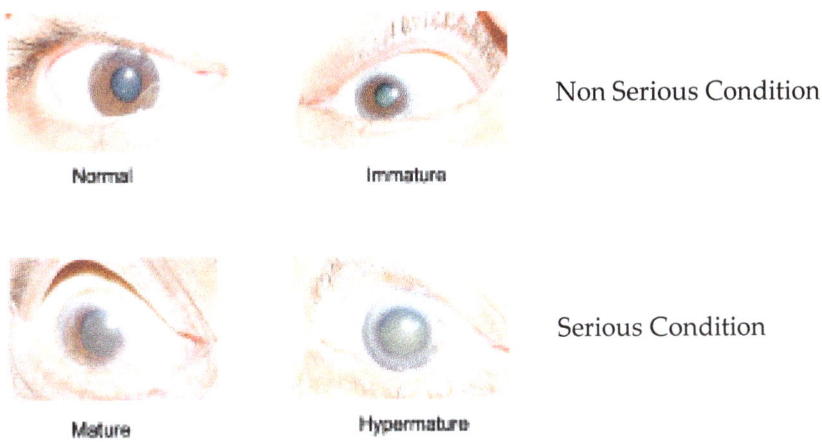

Figure 1. Example of eye images

In our method, we extracted all information about cataract from pupil area only because all information about cataracts comes from the lens only. This is based on the fact that the opacities as an important sign of cataracts occur in the lens. However, when using a compact digital camera, we found problems such as insufficient image quality and uncontrolled illumination. For example, if we employ intensity value for screening cataract, i.e. higher intensity corresponds to a serious condition; it would fail for a cataract eye image taken under low illumination as shown in Figure 3. It appears that a non-serious condition eye image has an average intensity about 155 inside a pupil while a serious condition eye image only has an average intensity about 55 inside a pupil. In order to develop a robust cataract screening techniques, we proposed to use specular reflection analysis as the core method for cataract screening because specular reflection always brighter than surrounding area and it is not depend on illumination condition. We also were considering texture information as the supporting method.

This chapter will discuss step by step instructions on the use of digital cameras as the main equipment for detecting cataract, complete with an explanation of image processing techniques for the analysis of digital images produced by digital cameras.

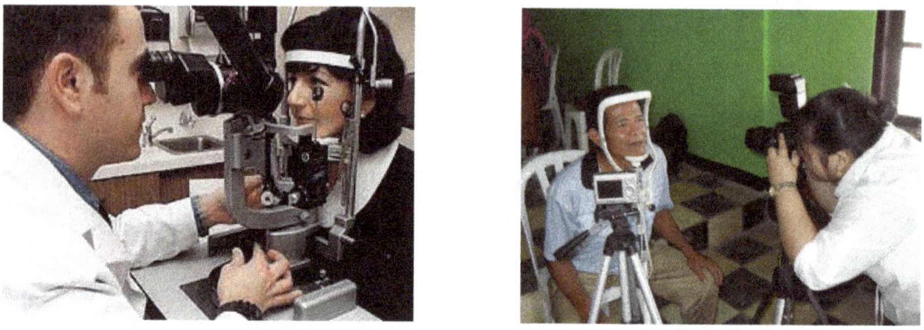

(a) Slit-lamp (b) Digital camera

Source: http://www.mrcopth.com/examinationtechniques
Source: Private documentation

Figure 2. Examination using (a) slit lamp (b) our system

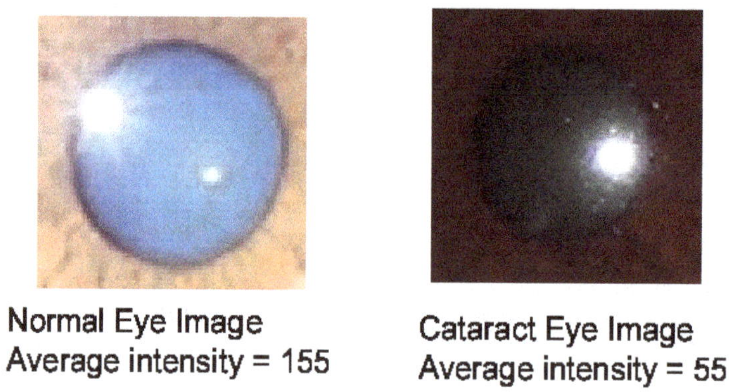

Figure 3. Example of photographs under uncontrolled illumination

2. Images processing analysis

2.1. Definition of pupil

As discussed in Section 1, we extracted all information inside the pupil including specular reflection and texture appearance because all information about cataract is taken from the pupil region only. The pupil of the eye is simply a hole in the iris through which one can peer into the eye. It appears black because of the darkness inside [3][4]. Based on these definitions, we can conclude that the color of the pupil is universal; it does not depend on ethnicity, although the color of the iris is different for different ethnicity, as shown in Figure 4.

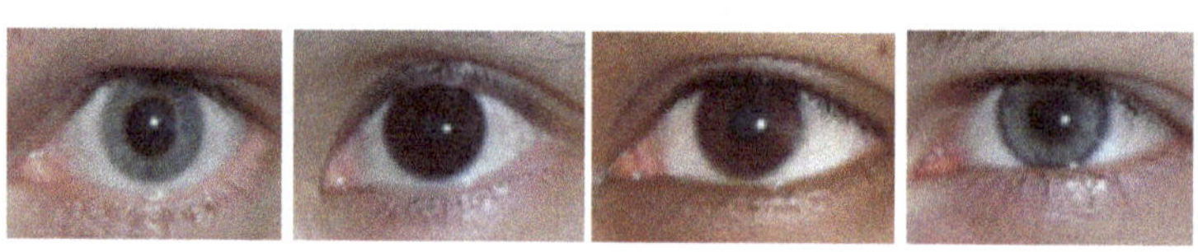

Figure 4. Figure 4. Color of pupil does not depend on ethnicity

The pupil gets wider in the dark but narrower in light. When narrow, the diameter is 3 to 4 millimeters. In the dark it will be the same at first, but will approach the maximum distance for a wide pupil of 5 to 8 mm depending on a person's age [5]. There are some definitions regarding pupil size in Figure 5.

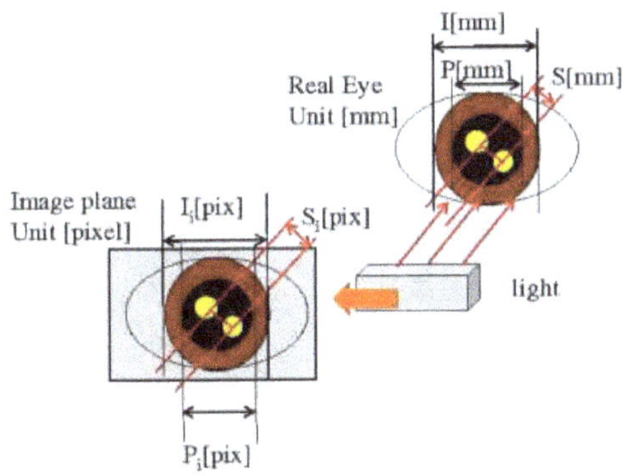

Figure 5. Definitions of pupil

The pupil's size always changes while the iris's size is fixed, therefore, to make pupil size independent in various conditions, in this paper we will use a ratio between pupil and iris as a unit to express size measurement, indicated by the symbol P_r and ex pressing by Equation 1.

$$P_r = \frac{P_i}{I_i} \approx \frac{P}{I} \tag{1}$$

2.2. Pupil localization

In general, the algorithm used in pupil localization is using 3 stages. Before performing these steps, the original image size changed to 50%. This is done to simplify the image processing operations.

1. Masking Step, namely the separation process of facial images based on skin color. How this is done by utilizing the luminance component and Cb and Cr to form the face of the box based on skin color as described in Figure 6.

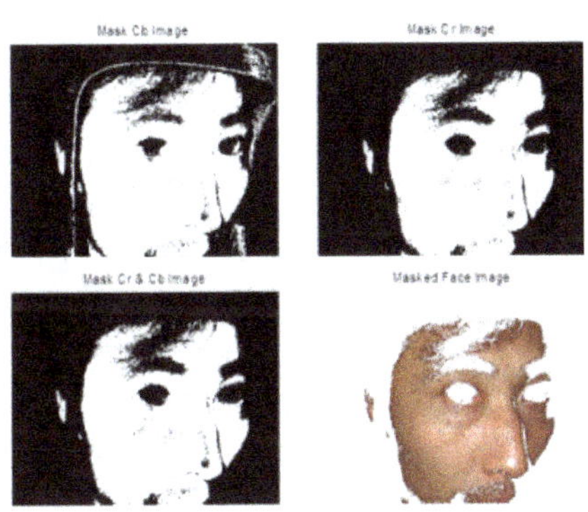

Figure 6. Face masking process

2. Region of eye Step, when it was getting a face image in the box and then take the eye area. Cutting the eye area is based on the normal form has a face that the proportion of 1 / 3 the length of a human face [6] as described in Figure 7.

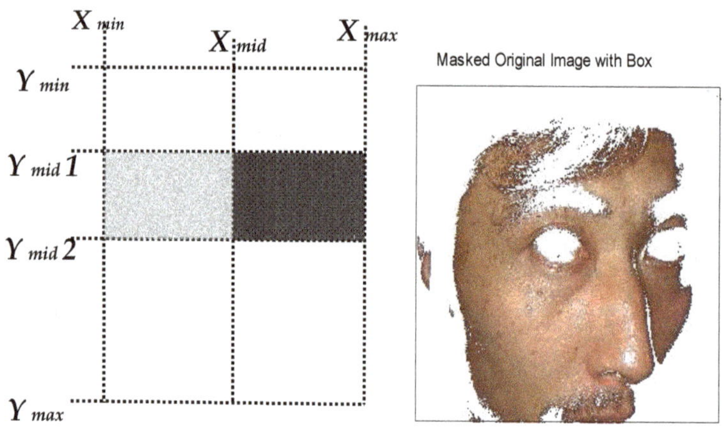

Figure 7. Estimation of eye area

3. Pupils Step, at this stage to use Lab color characteristics to determine the image of the pupil. Then using a fixed radius circle Hough to determine the center point of the circle which is the center point of pupil candidates as described in Figure 8.

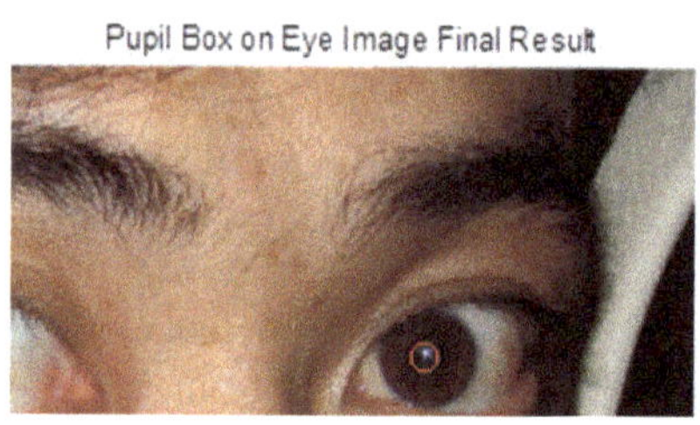

Figure 8. Pupil circle

2.3. Specular reflection analysis

The core of our method is specular reflection analysis. We develop our algorithm refer to the working principles of ophthalmoscope and slit lamp. An ophthalmoscope is an instrument that enables a doctor to examine the inside of a person's eye. The instrument has an angled mirror, various lenses, and a light source. A slit lamp is an instrument that enables a doctor to examine the entire eye under high magnification and that allows measurement of depth. The slit lamp focuses a bright light into the eye. Both equipments have a similarity for diagnosing cataract.

Figure 9 describes the principle work of the specular reflection method. Light hits the frontal surface of the lens and makes a reflection called frontside reflection. But actually light also hits the rear side of the lens. For a non serious condition, there is not a whitish color inside the lens so it will be reflected again, which is called backside reflection. For a serious condition especially, because there is a lot of clouding in the lens, light will not be reflected again. The different characteristics are shown in Figure 10. Based on the reflection theorem, the direction of the normal vector always goes to the center of the pupil, so when we look at the image appearance we can find the relationship of the location between the two reflections and the center of the pupil; they are on a single line

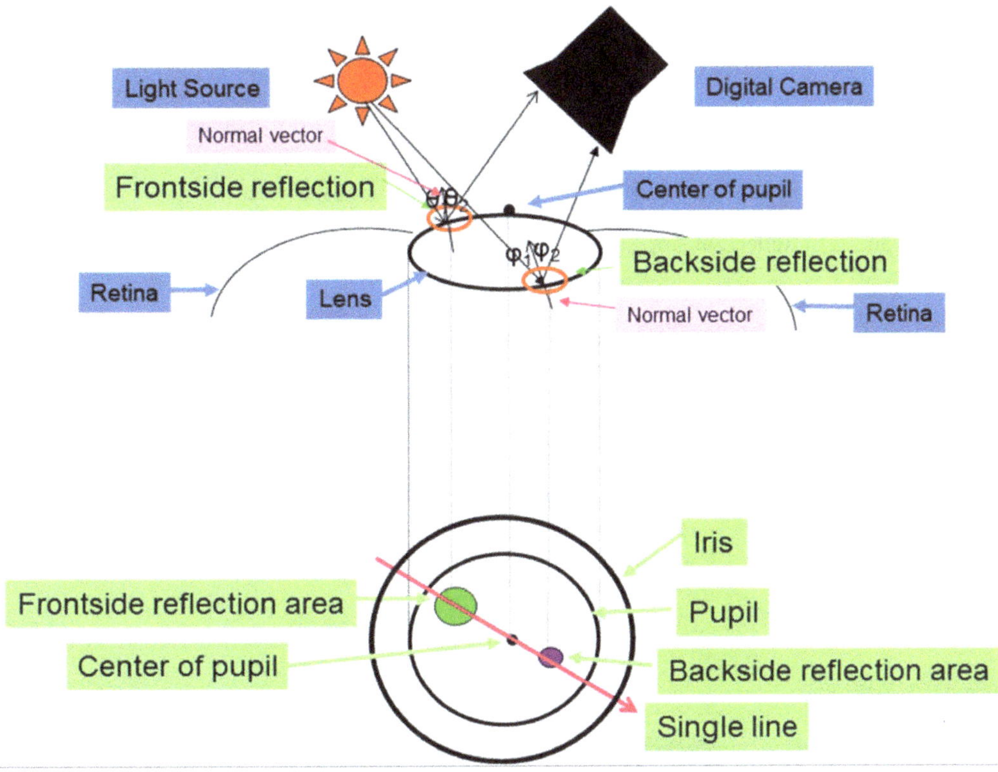

Figure 9. Model of reflection characteristics in eye

Using the relationship between both reflections, we conducted a search to find the backside reflection, as depicted in Figure 11. Using coordinate of the center and the radius of frontside reflection, we then searched for the backside reflection by searching for areas of higher intensity beside frontside reflection compared with their immediately surrounding areas in a line that expressed by Equation 2

$$A = d + r - \delta \tag{2}$$

Where A is the length of backside reflection searching, d is the distance between center of pupil and center of frontside reflection, r is the radius of pupil and δ is the radius of backside reflection.

In fact, the shapes of specular reflections are varied as described in Figure 12. As shown in Figure 12, some variations of the specular reflections shape are circle, cube, rectangular and ellipse, although we used the same flash light during taking photographs. Therefore, during searched for backside reflections area as described in Figure 11, we considered to assume various shapes of specular reflections and did intensity searching based on the shape that we assumed before as shown in Figure 13.

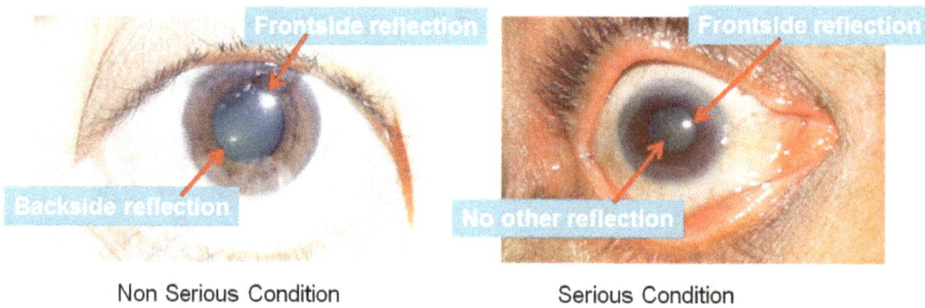

Figure 10. Example of Reflection Appearance

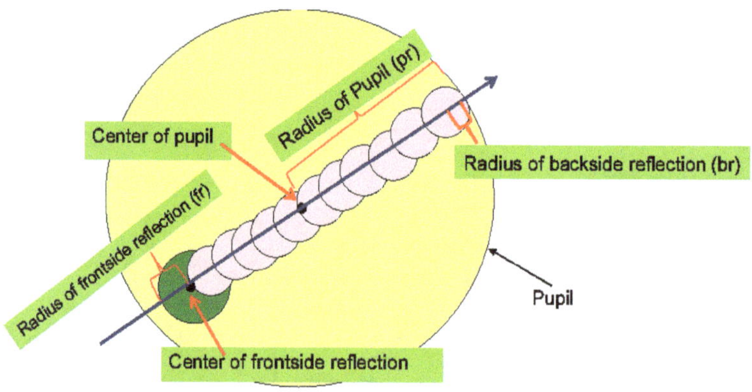

Figure 11. Searching backside reflection area data

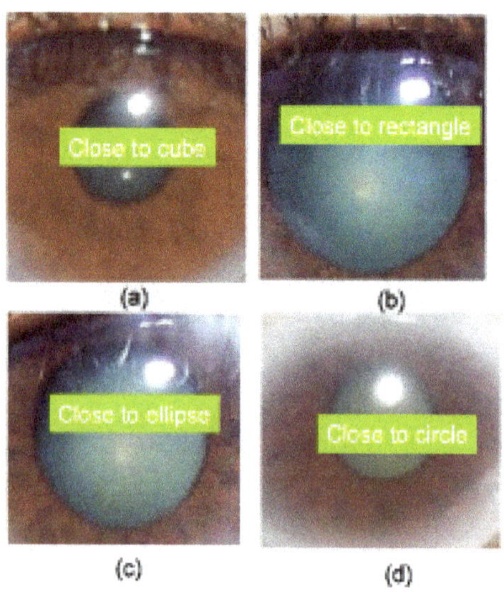

Figure 12. Various shapes of specular reflections inside the pupil

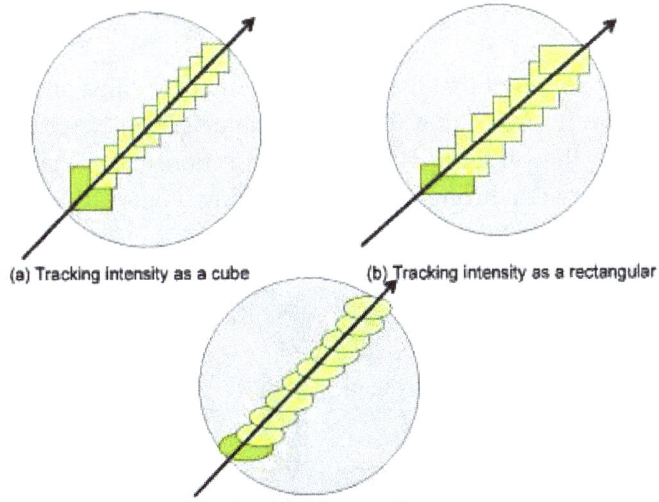

Figure 13. Intensity tracking using various shapes of specular reflections

We apply Eq. 2 which the value of δ is determined by following the assumption of specular reflection as shown in Figure 14.

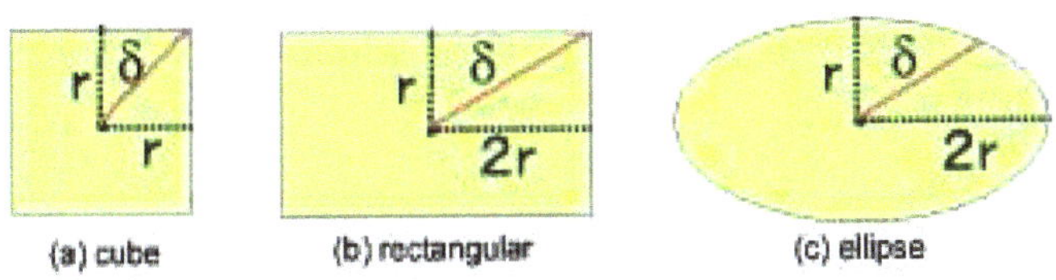

Figure 14. The size using for intensity tracking

Then, we compare the performance of each shapes of specular reflections in order to provide a recommendation on the tendency of specular reflection's shape that can give the best results for cataract screening sistem we apply an Eq.4.

Based on the result of intensity tracking as shown in Figure 11, we implemented a differential function in a discrete system to develop an automatic screening between the serious condition and not serious condition based on intensity tracking result and expressed by Equation 3.

$$D = I(s) - I(s-1)\ldots \tag{3}$$

Where I is intensity and S is a distance between center of frontside reflection and the next circle that will be investigated. During intensity searching, if $D(S) > 0$ it means there is an increasing intensity value. Otherwise if $D(S) < 0$ it means there is a decreasing intensity value. Based on the discussion in above paragraph, that non serious condition always have a great increasing intensity that indicated existence of backside reflection but it doesn't mean that serious condition didn't have increasing intensity during intensity tracking. Because we have variations of the numbers of intensity searching so we define normalized number of increasing value determined by Equation 4.

$$P_n = \frac{P}{n} \tag{4}$$

Where P is the numbers of point that has increasing intensity value and n is the numbers of point along an intensity tracking line. The main characteristic of serious and non-serious conditions depends on the presence of backside reflection in an image that is shown by increasing intensity in an area during intensity searching. Figure 15 shows the examples of the result of intensity tracking for serious and non-serious.

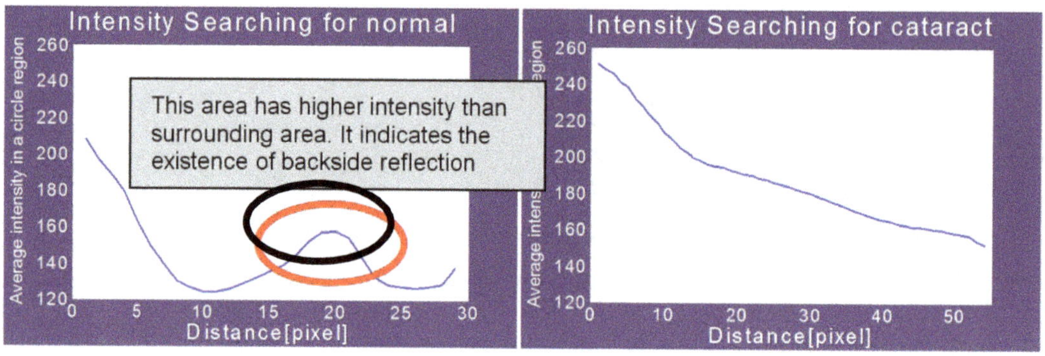

Figure 15. Analyzing backside reflection

2.4. Texture analysis

2.4.1. Uniformity

An important approach to region description is to quantify texture content. In statistical texture analysis, the descriptor measures properties such as smoothness, coarseness and regularity. Basically, there are two kinds of textures inside the pupil; smooth and coarse. This can be calculated by the uniformity value expressed in Eq.5. Where U is the value of uniformity, H is probability histogram of the intensity levels in a region, and N is the number of pixel in an image, Let i = 0, 1, 2, …., , L − 1, be the corresponding histogram, where L is the value of possible intensity. Uniformity will be maximum when all gray levels are equal [7]. Whitish color inside the lens has two kinds' distributions. First, whitish color spread smoothly inside the pupil. In the early stage, this kind of cataract has a thin layer of whitish color and covers the whole lens surface gradually until the whitish color layer becomes thick. Second, whitish color spread uneven inside the lens. It will appear a coarse texture inside the pupil. Almost all non serious conditions have a smooth texture with a high value of uniformity.

$$U = \sum_{i=0}^{L-1} \left(\frac{H(i)}{N}\right)^2 \qquad \text{……..(5)}$$

For example, in a 3 x 3 region and belongs to a smooth texture as shown in Figure 16 , the uniformity is shown in calculation below:

$$U = \left(\frac{9}{9}\right)^2 = 1$$

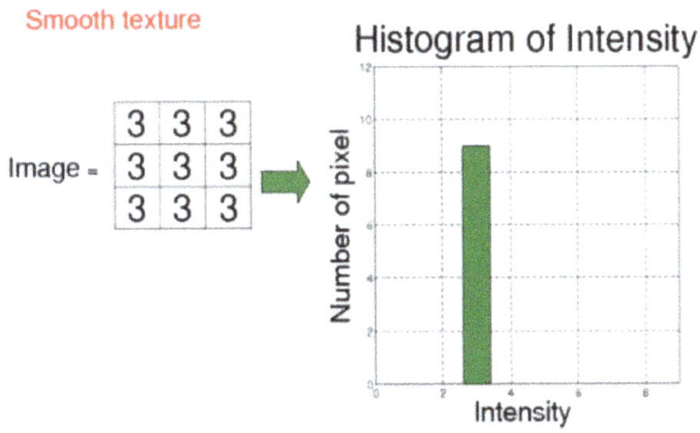

Figure 16. Example of Smooth Texture

Another example, in a 3 x 3 region and belongs to a coarse texture as shown in Figure 17, the uniformity is shown in calculation below:

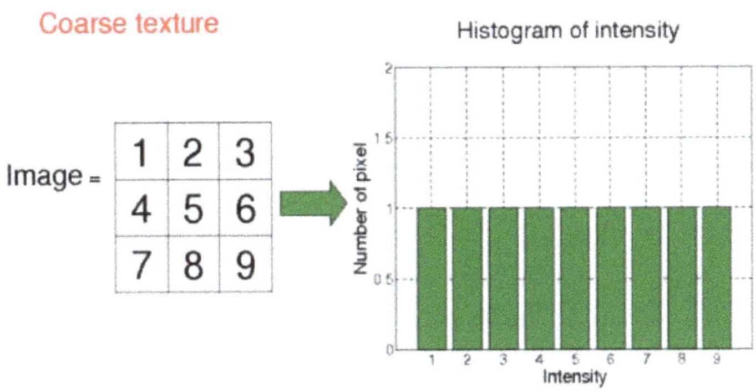

Figure 17. Example of coarse Texture

$$U = \left(\frac{1}{9}\right)^2 + \left(\frac{1}{9}\right)^2 + \left(\frac{1}{9}\right)^2 + \left(\frac{1}{9}\right)^2 + \left(\frac{1}{9}\right)^2 + \left(\frac{1}{9}\right)^2 + \left(\frac{1}{9}\right)^2 + \left(\frac{1}{9}\right)^2 + \left(\frac{1}{9}\right)^2 = 0{,}111$$

Figure 18(a) shows an image of eye in serious condition with a high value of uniformity caused by the whitish color is spreading smoothly inside the pupil. In the early stage, this kind of cataract has a thin layer of whitish color and covers the whole lens surface gradually until the whitish color layer becomes thick. Figure 18(b) shows an image of an eye with a coarse texture because the whitish color is spreading unevenly inside the pupil. Figure 18(c) shows an image of an eye in non-serious condition. Almost all non-serious conditions have a smooth texture with a high value of uniformity.

2.4.2. *Average intensity*

The equation to measure an average intensity expressed in Equation 6, where m is mean (average) of intensity, I is possible intensity, and N is number of pixel in an image [7]. It will be very simple intuition that cataract eyes have brighter intensities than normal eyes.

$$m = \sum_{i=0}^{L-1} \left(\frac{I(i)}{N}\right) \tag{6}$$

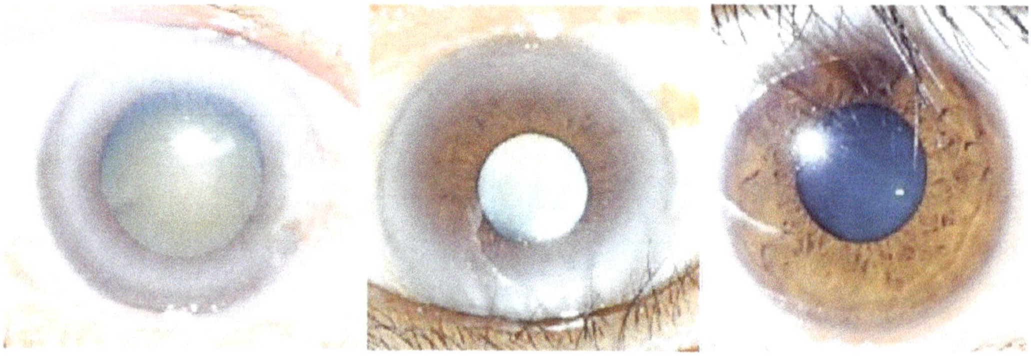

(c) Serious (b) Serious (a) Non- Serious

Figure 18. Example of Texture Appearance

For example, in a 3x3 region as shown in Figure 19 , the average intensity is shown in calculation below :

$$m = \frac{3+3+2+1+2+5+7+1+4}{9} = 3,11111$$

Image =

3	3	2
1	2	5
7	1	4

Figure 19. An example of average intensity

The whitish color inside a pupil has a corresponding with increasing intensity. Figure 20 shows an eye normal image and a cataract eye image. It appears that a cataract eye image has a higher intensity than a normal eye image. By assuming that a serious condition has a higher intensity than a non-serious condition, we distinguish both conditions.

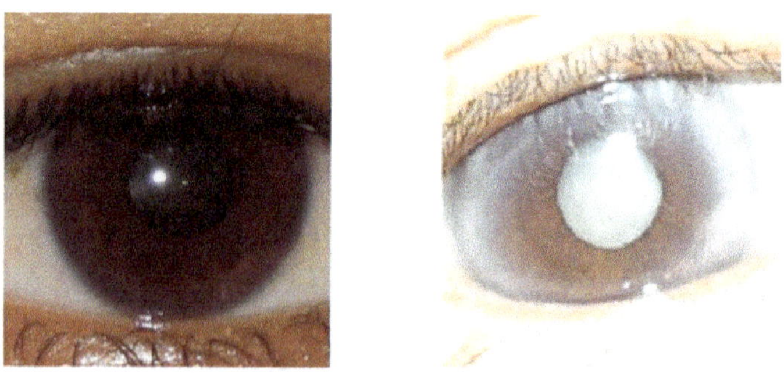

Normal Cataract

Figure 20. Intensity difference between normal and cataract

3. Diagnosing by classification

To build the system, we used Matlab R2007B with image processing toolbox. Also, for building a classifier to classify between serious and non-serious condition, we use SVM toolbox developed by Canu [3]. In order to make a classification for cataract screening we need two kinds of data: training data and testing data. Training data used to train the system to recognize the characteristics of a serious condition and non-serious condition so the system can determine the threshold for distinguishing between two conditions automatically. While testing data used to evaluate system performance refer to the characteristics obtained in the training data.

To test the performance of our system, we use several parameters. The first is True Positive Rate (TPR). TPR determines a classifier or a diagnostic test performance on classifying positive instances correctly among all positive samples available during the test. The second is FPR (False Positive Rate). FPR, on the other hand, defines how many incorrect positive results occur among all negative samples available during the test.

Criterion values for getting TPR and FPR parameters are described in Figure 21.

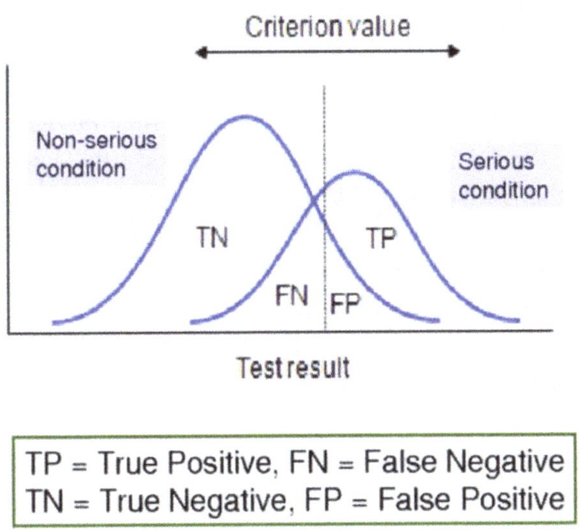

Figure 21. Parameter for measuring performance

To evaluate the overall system performance, we use cross validation techniques in which we did evaluation several times until all data were evaluated.. So that all images produced by various kinds of cameras are grouped into two groups. The first group is the images that show the serious conditions, while the second group is the images that show the non-serious conditions. We did some testing times by taking 90% of data as training data and 10% of data as testing data. Data changed each time, until finally all data used as training data and testing data. Figure 22 shows a summary of performance our algorithm. The result shows that current method has a good performance than other method.

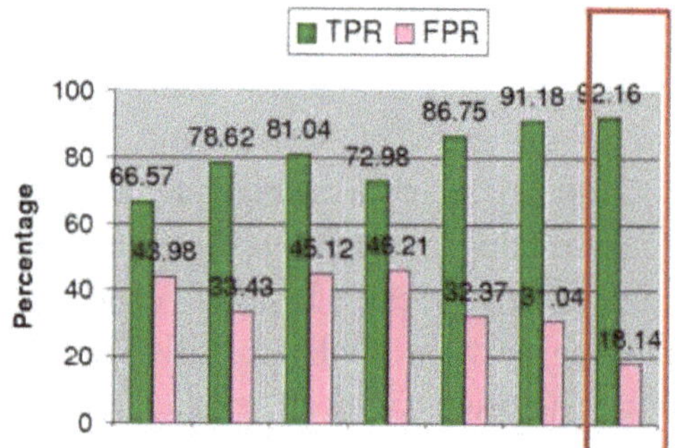

Average instensity	V			V	V		V
Texture uniformity		V		V		V	V
Specular reflection			V		V	V	V

proposed

Figure 22. Performance comparison for each method

4. Practical screening system and data acquisition

As discussed in subsection 2.3, the core of our method is specular reflection analysis. Referring to the reflection theorem, light hits the frontal surface of the lens and makes a reflection called frontside reflection. However, light also hits the rear side of the lens. For a non-serious condition, there is not a whitish color inside the lens, therefore, it will be reflected again, which is called backside reflection. For a serious condition especially, because there is a lot of clouding in the lens, light will not be reflected again. In order to investigate the availability of frontside reflection and backside reflection inside the lens, and also to obtain a minimum distance between two reflections that can be observed by our algorithm, we did a simulation. Refer to the experiments, our algorithm can observe availability of two reflections with minimum ratio between distance and iris of about 0.125. It is an important value because if our algorithm fails to investigate availability of the two reflections, will face problems. First, patient really has a serious condition. Second, it is caused by a wrong position between camera and patient during taking a photograph.

Regarding these problems, we have to make sure that we put camera and patient in an appropriate position. Therefore, a simulation of the angle's position is very important. In our simulation, we assume that a light is attached in camera. The purposes are:

1. Getting an optimal position of angle between camera and lens.
2. Getting an optimal pupil size to get an appropriate distance between two reflections.

The lens has an ellipsoid, biconvex shape. It is typically circa 10 mm in diameter and has an axial length of about 4 mm [5]. An iris is a colored disk inside the eye with diameter of about 12 mm [5]. Figure 23 describes the shape and size of the lens, pupil and iris in our simulation.

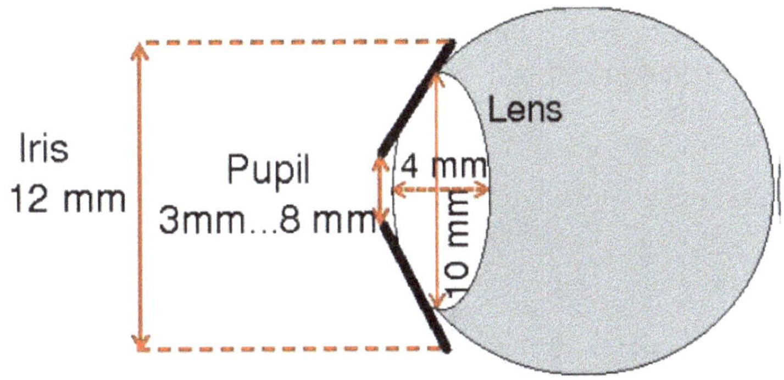

Figure 23. Typical shape and size of pupil

In this part, there are three conditions. First is a condition where the reflection does not occur inside the lens. Second is a condition where only a frontside reflection occurs and can be observed inside the lens. Third is an appropriate condition where a frontside reflection and backside reflection occur and can be observed in an image plane. Figures 24-26 show each condition, respectively.

During simulation, we change the position of the camera with light attached based on angle (φ) between camera and lens. It starts from angle 1° to angle 180°. Figure 24 shows that the position of light cannot reach the lens because light hits the surface of the iris; therefore, there is no reflection in the lens

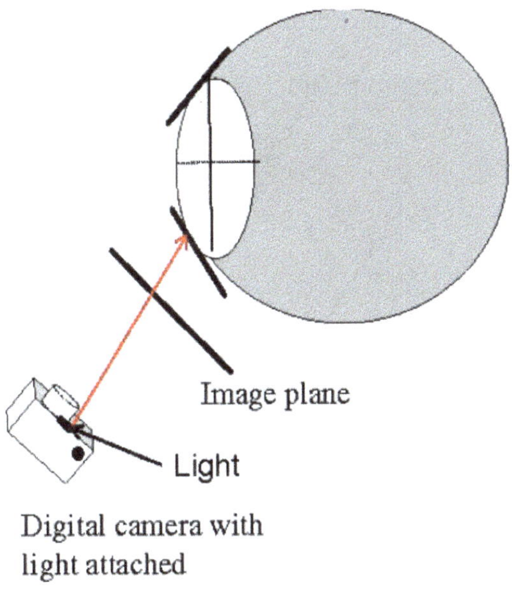

Figure 24. Condition in which no reflection occurs

Figure 25 shows that light hits the frontal surface of the lens therefore, a reflection occurs and is observed. However, when the light hits the rear side of the lens, a reflection occurs but it cannot be observed in the image plane. Therefore, in this condition, only frontside reflection is observed in the image plane. Figure 26 shows an appropriate condition in which both reflections occur and are observed in the image plane. This kind of parameter will be useful for distinguishing between serious and non-serious conditions.

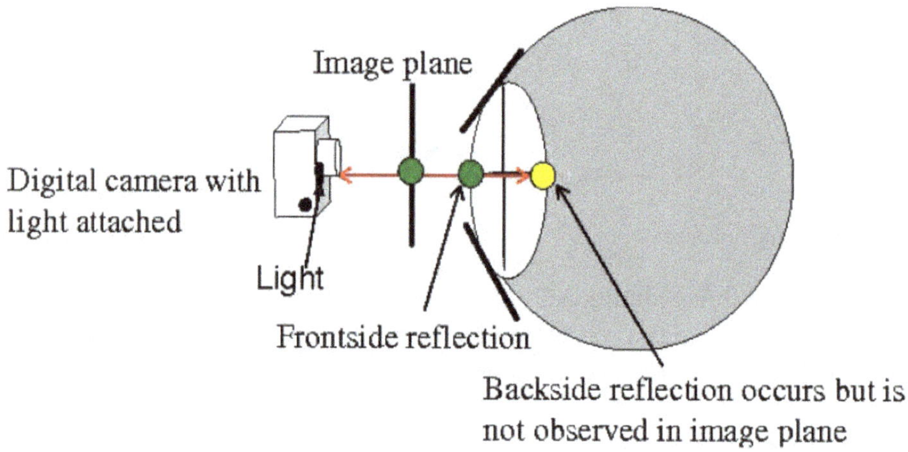

Figure 25. Condition in which only frontside reflection occurs and is observed in an image plane

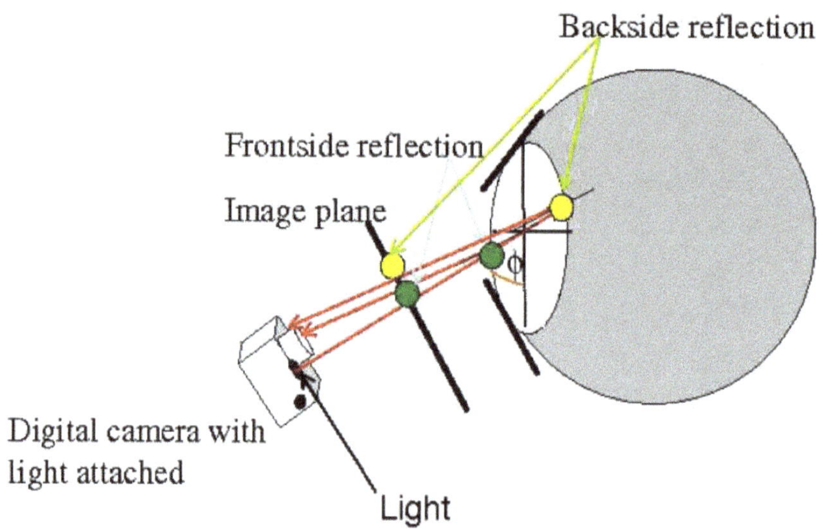

Figure 26. An appropriate condition in which both reflections occur and are observed in an image plane

In the real condition, As already discussed in the section 1, that our system is expected to be used by all people in all places, so that the equipment will be used in our system must also be simple as shown in Figure 28. Brief description about the function of equipment is described in the following paragraph.

3. Chin rest - This is equipment for patient to lean forward and place his or her in the chin rest and forehead against the bar. We use a simple chin rest created manually by using a board that is placed on something that could make it stand upright. The main goal is

to put the patient's chin so that patients feel comfortable during taking a photograph. On the other hand, by using a chin rest so will allow a user to get the right eye image during taking a photograph because the patient does not move his head movement that will result in the patient's eye movement. We should be emphasized here that this tool is not absolutely necessary in our system, if users can take photograph that make an appropriate input image and the patient feel comfortable, not moving their head so that the position of the eyes in a state of permanent, then the use of these tools are not needed.

4. Tripod - Tripods are used for both still and motion photography to prevent camera movement. The main purpose of using a tripod in our system is to make it easier to get good quality photo because the camera will be in a fixed position and not moving so the possibility of blur can be prevented. Another reason is to get more accurate angular position between the camera and the patient because they will affect the existence of specular reflection inside a pupil as be described in above paragraph. It should be noted here that as well as the use of chin rest, the use of a tripod in our system is not an absolute thing. If users able to get an appropriate input image without using a tripod therefore this equipment is not required in our system.
5. Digital Camera - This is the most important equipment in our system because all the input images are taken from a digital camera. In our system, we use all types of digital cameras from various brands available such as Canon and Nikon. We do not consider about the performance of cameras such as the number of pixels, zooming capabilities,and other facilities. Most important for our system is the camera has flash facility as a light source to get specular reflections, has a macro facility to get a good enough quality when taking photographs for the pupil of the eye area. Referring to Figure 2, it can be said that the performance of each camera is almost evenly.

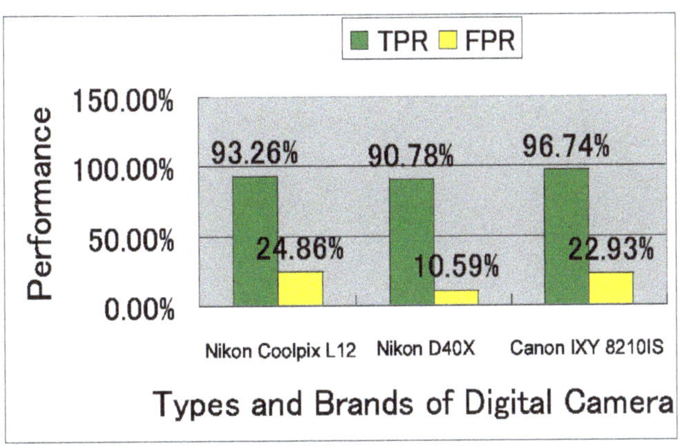

Figure 27. System performance based on types and brands of digital camera

6. Scale - This is equipment to provide guidance angle camera placement. We use a kind of plastic mats that have been marked to measure the angle between the patient and the camera.
7. Personal Computer

The main function is an interface for analyzing of input images that have been obtained in the data acquisition session. Our method written in the form of graphical user interface (GUI) so that user easily uses it just by pressing the command buttons available. Users do not need to analyze the complicated result because our methods give results about the patient's condition which he included in serious or non serious condition.

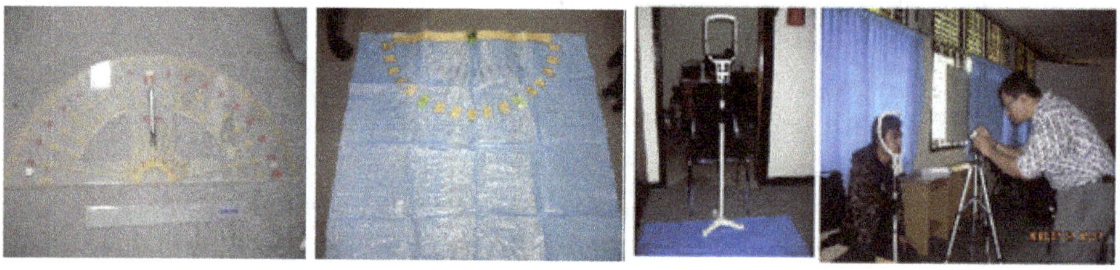

Figure 28. Equipment were used in our system

Figure 29 and Figure 30 describe about the implementation of data acquisition in the real condition.

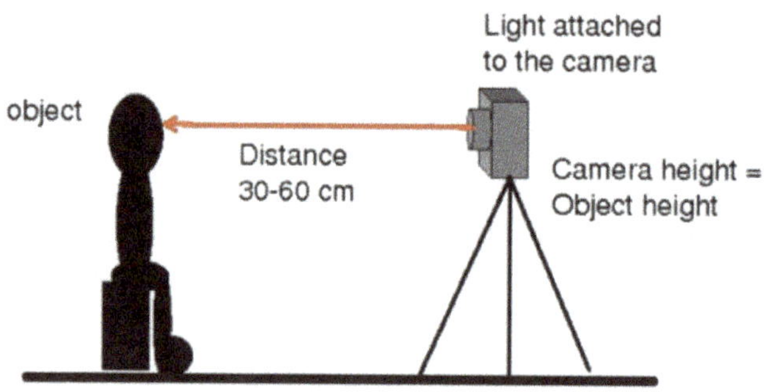

Figure 29. Side view of camera configuration

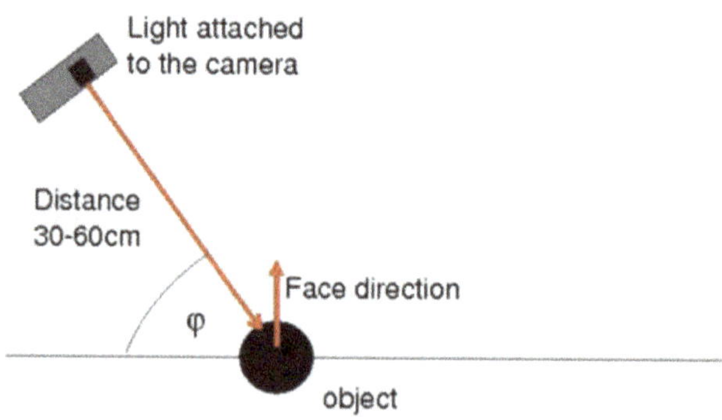

Figure 30. View from above camera configuration

5. Conclusion

Regarding the conditions in developing countries which have limitations both of eye doctors and health facilities, using simple equipment such as digital camera for cataract screening is promising and sufficient. Because digital camera is small and easily carried out, easy to use and inexpensive. Also, the method for supporting digital camera has a good performance for distinguishing between serious and non-serious condition; therefore, it is very useful for determining people who need a surgery as soon as possible.

Author details

Retno Supriyanti
Faculty of Science and Engineering, Jenderal Soedirman University, Indonesia

Hitoshi Habe and Masatsugu Kidode
Graduate School of Information Science, Nara Institute of Science and Technology, Japan

Acknowledgement

We Would like to thank the head and staffs of the Kamandaka Eye Clinic in Purwokerto Indonesia, Students and staffs of Electrical Engineering Dept, Jenderal Soedirman University Indonesia.The staffs of NAIST Japan, all members of the Advanced Intelligence Laboratory at NAIST, and members of the elder peoples house (CHOMEISHO) in Ikoma Japan , for their permission and willingness have photographs taken of cataract and normal patients. Also, this work is partly supported by the Konika Minolta Imaging Science Foundation and the Foundation for NAIST, also DIPA Jenderal Soedirman University through International Research Collaboration Project.

References

[1] Ilyas, Sidharta, 2005 "Eye Diseases", Balai Penerbit FKUI, Jakarta.

[2] Brian Gary, Hugh Taylor, 2001, "Cataract Blindness – challenges for 21st century", Bulletin of the World Health Organization.

[3] Medical Encyclopedia. 2007, Pupil. Available : http:// www. nlm. nih. gov/ medlineplus / ency/ article, accessed 2007 july 20.

[4] Eyemakeart. 2009, Anatomi mata. Available: http://eyemakeart.com/anatomi-mata/, accessed 2009 July 20..

[5] Taylor.Karen,2001, "Forensic Art and Illustrations ", CRC Press LLC, Florida.

[6] David B.L. Bong dan Kok Houi Lim, 2009, "Application of Fixed-Radius Hough Transform In Eye Detection". International Journal of Intelligent Information Technology Application, 2(3):121-127.

[7] Gonzales, RC, and R.E. Woods. 2002, "Digital Image Processing. 2nd ed." New Jersey: Prentice Hall, Inc.

[8] Canu. S, Y. Grandvalet, V. Guigue, and A. Rakotomamonjy. 2005, SVM and kernel methods matlab toolbox. Perception Systmes et Information, INSA de Rouen, Rouen, France.

7

Recent Advances in Ocular Nucleic Acid-Based Therapies: The Silent Era

Covadonga Pañeda, Tamara Martínez, Natalia Wright and Ana Isabel Jimenez

1. Introduction

The central dogma of biology describes the transfer of biological information from DNA through to protein (1). In the first phase, known as transcription, DNA is converted into a complementary sequence of messenger RNA (mRNA). This mRNA allows the genetic message to be communicated outside of the cell nucleus, to other areas of the cell, where it is then translated into protein by ribosomes. Post-transcriptional regulatory events take place after an RNA molecule is formed; thereafter the resulting RNA molecule is decoded to produce a specific protein. Protein production depends on the length of survival of RNA in a cell and the efficiency of its utilizations.

Since Paterson et al. first demonstrated the utility of nucleic acids in modulating gene expression over 30 years ago (2), and in 1978 Zamecnik and Stephenson showed the capacity of antisense molecules to inhibit viral replication (3, 4), nucleic acids have emerged as a potent force both as R&D tools and as therapeutic agents.

Indeed, the field of nucleic acid therapeutics has evolved considerably with numerous gene targets and methods having been applied *in vitro* and *in vivo* in a variety of contexts with varying degrees of success. Strategies have included ribozymes, DNA enzymes (DNAzymes), antisense oligonucleotides (ASON), decoys, aptamers and siRNAs, all of which attenuate gene expression by interfering with cytosolic mRNA or translated protein. Currently, a number of these approaches are being evaluated in human and animal trials and are poised to offer considerable inroads and additions to our current therapies.

Ribozymes are catalytically active RNA molecules capable of site-specific cleavage of target mRNA and can occur naturally (5). They must contain antisense sequences that will bind to the target, and also a sequence that will fold into a structure with ribonuclease activity. Such sequences are found in natural hammerhead or hairpin ribozymes. Consequently, ribozymes don't depend on cellular nucleases for activity (6). The possibility of designing ribozymes to cleave any specific target RNA has rendered them valuable tools in both basic research and therapeutic applications.

DNAzymes, like ribozymes, may be perceived as gene-specific molecular scissors. They appeared as a development in the study of ribozymes using analogous deoxyoligonucleotides, given that catalytic DNA has not been observed in nature (7). All existing molecules have been derived by *in vitro* selection processes similar to those used to identify aptamers (see below). The most well-characterized DNAzyme is the "10-23" subtype comprising a cation-dependent catalytic core of 15 desoxyribonucleotides that binds to and cleaves its target RNA. This core is flanked by complementary binding arms of 6 to 12 nucleotides in length that confer target mRNA Specificity (8).

ASONs are single-stranded segments of DNA or RNA generally 15 to 25 nucleotides in length designed to mirror specific mRNA sequences and block protein production. Although their precise mechanism of action is not fully understood, their function is mediated by interaction with target mRNA via hydrogen bonding, blocking translation into protein by steric hindrance of ribosomal movement or by activation of endogenous RNase H for targeted destruction of the DNA/RNA heteroduplex, resulting in mRNA degradation (9). Unmodified ASONs molecules are prone to degradation, and their negative charge makes cellular membrane penetration inefficient. As such, these molecules have evolved with a variety of modifications that enhance stability and efficacy. Around 50 clinical studies have used antisense strategies spanning a variety of disease processes, including cancer, cardiovascular disease, inflammation and infection (10). Fomivirsen or Vitravene®, which targets the immediate-early RNA encoded by human cytomegalovirus (CMV) DNA, has been approved by the FDA for use in humans for treatment of CMV retinitis (11).

In contrast to antisense approaches that target mRNA, oligonucleotide decoys are short, double-stranded DNA molecules that contain binding elements for a variety of protein targets that competitively inhibit promoter binding and gene expression. Although several types of decoys have been developed there are important issues to take into account affecting the potential clinical use of these molecules, including susceptibility to nuclease degradation, propensity to induce a host immunological response, and cell transfection difficulties with higher concentration requirements (12). Currently, decoy oligonucleotides are not pursued as aggressively as other forms of therapeutic oligonucleotides (13).

Aptamers are single-stranded oligonucleotides which may fold into complex secondary and tertiary structures and bind their target protein with high affinity and specificity, inhibiting its function. They are derived by *in vitro* selection from a combinatorial library of nucleic acid sequences (14). Recent developments demonstrate that aptamers are valuable tools for diagnostics, purification processes, target validation, drug discovery and therapeutics. Macugen® is an aptamer approved by the FDA for treatment of wet AMD (15).

RNA interference (RNAi) is one of the gene silencing strategies which has received most attention in recent times. Its initial discovery in 1998 by Nobel laureates Fire and Mello (16) in *Caenorhabditis elegans*, led to the subsequent finding of the mechanism in mammalian cells and the understanding that it was triggered by small double stranded RNA duplexes of 19-23 nucleotides in length (17). In the following decade siRNA (short interfering RNA) have become widely used tools for silencing gene expression, as they make use of a naturally occurring regulatory mechanism that uses these molecules to direct homology-dependent mRNA degradation via a multienzymatic complex termed RISC (RNA-induced silencing complex). Cells use their own small RNA duplexes as a form of gene regulation. These novel molecules have enormous therapeutic potential and at present there are close to 20 compounds which have reached clinical trials (18).

2. Ocular diseases addressable by nucleic acid–based drugs

2.1. Glaucoma

Glaucoma is the second leading cause of blindness globally (19). By year 2020 almost 80 million people are estimated to be affected by primary open-angle glaucoma (POAG), the most common type of glaucoma. Glaucoma is defined as the process of ocular tissue destruction caused by a sustained elevation of intra ocular pressure (IOP) above its normal physiological limits (20). In open angle glaucoma (OAG), elevated IOP causes a progressive optic neuropathy due to loss of retinal ganglion cells that ultimately leads to blindness (21). In angle-closure glaucoma the sudden high rise in IOP often renders the eye blind. Blindness in glaucoma is caused by a degenerative process of the retina and optic nerve, but is functionally associated with impairments in the balance between aqueous humor (AH) secretion and outflow. Mechanistically, the changes observed in the trabecular meshwork include loss of cells as well the deposition and accumulation of extracellular debris including protein plaque-like material (22). The loss of vision is not usually evident until significant nerve damage has occurred. For this reason, up to half of glaucoma sufferers are unaware of their condition. Because of this, early diagnosis and treatment is crucial in halting the progression of this pathological condition (23). Risk factors associated with glaucoma include high intraocular pressure, advanced age, family history of glaucoma, African ancestry myopia, hypertension, morphologic features of the optic disc, thinness of the cornea, eye trauma, concomitant use of drugs, diabetes mellitus, hypothyroidism, cardiovascular and haematological abnormalities (24-28). Treatment of glaucoma is mainly focused on lowering IOP. The first line of treatment is medication, followed by surgical and laser treatment. Pharmacological compounds for treating glaucoma fall into four main classes of drugs: parasympathomimetics, antagonists of α and β-adrenoreceptors, inhibitors of carbonic anhydrases and prostaglandin analogues. Clinicians prescribe medications in a stepwise manner to achieve the target goal of IOP and maintain a balance between medication effectiveness, tolerability and safety. Beta blockers and prostaglandins are the standard first line treatment for POAG (29). Both groups of drugs are very efficient in lowering IOP but beta blockers are not recommended in patients with cardiovascular and respiratory problems and prostaglandin-analogs have local tolerability issues (30, 31). Second-line drugs of choice include alpha-2-adrenergic agonists and carbonic anhydrase inhibitors. When IOP is not adequately regulated with monotherapy it is common to combine different antiglaucoma drugs, these combinations appear to have the advantage of greater efficacy, better cost and safety, but limit the individualization of dosing. The efficacy of current IOP-lowering therapies is relatively short lived, requiring repetitive dosing throughout the day and in some cases the efficacy decreases with time. Such negative effects may lead to decreased patient compliance or to the end of treatment. If no efficacy in reducing IOP is achieved with any of these drugs, laser therapy may be applied to the trabecular meshwork in order to increase AH outflow. The last therapeutic resource is surgical intervention to create a new route for AH outflow (32).

Novel nucleic-based therapies seek improving the limitations of current antiglaucoma treatment. These are the goals pursued by Sylentis' SYL040012, an siRNA-based drug for the treatment of glaucoma, currently in phase II clinical trial. SYL040012 is a chemically synthesized double-stranded oligonucleotide, specifically designed to target and inhibit synthesis of β_2-adrenergic receptors. The compound has proven efficacious in inhibiting the expression of its target in cell cultures and in lowering IOP in normotensive and hypertensive rabbits (Martínez et al, unpublished results). The efficacy of SYL040012 in reducing IOP is similar to that of commercially available drugs (34). On the other hand, when commercial drugs are used, sustained reduction of IOP relies on the continuous application of the drugs. This is not the case with SYL040012, whose effect in animal models not only lasts 15 times longer than the effect of current treatments, but is also able to maintain the reduction in IOP levels even when the compound is not administered for a period of up to 72 hours. This feature is very attractive since it would protect against the eventual optic damage caused by a reboot effect on IOP in case of poor compliance with the treatment. Moreover, SYL040012 is stable up to 24 h in rabbit aqueous humour, but stability rapidly decreases in rabbit serum. The stability properties of SYL040012 support the use of a siRNA-based therapeutic approach for glaucoma since the compound should be stable enough to exert its effect in the eye but should be rapidly degraded when reaching general circulation, hence anticipating low systemic side effects.

Using a completely different approach, Quark pharmaceuticals is developing QPI-1007, a synthetic chemically modified siRNA designed to temporarily inhibit the expression of the pro-apoptotic protein Caspase 2. QPI-1007 is currently undergoing clinical trials for optic nerve atrophy and non-arteritic ischemic optic neuropathy, but the company has expressed interest in developing adequate delivery systems for the potential use of this drug as a neuroprotectant for glaucoma (35).

2.2. Age-Related Macular Degeneration (AMD)

Age-related macular degeneration (AMD) is the leading cause of severe vision loss in the Western world, it occurs primarily among individuals over 50 years of age (36). AMD was a rare disorder in the 19th century but increase in life expectancy together with changes in life-style have enormously affected the prevalence of this disease (37). According to the 2005-2008 National Health and Nutrition Examination Survey 6.5% of the US population over 40 years of age had signs of AMD (38). Extensive epidemiologic and genetic studies indicate that development of AMD is the result of a combination of several aspects such as genetic predisposition and environmental factors. Tobacco smoking seems to be the most consistent and modifiable risk factor (39). Other risk factors include hypertension, cardiovascular disease and high body mass index (40). Among the genetic factors that confer susceptibility to developing AMD are variants in several genes encoding complement pathway proteins (41).

The underlying cause for AMD seems to be accumulation of residual material produced by the renewal process of the external part of the photoreceptors of the retina in the retinal pigment epithelium (RPE). The accumulation of this undegraded material, known as *drusen* in the RPE leads to production of inflammatory mediators that cause photoreceptor degeneration in the central retina, or macula (42). The center of the macula, named fovea, mediates high acuity vision; hence its degeneration causes severe vision loss. In the early stages of the disease the accumulations of *drusen* are small and often observed along with hypo- or hyperpigmentation of the RPE. As the disease progresses both the size and the amount of *drusen* increase. Advanced AMD is characterized by the presence of large or several medium size *drusen* and loss of central vision and can take two forms: dry or wet. The dry form is characterized by a sharply delineated area of RPE atrophy along with loss of photoreceptors and changes in pigmentation of the RPE. In the wet form, or choroidal neovascularisation (CNV), fragile blood vessels of the choriocapillaris grow into the RPE and frequently leak blood and fluid that accumulate between RPE and the choriocapillaris. As a result of these abnormal growths, dense scars are formed in the macula. Detachment of the RPE is also a frequent feature of this form of AMD. The wet form is more severe than the dry form and sometimes dry AMD can develop into wet AMD.

Great advances have been made in recent years in the treatment of wet AMD; on the other hand treatment options for dry AMD are currently limited to dietary supplements and life-style changes. Several pharmaceutical companies are developing compounds for dry AMD by targeting different aspects of the physiopathological progress of the disease. As mentioned above, inflammatory mediators are generated during the process leading to dry AMD, for this reason it has been suggested that antioxidants may play a role in minimizing progression of the disease. The Age-Related Eye Disease Study (AREDS) demonstrated that oral supplementation of antioxidants in patients with unilateral intermediate or advanced AMD reduced vision loss by 19%. In addition these patients showed a decrease of 25% in the chances of developing AMD in the other eye (43, 44).

Other therapeutic approaches for dry AMD currently in clinical development are aimed towards reducing the accumulation of toxic metabolites, diminishing activation of the complement system or avoiding loss of neurons in the retina using neuroprotectants.

As of March 2012 there were approximately 10 clinical studies for pharmaceuticals under development to treat dry AMD registered at www.clinicaltrials.gov with status "recruiting" or "active". Among these clinical trials, only one is using an oligonucleotide based approach to treat dry AMD. ARC1905 is a pegylated aptamer that is currently in phase I study sponsored by Ophtotech Corporation. This compound antagonizes the cleavage of complement component C5 into C5a and C5b, thus inhibiting complement activation.

ARC1905 has shown to be safe when administered by intravitreal injection in combination with ranibizumab for wet AMD (45).

Perhaps one of the facts preventing more oligonucleotide based therapies being developed for dry AMD is that doublestrand RNAs as short as 21 base pair are able to bind and activate Toll Like Receptor 3; and activation of this receptor has been associated with progress of dry AMD (46, 47).

Wet AMD is characterized by the invasion of leaky blood vessels into the RPE. This mechanism is mediated by the action of vascular endothelial growth factor (VEGF). The biological activity of this growth factor has been the target of several therapeutic strategies in the past few years and the pharmaceuticals developed under these programs are the current first line treatment for wet AMD.

Pegaptanib sodium (Macugen®) is a 28-base pegylated aptamer designed to target VEGF (48) by Gilead Pharmaceuticals, licensed to Eyetech Pharmaceuticals/OSI. This drug was approved by the FDA in December 2004 for the treatment of all subtypes of wet AMD by intravitreal injection every six weeks. Pegaptanib specifically binds to $VEGF_{165}$, the most pathogenic of the four isoforms of VEGF that are generated by alternative splicing of a common mRNA. The union of pegaptanib to VEGF prevents activation of either of the two receptors for VEGF (VEGFR-1 and VEGFR-2) present on the surface of epithelial cells; hence inhibiting its biological activity. The VEGF Inhibition Study in Ocular Neovascularizations trial demonstrated that pegaptanib sodium injection reduced the risk of moderate vision loss from 70% to 55% and of severe vision loss from 22% to 10% without serious systemic effects and a low rate of serious ocular adverse events (49).

In July 2006 the second drug based on anti-VEGF therapy was approved by the FDA. Ranibizumab (Lucentis®) is a recombinant, humanised, monoclonal anti-VEGF antibody fragment with high affinity for all isoforms of VEGF developed by Genentech that is administered by intravitreal injection. Two clinical trials (MARINA and ANCHOR) support the safety and efficacy of ranibizumab for wet AMD (50, 51). The results of these trials showed that almost 95% of patients receiving the drug avoided moderate visual loss versus the 62.2% that managed to do so in the control group (receiving veteporfin). In addition, ranibizumab was not only able to stall progression of wet AMD but even to improve visual acuity in 35.7% of the patients treated with the low dose and in 40.3% of the patients treated with the high dose.

The third anti-VEGF compound currently used in the clinic for treatment of wet AMD is bevacizumab (Avastin®). Bevacizumab is a full-length monoclonal antibody that binds to and inhibits all isoforms of VEGF also developed by Genentech. Bevacizumab is in fact the full length antibody that was modified to develop ranibizumab. Ranibizumab was developed because preliminary results indicated that the size of the full length antibody would not allow for appropriate distribution within the retina. Additionally, the longer half life of bevacizumab raised concerns in terms of systemic toxicity. Bevacizumab is currently approved for the treatment of metastatic colorectal cancer and several other malignancies, and it is used off-label for wet AMD (52). The reduced cost of bevacizumab compared to ranibizumab has extended the off-label use of this drug, for this reason several clinical trials have started in the last four years in order to gather evidence on the efficacy of bevacizumab in wet AMD (53, 54).

In addition to pegaptanib, several other attempts have been made to treat wet AMD with oligonucleotides. Bevasiranib was the first small interfering RNA agent developed for this condition. Developed by OPKO Health, this agent is a naked 21-nt siRNA designed to target VEGF administered by intravitreal injection (55). The results of clinical trials conducted for phases I and II were positive and OPKO Health initiated a phase III clinical trial to examine the safety and efficacy of the combination of bevasiranib with ranibizumab. In March 2009 OPKO terminated the phase III trial because the primary endpoint was not likely to be met: improved efficacy over ranibizumab.

Following the same VEGF-inhibition strategy Sirna Therapeutics (now Merck) developed Sirna-027; a modified siRNA that targets one of the receptors for VEGF, VEGFR-1 (56). In vivo studies demonstrated that Sirna-027 was able to reduce the mRNA and protein levels of VEGFR-1 and to reduce the areas of neovascularation in a mouse model of ischemic retinopathy. An inverted sequence with the same chemical modifications as Sirna-027 was used as control and was shown not to have an effect on any of the parameters analysed (56). The control used in this study demonstrated that the effect of Sirna-027 was sequence specific; this was relevant due to the controversy generated by the results of a study published in 2008 that stated that angiogenesis could be suppressed by 21-nt siRNAs in a sequence-independent manner via TLR3 (57). Further clinical development of Sirna-027 was sponsored by Merck in collaboration with Allergan but, again, clinical trials for this compound were halted because the primary endpoint of efficacy trials was not met.

Using a different strategy Quark developed PF-655, now developed in collaboration with Pfizer, a 19-nt 2'O-methyl-stabilized siRNA designed against RTP801, a newly discovered target that is rapidly and sharply upregulated in hypoxia and promotes apoptosis of neural cells (58, 59). In addition to its anti-apoptotic effect, this compound cooperates with VEGF inhibitors to reduce retinal neovascularisation. Although full results of the clinical trial have not yet been made public, in March 2011 Quark announced that their compound was not superior to ranibizumab, thus expectations for the phase IIb initiated by Quark alone are somewhat low.

With two of the candidates already halted and a third most likely to be so, the fate of siRNAs in AMD is at least uncertain. Reports supporting that siRNAs 21 nt or longer activate TLR3 have certainly had a say in the matter. Activation of TLR3 in the RPE seems to induce RPE cell death and contribute to development of dry AMD (47), therefore tackling any form of AMD with double stranded RNA has to be achieved with shorter compounds and target specificity should be thoroughly studied.

2.3. Diabetic retinopathy

Diabetic retinopathy (DR) is a microvascular complication secondary to diabetes mellitus that leads to structural and functional changes in the retina, this complication is the leading cause of visual loss in working-age individuals (60). The overall prevalence of this complication among individuals with diabetes is 34.6% (61) and it accounted for 2.4 million cases of blindness worldwide in 2002 (60). Hyperglycemia is a decisive factor in the development of DR because of its damaging effects *per se;* it also serves as a biomarker for control on the disregulation of metabolism that occurs in diabetes.

In the initial phases of DR the vessels that irrigate the retina show microaneurysms and small leakages, this initial step of the disease is frequently referred to as nonproliferative DR. The changes observed in this phase are result of thickening of the capillary basement membrane as well as apoptosis and migration of pericytes. As the disease progresses the capillaries become permeable due to loss of interaction between endothelial cells and pericytes, and eventually macular edema can develop due to accumulation of fluids in the macula. The progressive occlusion of capillaries in the retina leads to tissue ischemia. As a result of the hypoxia caused by ischemia angiogenic factors such as VEGF are upregulated and capillaries grow into the retina, this stage is also known as proliferative DR (62). The new veins formed in response to the changes seen in the diabetic retina are fragile and permeable and some of them can break through the optic nerve leaking into the vitreous cavity or into the preretinal space. The process of neovascularisation is also associated with accumulation of a fibrous component that when contracted can lead to retinal detachment severely impairing vision (63).

Currently, the gold-standard for treating DR is laser photocoagulation (64); this procedure seeks to mitigate damage but has no effect on the underlying causes of the disease. In addition, steroids can be intravitreally administered into the eye to reduce accumulation of fluids within the retina. Sometimes, the accumulation of blood in the vitreous humour can physically impede laser photocoagulation; in these cases a vitrectomy can be performed in order to remove the blood accumulated in the vitreous prior to laser photocoagulation.

As mentioned previously, the action of angiogenic factors plays an important role in the development of DR. In this sense, several VEGF-inhibitors currently used for the treatment of AMD, are being studied for DR (see section 2.2 for details). Most of them are in late clinical trials and are expected to reach market authorization shortly.

In the oligonucleotide-based field, some of the compounds initially developed for AMD have undergone clinical trials for different forms of diabetic retinopathy as well. Opko Health's bevasiranib is one of these cases. A phase II clinical trial for diabetic macular edema was completed in 2008, and although positive results were reported, further development has not been announced. iCo Therapeutics is using a different approach with their lead compound iCo-007. iCo-007 is a chemically modified ASON inhibiting c-raf; a downstream mediator of several growth factors, including VEGF. In 2011 a phase II clinical trial was started for diabetic retinopathy in which two different doses of iCo-007 are to be assayed, either as a monotherapy or in combination with ranibizumab or laser photocoagulation. Preliminary results of this trial are expected in the second half of 2012. Another antisense alternative is being developed by Antisense Therapeutics, in this case a novel antisense compound ATL1103 which targets growth hormone receptor and has successfully completed a phase I clinical trial. This compound is being developed for treatment of acromegaly and also diabetic retinopathy (65).

2.4. Dry eye pain

Dry eye disease (DED) or keratoconjunctivitis sicca (KCS) is a multifactorial ocular condition resulting from tear film instability that can eventually lead to ocular surface damage. Typical symptoms of DED include ocular discomfort, visual disturbance, itching, burning, sensation of foreign body, light sensitivity; inflammation and pain. Factors contributing to DED are insufficient tear secretion; excessive evaporation and alteration in the composition of the tear film. The tear film has three essential components: aqueous layer, secreted by the lachrymal glands; mucus layer, produced by the globet cells of the conjunctiva and by epithelial cells of the cornea and conjunctiva and finally a lipid layer, secreted by the meibomian glands. Changes in the tear film can be temporary causing an acute form of DED or long-lasting leading to chronic DED; damage to the ocular surface is usually more severe in the chronic forms than in the acute ones. DED is frequent in some conditions such as Sjögren's disease, or lachrymal gland dysfunction, but it can also be caused by vitamin deficiency, contact lens wear and use of several prescription drugs. As such, it is not surprising that DED is a very frequent condition; the prevalence varies tremendously depending on the study, and the condition is more frequent in patients with autoimmune diseases, postmenopausal women and elderly population (66).

Treatment of DED depends on the etiology of the condition. The first line treatment is usually use of lubricants such as artificial tears and avoidance of preservatives such as BAK if other eye treatments are required. Other treatment options include procedures that favour tear retention: punctal occlusion, moisture chamber spectacles and contact lenses; pharmacologic agents that stimulate tear secretion or anti-inflammatory therapy.

Although some advances have been made towards alleviating some of the symptoms of DED, pain associated to this condition is not usually addressed. Sylentis is currently developing an siRNA, SYL1001, for the treatment of pain associated to DED. The compound targets TRPV1, a very well known target for pain, which is highly expressed in the cornea and trigeminal ganglion. SYL1001 is applied in eye drops, contains no preservatives and has recently shown favourable local and systemic tolerance results in a phase IA study.

2.5. Corneal neovascularitation associated with corneal graft rejection

Optimal vision is contingent upon transparency of the cornea. Corneal neovascularization, trauma and surgical procedures such as photorefractive keratectomy and graft rejection after penetrating keratoplasty (PKP) can lead to corneal opacification (67). Corneal neovascularization, regardless of the underlying cause, leads to decreased vision, recurrent corneal erosion, and incompetent barrier function thus presenting a serious clinical problem for which treatment is poor (68). When transparency of the native cornea cannot be maintained at a functional level corneal transplantation is often the next intervention. Once transplanted, the major cause of corneal graft failure is allograft rejection. Despite this fact, corneal transplantation has a very high success rate. Over 90% of low-risk corneal transplants retain clarity years after transplantation using only local immunosuppression. Blocking access of the host immune system to the donor cornea is the first line of defense against corneal allograft rejection, of which corneal avascularity is an essential component. Corneal graft rejection is primarily a cell-mediated immune response controlled by T cells (69). Normal corneal immune privilege can be eroded by neovascularisation, especially if it is accompanied by ocular inflammation and increased intraocular pressure. New vessels generated by neovascularisation provide a route of entry for immune-mediating cells to the graft, while the growth of new lymphatic vessels enables the exit of APCs and antigenic material from the graft to regional lymph nodes. The cornea consequently becomes infiltrated with and sensitized to immune reaction mediators. Therefore, neovascularisation may induce an immune response that can lead to immunological corneal graft rejection (70, 71). In normal low risk grafts it is a general practice to avoid exposing suture knots and ends which may stimulate neovascularization, and to treat neovascularization aggressively using topical steroids (67).

Due to the crucial role of VEGF in neovascularisation (see section 2.2), many have suggested that VEGF inhibition may prevent corneal transplant rejection. Despite the efforts made in recent years on the use of anti-VEGF compounds for corneal rejection it is still not clear whether the treatment is adequate (72, 73).

Several nucleic-based therapies are currently being developed with the hope of filling this uncovered therapeutic gap. Although the molecular mechanisms that control neovascularization are not well understood, inflammation has been found to frequently precede corneal neovascularisation. For this reason, many studies have concentrated their efforts on targeting humoral and corneal-derived inflammatory mediators. Among these mediators are arachidonic-acid derived eicosanoids of the cytochrome P450 monooxygenase (CYP) pathways. Seta and collaborators designed specific siRNAs targeting CYP4B1a, CYP4B1b and CYP4B1c and demonstrated that silencing the expression of CYP4B1 diminished corneal vascular response and greatly attenuated VEGF mRNA levels in an animal model of inflammatory neovascularization (68). One of the most advanced nucleic-based therapies is GS-101 (Aganirsen). GS-101, developed by the Swiss company GeneSignal, is a 25-mer phosphorothioate ASON that inhibits the expression of Insulin Receptor Substrate-1 (IRS-1). IRS-1 is a cytoplasmic adapter protein without intrinsic kinase activity. The main function of this protein is to recruit other proteins to their receptors and induce the organization of intracellular signalling cascades (74). IRS-1 interacts with the VEGF-receptor complex in angiogenesis (75) and it promotes lymphangiogenesis by interacting with integrins (76, 77). Downregulation of IRS-1 results in prevention of neovascular growth and has been reported to prevent the angiogenic process in preclinical *in vivo* and *in vitro* experiments (78, 79). Phase I clinical studies demonstrated excellent safety and tolerability of GS-101 when applied as eyedrops three times a day. In April 2007 the EMA granted orphan drug designation for GS-101 for the treatment of corneal graft rejection associated to corneal neovascularisation. After successfully completing a phase II trial GS-101 is about to enter phase III clinical trials (80).

2.6. Ophthalmic infections

There are several sight-threatening diseases caused by viral infections. Infections caused by virus imply the use of the cellular machinery by the virus to replicate. Hence, all infected cells will have foreign nucleic acids encoding viral specific proteins inside them. Given that oligonucleotide based therapies pursue downregulating expression of genes it seems obvious to target viral specific genes. In the following section several approaches using this rationale will be explained focusing on antivirals developed for treating viral infections in the eye. The first success case of oligonucleotide-based therapies came precisely in this field, fomivirsen was the first compound based on oligonucleotides to be approved by the FDA.

Citomegalovirus-induced retinitis is among the most common opportunistic infections in severely immunocompromised patients (81). In AIDS patients, CMV infection is associated with gastrointestinal disorders and retinitis. An estimated 15 to 40% of AIDS patients will suffer CMV-induced retinitis. This condition if left untreated leads to blindness within six months (82). Three systemic compounds are available for the treatment of this disease: ganciclovir, foscarnet, and cidofovir. The mechanism of action of these three compounds is inhibition of the CMV DNA polymerase. However, these treatments have some drawbacks such as limited efficacy, poor oral bioavailability, toxicity and emergence of multidrug resistant strains due to mutations in the target gene (83). Because of this, effective therapy usually implies alternation between the three available antivirals or different combinations of them, along with intraocular drug injections. This approach, known as highly active antiretroviral therapy (HAART), reduces 55%-95% the number of new cases of CMV (81). Without acute therapy, retinitis spreads throughout the entire retina causing total retinal destruction and blindness; without chronic suppressive maintenance therapy relapse of the retinitis occurs promptly (84). Looking for an alternative approach Isis Pharmaceuticals Inc. developed an ASON that targets the *immediate-early* (*IE*) gene of human CMV. Fomivirsen, (Vitravene®) is a phosphorothioate oligonucleotide (ISIS-2922) developed by Isis in partnership with CIBA vision, for the treatment of newly diagnosed and advanced CMV retinitis in AIDS patients and was the first oligonucleotide based drug approved by the FDA in 1998. Administered by intravitreal injection it has shown good clinical activity against this disease (85).

Acute Retinal Necrosis (ARN) is a type of retinitis that affects both healthy and immuno-compromised patients (86). This inflammatory disease is caused by several members of the herpesvirus family including herpes simplex virus (HSV-1), varicela zoster virus (VZV) and citomegalovirus (CMV) (87, 88). The disease usually starts with signs of uveitis: red eyes, light sensitivity, eye pain and blurred vision. Detailed examination of the eyes of these patients show infiltration of inflammatory cells in the anterior and posterior segments in all retinal layers (89). As the disease progresses retinal necrosis and occlusive arteriolar retinopathy are found. Current treatment for this condition includes antiviral therapy and topical cortosteroids (89). There is no treatment that can prevent the establishment or persistence of latent infection. Reactivation of HSV-1 infections, are currently controlled clinically with long term administration of acyclovir or its derivatives.

Antiviral drugs can quell symptoms resulting from reactivation outbreaks but cannot eliminate latent virus. Furthermore, long-term usage of antiviral drugs can lead to development of drug-resistant viruses (90). Several authors have designed specific ASON targeting the proinflammatory cytokine tumor necrosis factor alpha (TNFα) (91, 92). TNFα is known to possess many cell-activating and proinflammatory activities. TNFα mRNA and protein are up-regulated in eyes infected with HSV-1 (93). Moreover, experiments using DNA microarrays have shown that TNFα and its receptors are upregulated in eyes of mice with HSV-1 retinitis (94). The results of these experiments show that either intravitreal or subconjunctival injections of TNFα-ASON provide local therapeutic effects without systemic adverse effects. Another strategy uses morpholino oligomers specifically designed to reduce viral mRNA trough steric blocking. Moerdyk-Schauwecker and collaborators have developed five phosphoro- diamidate morpholino oligomers (PMO) that target three HSV-1 genes: *ICP0, ICP4* and *ICP27.* Their experimental results demonstrated that PMO targeting HSV-1 mRNAs not only inhibited viral replication in cell cultures but also in mouse models of the disease (90).

HSV-1 not only causes ARN it is also responsible for Herpetic Stromal keratitis (HSK) a well- defined immune mediated blinding corneal disease (95). There is profound evidence that the corneal inflammation in HSK is orchestrated by CD4+ T cells and is accompanied by uncontrolled development of blood vessels within the eye (96). The corneal infiltration contains abundant polymorphonuclear cells. These cells, although important for controlling virus replication, are also responsible for damage to the cornea (97, 98). Due to the relevant role of TNF-α and IFNγ in the progress of HSK, targeting TNF-α and IFNγ has been proposed as a therapeutic approach (99). Wasmuth and collaborators demonstrated that topical administration of ASONs targeting either TNF-α or IFNγ were capable of reducing their target in mice infected by HSV-1 without altering antiviral immune response (100, 101). In addition to the production of proinflammatory cytokines, neovascularization of the cornea is observed in this pathogenesis. As in other diseases in which neovascularisation plays a role, VEGF seems to be at least in part, responsible for the process. Validation of this theory has been performed by inhibiting HSV induced angiogenesis in mice with either a VEGF neutralizing antibody or an siRNA designed against this target (102).

Acute Hemorrhagic Conjuntivitis (AHC) is a highly contagious eye disease caused primarily by enterovirus 70 (EV70) or coxackievirus A24 (CVA24) infection. Thus, several authors attempted to develop novel siRNA-based anti-AHC agent effective against both EV70 and CVA24. Resulting siRNAs showed excellent cytoprotective effects and dramatic decreases in viral replication and protein synthesis in primary human conjunctival cells, MRC5 and HeLa cells (103) or in Rabdomyosarcoma cells (104).

2.7. Chronic optic nerve atrophy and ischemic optic neuropathy

Ischemic optic neuropathy is defined as vision loss due to lack of blood supply to the optic disc (infarction). Decreased visual acuity and visual field are usually the only symptoms of ischemic optic neuropathy regardless of the underlying cause. Ischemic optic neuropathy is primarily of two types: Anterior (AION) and posterior (PION) involving the optic nerve head (ONH) and the rest of the optic nerve, respectively (105). AION can be arteritic (A-AION) and non-arteritic (NA-AION). In the management of AION, it is crucial to identify the form of AION. A-AION is an ophthalmic emergency and requires urgent treatment with high-dose steroid therapy to prevent further visual loss to both the affected eye and the sometimes asymptomatic Contralateral eye. NA-AION is the most common form of the disease and it is usually detected due to unilateral painless visual loss along with edema to the optic nerve. It is more frequent in patients between 40 and 70 years of age and vision loss is usually less severe than in the A-AION. Systemic risk factors particularly nocturnal arterial hypotension, play major roles in the development of NA-AION. NA-AION patients treated with high doses of systemic steroid therapy showed significant improvement in visual acuity and visual field. (106).

Given that the loss of vision in these conditions is due to loss of retinal ganglion cells (RGC) neuroprotection seems a rational approach. Focusing on this line of thought, Quark Pharmaceuticals is currently developing a nucleic-acid based therapy, specifically a siRNA-based therapy: QPI-1007. QPI-1007 is a synthetic siRNA designed to temporarily inhibit expression of the pro-apoptotic protein caspase 2 that is currently in clinical trials for the treatment of NA-AION. Ahmed and colleagues in collaboration with Quark pharmaceuticals have shown that caspase-2 contributes loss of RGC in rat models of the condition and have demonstrated that intravitreal injections of QPI-1007 are effective in protecting against the death of RGC (35). Quark Pharmaceuticals is conducting a Phase I-dose escalation safety study using QPI-1007 in patients suffering from Optic Nerve Atrophy and NA-AION. Caspase 2 isn't the only interesting target that offers a potential avenue for treatment in optic neurophaty. Helen and collaborators have focused on the action of another protein: connexin 43 (Cx43). Preclinical results show that an ASONs designed to specifically reduce upregulated levels of Cx43 in a model of optic ischemia has therapeutic potential (107)

2.8. Inherited ocular diseases: Retinitis Pigmentosa (RP) and Ocular Albinism (OA)

Retinitis pigmentosa (RP) is a class of diseases involving progressive degeneration of the retina and a leading cause of inherited blindness. RP is a heterogeneous disorder that starts in mid-periphery and advances towards the macula and fovea. Typical symptoms include night blindness followed by decreasing visual field, leading to tunnel vision and eventually legal blindness or in many cases complete blindness (108). This disorder involves photoreceptor-cell degeneration and affects ~ 1 in 3000 people (109). On the cellular level the rod photoreceptor system is predominantly affected but in later stages of the disease cone photoreceptors can also be affected (108). More than 40 causative genes have been implicated in RP, although mutations in rhodopsin gene (RHO) account for 15% of all types of RP. Great efforts have been made to explore new gene therapies for RP, but inter and intragenic heterogeneity represent significant barriers to therapeutic development. For example more than 100 mutations in the human RHO gene, which encodes the photosensitive pigment in rod photoreceptors, have been identified in autosomal dominantly inherited RP (110). Development of therapies for each individual mutation would be technically difficult to achieve and not economically viable; thus a therapeutic approach that circumvents mutational diversity would be of great value. At present, there is one treatment which has reached the clinic for the treatment of Leber's congenital amaurosis form 2 (LCA2), a type of RP, based on adenoviral (AAV) delivered gene therapy. Three years ago, Maguire and colleagues reported results in 12 patients who were treated with gene-replacement therapy. LCA2 is associated with mutations in *RPE65*, which encodes a protein requisite for the isomerohydrolase activity of the retinal pigment epithelium. This activity produces 11-*cis*-retinal, the natural ligand and chromophore of the opsins of rod and cone photoreceptors, the opsins cannot capture light and transduce it into electrical responses to initiate vision. In this study patients received one subretinal injection of AAV2-hRPE65v2 (a viral vector encoding RPE65 protein). Visual improvement was observed in all 12 patients with the greatest gains among younger patients (111).

Still in early research stages are different approaches to the treatment of RP based on the administration of AAV-delivered RNA interfering compounds. Amongst these, both the University of Florida and Smurfit Institute of Genetics have achieved interesting results *in vivo* by silencing the expression of RHO in mouse models (112). More recent studies by Jiang and collaborators show how using an AVV2/8 vector to develop an RNAi-based therapy in a dominant retinal degeneration mouse model expressing bovine GCAP1 (Y99C), significantly improved photoreceptor survival, delaying disease onset and increasing visual function (113). There are also several studies that target inosine 5'-monophosphate dehydrogenase 1 (IMPDH1) with viral delivered siRNA for the treatment of RP10 form of autosomal dominant RP(114). Another interesting approach based on RNAi therapy uses siRNAs to facilitate transplantation of rod photoreceptors, by disrupting junctional proteins and enhance donor cell integration in the retina (115).

Ocular albinism type 1 is a group of X-linked or autosomal genetic disorders characterized by partial or total lack of melanin pigmentation in the eyes due to mutations in genes encoding proteins involved in melanogenesis. Eyes may be severely affected with photophobia and reduced visual acuity. Nystagmus or strabismus, are often associated and the irides and fundus are depigmented. Many forms of albinism, more or less severe, have been described. Some forms also affect skin and hair. As in other forms of albinism, these patients suffer loss of stereoscopic vision due to reduction of the ipsilateral component of the optic tract (116). General prevalence of albinism is 1/15,000 inhabitants. Treatment is exclusively symptomatic. Vetrini and collaborators have described an intronic point mutation in ocular albinism type 1 (OA1) gene in a family with the X-linked form of ocular albinism. Interestingly the mutation creates a new acceptor splice in intron 7 of the OA1 gene leading to aberrant protein expression. In addition to low levels of normally spliced mRNA product of the OA1 gene, patient samples contained aberrant spliced mRNA. OA1 expression was rescued in the patient's melanocytes with an antisense morpholino modified oligonucleotide (MO) complementary to the mutant sequence. The MO was able to rescue OA1 expression and restore the protein level in the patient's melanocyte by skipping the aberrant inclusion (116).

Compound	Indication	Company	Type of compound	Target	Stage
SYL040012	Glaucoma	Sylentis	Naked siRNA	ADRB2	Ph II
QPI-1007	Glaucoma	Quark Pharmaceuticals	Modified siRNA	Caspase 2	R&D
	NA-ION				Ph I
ARC1905	Dry AMD	Ophthotech Corporation	Pegylated aptamer	Complement component C5	Ph I
	Wet AMD (in combination with ranibizumab)				Ph I
E10030	Wet AMD (in combination with ranibizumab)	Ophthotech Corporation	Aptamer	PDGF	Ph II
Pegaptanib	Wet AMD	Eyetech/OSI Eyetech/Pfizer	Pegylated aptamer	VEGF	Approved
	Diabetic Macular Edema				Ph III
Bevasiranib	Wet AMD	OPKO Health	Naked siRNA	VEGF	Ph III (Term.)
	Diabetic Macular Edema				Ph II
Sirna-027	Wet AMD	Merck/Allergan	Modified siRNA	VEGF	Ph II (Term.)
PF-655	Wet AMD	Quark/Pfizer	Modified siRNA	RTP801	Ph IIb
iCO-007	Diabetic Macular Edema	iCO Therapeutics	Modified antisense	c-raf	Ph II
ALT1103	Diabetic retinopathy	Antisense Therapeutics	Antisense	GHR	R&D
SYL1001	Dry eye pain	Sylentis	Naked siRNA	TRPV1	Ph I
GS-101	Corneal graft rejection associated to corneal neovascularization	GeneSignal	Phosphorothioate antisense	IRS-1	Ph III
Fomivirsen	Advanced CMV infection in AIDS patients	Isis/CIBA	Phosphorothioate antisense	IE gene CMV	Approved

Table 1. Compounds based on oligonucleotides under development for the treatment of ocular diseases.

3. Safety issues

3.1. Immunotoxicity

As part of the defensive duties of the innate immune system it needs to discriminate between foreign and endogenous genetic material. Destruction of exogenous genetic material is an essential part of protection against microorganisms, but can be a hurdle when trying to introduce synthetic genetic material for therapeutic purposes. The immune system responds to microbial RNA and DNA by producing type I interferon and proinflammatory cytokines. The chain reaction leading to production of these immune mediators is initiated by detecting conserved motifs of pathogens; this job is performed by several cell membrane and cytoplasmic receptors present at low levels in most cells. Toll-like receptors (TLR) are present in either the cell surface or in intracellular endocytic organelles and activation of these receptors leads to increase in the presenting capacity of dendritic cells and production of type I interferon. The TLRs responsible for detecting oligonucleotides are present exclusively in endosomes and are TLR3 that senses dsRNA (117), TLR7/8 that sense ssRNA (118) and TLR9 that senses ssDNA (119). TLRs are mainly expressed in immune cells; but foreign material has to be detected in non-immune cells as well; this task is performed by cytosolic sensor proteins. The dsRNA-dependent protein kinase (PKR) is a cytoplasmic sensor of RNA. Upon activation by binding to dsRNA, PKR forms a homodimer that acquires phosphorilation activity. Among the phosphorilation targets of PKR is eIF-2α; phosphorilation of this transcription factor leads translation inhibition and apoptosis (120). A second cytosolic sensor of dsRNAs is 2′-5′ oligoadenylate synthetase (OAS). Activation of this protein promotes the activation of ribonucleases that degrade endogenous and exogenous RNA, again leading the cell to apoptosis (121). Other cytosolic sensors of dsRNA are the retinoic acid-inducible gene-I (RIG-I)-like receptors (RLRs) (122). RLRs are DExD/H RNA helicases. Two members of this family, RIG-I and MDA-5, have in addition to the helicase domain, two caspase activation and recruiting domains. Binding of dsRNA to RIG-I or MDA-5 activates a complex signalling cascade that ultimately leads to interferon-β production and apoptosis (123). As reviewed above, the immune system is prepared to react when foreign biological material is detected inside the body; several strategies can be used to bypass or modulate the response of the immune system:

- Avoidance of sequence motifs or structures that are specifically recognized by the oligonucleotide sensors of the innate immunity. Lowering the number of uridines in a given RNA seems to lower the likelihood of an immune response; completely replacing the uridines by adenosines completely abrogates immune activation (124). Also, avoiding blunt ends on siRNAs could help reducing the immune response. RIG-I recognizes siRNAs with or without 2-base 3′ overhangs, but only those with blunt ends are able to trigger its ATPase activity and subsequent downstream signalling (125).
- Introducing chemical modifications in nucleotides and/or their backbones to avoid activation of the immune response. 2′OMe and pseudouridine are modifications frequently present in mammalian RNAs; these modifications help avoiding triggering the immune response. Other modifications such as 2′F and LNA can also help evade immune detection (124). Whenever modifications are introduced into an oligonucleotide the modified molecule should be tested in order to make sure that the silencing activity has not been abolished.
- Use targeted delivery of oligonucleotides (126) or delivery techniques that avoid the endosome routes for sequences that could activate TLRs. Use of inhibitors of

endosomal maturation such as chloroquine and bafilomycin A1 can also abrogate the immune response (125).

- Use of immunomodulators to impair or abolish the immune response.

Some of the first therapeutic approaches using oligonucleotides were made in the field of ophthalmology. The eye is an immune privileged site, and this fact is one of the rationales behind the election of this site for the first trials. Several overlapping mechanisms contribute to establishing and maintaining immune privilege: the eye has a high content of immunosuppressive factors; it has a low expression of MHCII, hence limiting antigen presentation; stromal cells of the iris, ciliary body and retina are able to convert immune T cells to regulatory (Treg) cells, and retinal epithelial pigment cells are able to inhibit primed T cells; and finally death receptors such as FasL and PDL-1 are expressed by stromal cells that are able to induce apoptosis in immune cells that enter the eye (127). These advantages should not be interpreted as a free pass in terms of immunity for oligonucleotide therapies in the eye. In this regard, it has been shown that some siRNAs are able to activate TLR3 in a sequence-independent manner. Activation of this receptor by dsRNA has been found to suppress angiogenesis (57) and to induce retinal cell death; thus promoting atrophic AMD (46).

3.2. Non immune off target effects

The interaction of therapeutic oligonucleotides with their intended target RNAs is, with the exception of aptamers, highly sequence-specific. However, binding of one of these molecules to a non-target sequence requires only homology with a few base pairs. The result of this undesired interaction could be the inhibition of an unintended gene or an *off target effect* (OTE). Off-targeting is mostly mediated by the interaction between certain regions of the therapeutic molecule and complementary sites in the unintended target rather than overall homology between the two molecules (128). Careful comparison of candidate sequences with the entire transcriptome, attempting to avoid long stretches of homology, still remain necessary but are inadequate on their own to predict the actual risk of OTEs. Use of chemical modifications and improvement in oligonucleotide design has been successfully employed to reduce the likelihood of OTEs.

The specificity of a sequence can be improved taking into account some important designing parameters such as thermodynamic stability of the duplex and 5′ and 3′-ends, the Tm value of the interaction region between the therapeutic oligonucleotide and possible off-targets (129) When dealing with knock down of mRNAs using siRNAs or antisense oligonucleotides the target position should be selected choosing regions that are as far away as possible from the initiation codon (130). The silencing effect of oligonucleotides is in general concentration-dependent, considerable success in reducing siRNA/antisense off-targeting has been achieved optimizing doses of the therapeutic oligonucleotide (131). Improvements in specificity achieved by altering sequences and/or introducing chemical modifications as well as in delivery of the molecule have also shown to have an impact on reducing potential off-target effects. Placing a 2′OMe at position 2 of the guide strand of a siRNA (132), or incorporating a destabilizing UNA at position 7 are examples of modifications that reduce OTEs (131).

3.3. Oversaturation of endogenous RNAi-silencing complex (RISC)

Bioactive drugs that rely on cellular processes to exert their functions face the risk of saturating endogenous pathways. This may be the case with RNAi-based drugs. Naturally occurring, small RNAs have undergone the process of evolution because of selection pressure and they exist in a perfect balance with their precursors and targets, as well as with the associated machinery involved in this process. Gene Silencing is performed by introducing artificially synthesized small RNAs into the cell or by expressing siRNAs/shRNAs within the cell, which enter the endogenous RNAi pathway at different levels. shRNAs and siRNAs are very similar to miRNA precursors before and after Dicer processing, respectively, relying on endogenous miRNA machinery to achieve target silencing. If the siRNA design parameters are not optimal they might cause an imbalance of the endogenous small RNA mediated pathways resulting in various and deleterious unwanted effects in the cells. It becomes therefore crucial to optimize the siRNA/shRNA design parameters and work at the lowest possible concentrations to mitigate the potential of side effects.

4. Advantages of RNAi-based therapeutics and challenges ahead

This new revolutionary technology presents many advantages for therapeutic development with respect to classical compounds, mainly:

- They are based on an endogenous mechanism, thus involving the administration of a type of molecule already present in the cells, and hence, in principle, less hazardous: cells should have the capacity to handle resulting breakdown products.
- As with antisense molecules before them, RNAi molecules can potentially address any pathological target, this means that even diverse intracellular molecules can be the object of these therapies. However, one must bear in mind that in practice, some genes are harder to target than others, and further more sophisticated algorithms must be developed to address this issue.
- Also in comparison to antisense, RNAi is considerably more potent (133) and consequently may be used at lower concentrations. It is believed also to have a more persistent pharmacological action than traditional drugs because it blocks protein synthesis and hence, the cell will have to re-synthesise the protein from scratch to return to its previous state. Thus allowing the use of lower or less frequent doses.
- Given the selectivity and specificity of these compounds, coupled with the fact of their *in silico* design and analysis they will have potentially less harmful side effects.
- Another main advantage from an industry perspective is their much shorter pharmacological development, the estimate being 2-3 years vs 4-6 years from proof of concept. This can be attributed among other things, to the fact that the compound can be designed against homologous regions of the human gene sequence between the

different animal models used for preclinical studies, thus simplifying toxicology studies.

- Finally, despite being novel entities they are easy to manufacture using a nucleotide synthesiser which simplifies large scale production. Additionally, this means the compounds are chemical entities rather than biological products, greatly helping the regulatory process for approval of these medicaments.

Nevertheless, RNAi still has certain hurdles to overcome before its full potential can be exploited. The main obstacle is delivery of siRNAs to the desired tissue, and although many advances have been made in this area, much work still remains for therapeutic possibilities to be fully exploited. On the other hand, in a clinical setting, RNAi can only be used to treat pathologies caused by expression or overexpression of a given protein or by the presence of exogenous organisms, as its mechanism works through suppression of protein expression; i.e. it is only of use when the therapeutic option requires a loss of function. Furthermore, although any gene is a potential target for RNAi, in practice not all mRNAs are as easily silenced and new more sophisticated algorithms will need to be developed to overcome this issue. And last but not least, as discussed in the previous section the issue of off-target effects resulting from siRNAs silencing unwanted genes can lead to important safety considerations when developing new medicaments.

From the perspective of ocular disorders, the eye is a relatively isolated compartment which makes it an ideal target organ for gene silencing. Local delivery of the compound to the eye limits exposure to the rest of the body and reduces the amount that is needed. siRNA injected into the vitreous cavity readily diffuses throughout the eye and is detectable for at least five days (56), the amounts used for intraocular injections are small compared to those used for systemic application and so as siRNA gets out of the eye it is diluted and is difficult to detect. This allows local silencing of a gene with little chance for an effect on the same gene outside the eye, reducing concern of remote effects in other tissues complicating observations in the eye. The sequence specificity of siRNA resulting in targeting of a single gene combined with local administration in the relatively isolated confines of the eye provides an ideal way to study eye-specific effects of gene disruption (34). While the development of siRNA-based therapies has promise for all tissues, the unique characteristics of the eye provide advantages which explain why the first siRNA compounds to advance through clinical trials were for the treatment of wet AMD, a disease affecting the back of the eye.

5. Prospects for current therapies based on nucleic-based strategies

The clinical progress of oligonucleotide drugs has been slow because realizing them requires inventing a new model for pharmaceutical development that allows large, highly charged molecules to be synthesized economically, distribute to target tissues, enter cells, and function within acceptable limits for toxicity. Oligonucleotides are large, unlike traditional small molecule drugs (<500-700 molecular weight), and much effort has been required to understand their properties and optimize them. However, considering RNAi was discovered just over a decade ago, this technology has advanced towards clinical trials with amazing speed. Both for antisense molecules and RNAi compounds initial most advanced therapies were developed taking advantage of the environment within the interior of the eye. One antisense oligonucleotide has been approved by the FDA in 1998: Vitravene® or fomivirsen developed by Isis Pharmaceuticals for the treatment of cytomegalovirus retinitis in immunocompromised patients. Initial most advanced siRNAs were designed to treat wet age-related macular degeneration (AMD) taking advantage of the relatively RNAse free environment of the interior of the eye. These therapies were based on intravitreal injection, a form of administration which allows bypassing on of the main rate-limiting issues for therapeutic oligonucleotides, that of delivery to the required target tissue.

Delivering oligonucleotides in whole organisms requires crossing many barriers. Degradation by serum nucleases, clearance by the kidney, or inappropriate biodistribution can prevent the oligonucleotide from ever reaching its target organ. Generally, the oligonucleotide must pass through the blood vessel wall and navigate the interstitial space and extracellular matrix. Finally, if the oligonucleotide succeeds in reaching the appropriate cell membrane, it will usually be taken up into an endosome, from which it must escape to be active. Antisense oligonucleotides are usually delivered in saline and rely on chemical modifications to enable uptake. Their phosphorothioate backbone binds to serum proteins, slowing excretion by the kidney (134). The aromatic nucleobases also interact with other hydrophobic molecules in serum and on cell surfaces; many types of cells in vivo express surface receptors that actively take up oligonucleotides.

Delivery is even more challenging for siRNAs, where all the aromatic nucleobases are on the inside, leaving heavily hydrated phosphates on the outside of the duplex. This hydrated surface interacts poorly with cell surfaces and is rapidly excreted in the urine. Hence, except for direct injection in targets such as the eye where they are also delivered in saline, researchers have invested heavily in the development of delivery vehicles for siRNA. Various delivery strategies include nanoparticles, cationic lipids, antibodies, cholesterol, aptamers and viral vectors for short hairpin RNAs. In this case, the delivery system most clinically validated is that based on SNALP (stable nucleic acid lipid particle) technology developed by Tekmira for systemic administration of siRNAs. However, although it is being used to formulate at least 4 different siRNAs currently undergoing clinical trials, it has yet to be used more extensively before victory can be claimed on the battle of delivery.

The field of oligonucleotide therapeutics has often swung from irrational optimism to irrational despair. This is true for industry, but in the laboratory as well, gene knockdown experiments have fallen in and out of favour with researchers. In reality, oligonucleotides are useful tools with strengths and weaknesses (135). The promise of RNAi as a powerful new approach for therapeutic treatment of diseases has propelled early stage clinical testing of siRNAs for a variety of diseases. However, it is still too soon to evaluate whether or not RNAi based therapeutics will live up to their expectations. Given the mood swings in this area, with big pharma investing large sums in the technology at one point and then backing out only two or three years later, the industry has been in a turmoil which is now beginning to even out. This relative calm should bring about maturity in the field with the science becoming more solid as we gain more knowledge of the biology of these compounds. From an industry perspective, it is foreseeable that Big Pharma's involvement will continue the later trend of product-specific licensing and co-development rather than the purchase of platform technologies from smaller biotech experts performed in the early days of the technology. This is also in line with structural changes in the industry towards the outsourcing of research (136).

Author details

Covadonga Pañeda*, Tamara Martínez, Natalia Wright and Ana Isabel Jimenez
Sylentis SAU, R&D department, PCM c/Santiago Grisolía, Madrid, Spain

References

[1] Crick F. Central dogma of molecular biology. Nature. 1970 Aug 8;227(5258):561-3.

[2] Paterson BM, Roberts BE, Kuff EL. Structural gene identification and mapping by DNA- mRNA hybrid-arrested cell-free translation. Proc Natl Acad Sci U S A. 1977 Oct;74(10):4370-4.

[3] Stephenson ML, Zamecnik PC. Inhibition of Rous sarcoma viral RNA translation by a specific oligodeoxyribonucleotide. Proc Natl Acad Sci U S A. 1978 Jan;75(1):285-8.

[4] Zamecnik PC, Stephenson ML. Inhibition of Rous sarcoma virus replication and cell transformation by a specific oligodeoxynucleotide. Proc Natl Acad Sci U S A. 1978 Jan;75(1):280-4.

[5] Bhindi R, Fahmy RG, Lowe HC, Chesterman CN, Dass CR, Cairns MJ, et al. Brothers in arms: DNA enzymes, short interfering RNA, and the emerging wave of small- molecule nucleic acid-based gene-silencing strategies. Am J Pathol. 2007 Oct;171(4):1079-88.

[6] Goodchild J. Therapeutic oligonucleotides. Methods Mol Biol.764:1-15.

[7] Schlosser K, Li Y. Biologically inspired synthetic enzymes made from DNA. Chem Biol. 2009 Mar 27;16(3):311-22.

[8] Santoro SW, Joyce GF. A general purpose RNA-cleaving DNA enzyme. Proc Natl Acad Sci U S A. 1997 Apr 29;94(9):4262-6.

[9] Bennett MR, Schwartz SM. Antisense therapy for angioplasty restenosis. Some critical considerations. Circulation. 1995 Oct 1;92(7):1981-93.

[10] Crooke ST. Progress in antisense technology. Annu Rev Med. 2004;55:61-95. [11] Persidis A. Antisense therapeutics. Nat Biotechnol. 1999 Apr;17(4):403-4.

[12] Lee IK, Ahn JD, Kim HS, Park JY, Lee KU. Advantages of the circular dumbbell decoy in gene therapy and studies of gene regulation. Curr Drug Targets. 2003 Nov;4(8):619- 23.

* Corresponding Author

[13] Tomita N, Morishita R, Tomita T, Ogihara T. Potential therapeutic applications of decoy oligonucleotides. Curr Opin Mol Ther. 2002 Apr;4(2):166-70.

[14] Thiel KW, Giangrande PH. Therapeutic applications of DNA and RNA aptamers. Oligonucleotides. 2009 Sep;19(3):209-22.

[15] Fraunfelder FW. Pegaptanib for wet macular degeneration. Drugs Today (Barc). 2005 Nov;41(11):703-9.

[16] Fire A, Xu S, Montgomery MK, Kostas SA, Driver SE, Mello CC. Potent and specific genetic interference by double-stranded RNA in Caenorhabditis elegans. Nature. 1998 Feb 19;391(6669):806-11.

[17] Elbashir SM, Harborth J, Lendeckel W, Yalcin A, Weber K, Tuschl T. Duplexes of 21- nucleotide RNAs mediate RNA interference in cultured mammalian cells. Nature. 2001 May 24;411(6836):494-8.

[18] Martinez T, Wright N, Pañeda C, Jimenez A, Lopez-Fraga M. RNA Interference-Based Therapeutics: Harnessing the Powers of Nature In: Rundfeldt C, editor. Drug Development - A Case Study Based Insight into Modern Strategies: InTech; 2011. p. 265- 312.

[19] Varma R, Lee PP, Goldberg I, Kotak S. An assessment of the health and economic burdens of glaucoma. Am J Ophthalmol. 2011 Oct;152(4):515-22.

[20] Quigley H. Glaucoma. Lancet. 2011;377((9774)):1367-77.

[21] Weinreb RN, Khaw PT. Primary open-angle glaucoma. Lancet. 2004 May 22;363(9422):1711-20.

[22] Marquis RE, Whitson JT. Management of glaucoma: focus on pharmacological therapy. Drugs Aging. 2005;22(1):1-21.

[23] Kaur IP, Kakkar S. Newer therapeutic vistas for antiglaucoma medicines. Crit Rev Ther Drug Carrier Syst. 2011;28(2):165-202.

[24] Gordon MO, Beiser JA, Brandt JD, Heuer DK, Higginbotham EJ, Johnson CA, et al. The Ocular Hypertension Treatment Study: baseline factors that predict the onset of primary open-angle glaucoma. Arch Ophthalmol. 2002 Jun;120(6):714-20; discussion 829-30.

[25] Kass MA, Heuer DK, Higginbotham EJ, Johnson CA, Keltner JL, Miller JP, et al. The Ocular Hypertension Treatment Study: a randomized trial determines that topical ocular hypotensive medication delays or prevents the onset of primary open-angle glaucoma. Arch Ophthalmol. 2002 Jun;120(6):701-13; discussion 829-30.

[26] Jonas JB, Martus P, Horn FK, Junemann A, Korth M, Budde WM. Predictive factors of the optic nerve head for development or progression of glaucomatous visual field loss. Invest Ophthalmol Vis Sci. 2004 Aug;45(8):2613-8.

[27] Kroese M, Burton H. Primary open angle glaucoma. The need for a consensus case definition. J Epidemiol Community Health. 2003 Sep;57(9):752-4.

[28] Martus P, Stroux A, Budde WM, Mardin CY, Korth M, Jonas JB. Predictive factors for progressive optic nerve damage in various types of chronic open-angle glaucoma. Am J Ophthalmol. 2005 Jun;139(6):999-1009.

[29] De Natale R, Le Pen C, Berdeaux G. Efficiency of glaucoma drug regulation in 5 European countries: a 1995-2006 longitudinal prescription analysis. J Glaucoma. Apr- May;20(4):234-9.

[30] Servat JJ, Bernardino CR. Effects of common topical antiglaucoma medications on the ocular surface, eyelids and periorbital tissue. Drugs Aging. Apr 1;28(4):267-82.

[31] Han JA, Frishman WH, Wu Sun S, Palmiero PM, Petrillo R. Cardiovascular and respiratory considerations with pharmacotherapy of glaucoma and ocular hypertension. Cardiol Rev. 2008 Mar-Apr;16(2):95-108.

[32] Francis BA, Singh K, Lin SC, Hodapp E, Jampel HD, Samples JR, et al. Novel glaucoma procedures: a report by the American Academy of Ophthalmology. Ophthalmology. 2011 Jul;118(7):1466-80.

[33] Martinez T, Gonzalez V, Panizo G, Wright N, Pañeda C, Jimenez A. In vitro and in vivo efficacy of SYL040012, a novel siRNA compound for treatment of glaucoma. Submitted. 2012.

[34] Campochiaro PA. Potential applications for RNAi to probe pathogenesis and develop new treatments for ocular disorders. Gene Ther. 2006 Mar;13(6):559-62.

[35] Ahmed Z, Kalinski H, Berry M, Almasieh M, Ashush H, Slager N, et al. Ocular neuroprotection by siRNA targeting caspase-2. Cell Death Dis. 2011;2:e173.

[36] Smith W, Assink J, Klein R, Mitchell P, Klaver CC, Klein BE, et al. Risk factors for age- related macular degeneration: Pooled findings from three continents. Ophthalmology. 2001 Apr;108(4):697-704.

[37] Rattner A, Nathans J. Macular degeneration: recent advances and therapeutic opportunities. Nat Rev Neurosci. 2006 Nov;7(11):860-72.

[38] Klein R, Chou CF, Klein BE, Zhang X, Meuer SM, Saaddine JB. Prevalence of age-related macular degeneration in the US population. Arch Ophthalmol. Jan;129(1):75-80.

[39] Thornton J, Edwards R, Mitchell P, Harrison RA, Buchan I, Kelly SP. Smoking and age- related macular degeneration: a review of association. Eye (Lond). 2005 Sep;19(9):935- 44.

[40] Clemons TE, Milton RC, Klein R, Seddon JM, Ferris FL, 3rd. Risk factors for the incidence of Advanced Age-Related Macular Degeneration in the Age-Related Eye Disease Study (AREDS) AREDS report no. 19. Ophthalmology. 2005 Apr;112(4):533-9.

[41] Khandhadia S, Cipriani V, Yates JR, Lotery AJ. Age-related macular degeneration and the complement system. Immunobiology. Feb;217(2):127-46.

[42] Bird AC. Therapeutic targets in age-related macular disease. J Clin Invest. 2010 Sep;120(9):3033-41.

[43] A randomized, placebo-controlled, clinical trial of high-dose supplementation with vitamins C and E, beta carotene, and zinc for age-related macular degeneration and vision loss: AREDS report no. 8. Arch Ophthalmol. 2001 Oct;119(10):1417-36.

[44] SanGiovanni JP, Chew EY, Clemons TE, Ferris FL, 3rd, Gensler G, Lindblad AS, et al. The relationship of dietary carotenoid and vitamin A, E, and C intake with age-related macular degeneration in a case-control study: AREDS Report No. 22. Arch Ophthalmol. 2007 Sep;125(9):1225-32.

[45] Cousins SW, Group OS. Targeting Complement Factor 5 in combination with Vascular Endothelial Growth Factor (VEGF) Inhibition for Neovascular Age Related Macular Degeneration (AMD): Results of a Phase 1 Study ARVO Meeting abstracts. 2010;51:1251.

[46] Yang Z, Stratton C, Francis PJ, Kleinman ME, Tan PL, Gibbs D, et al. Toll-like Receptor 3 and Geographic Atrophy in Age-Related Macular Degeneration. N Engl J Med. 2008 Aug 27.

[47] Zhou P, Fan L, Yu KD, Zhao MW, Li XX. Toll-like receptor 3 C1234T may protect against geographic atrophy through decreased dsRNA binding capacity. FASEB J. Oct;25(10):3489-95.

[48] Ruckman J, Green LS, Beeson J, Waugh S, Gillette WL, Henninger DD, et al. 2'- Fluoropyrimidine RNA-based aptamers to the 165-amino acid form of vascular endothelial growth factor (VEGF165). Inhibition of receptor binding and VEGF-induced vascular permeability through interactions requiring the exon 7-encoded domain. J Biol Chem. 1998 Aug 7;273(32):20556-67.

[49] Gragoudas ES, Adamis AP, Cunningham ET, Jr., Feinsod M, Guyer DR. Pegaptanib for neovascular age-related macular degeneration. N Engl J Med. 2004 Dec 30;351(27):2805- 16.

[50] Brown DM, Kaiser PK, Michels M, Soubrane G, Heier JS, Kim RY, et al. Ranibizumab versus verteporfin for neovascular age-related macular degeneration. N Engl J Med. 2006 Oct 5;355(14):1432-44.

[51] Rosenfeld PJ, Brown DM, Heier JS, Boyer DS, Kaiser PK, Chung CY, et al. Ranibizumab for neovascular age-related macular degeneration. N Engl J Med. 2006 Oct 5;355(14):1419-31.

[52] Avery RL, Pieramici DJ, Rabena MD, Castellarin AA, Nasir MA, Giust MJ. Intravitreal bevacizumab (Avastin) for neovascular age-related macular degeneration. Ophthalmology. 2006 Mar;113(3):363-72 e5.

[53] Patel PJ, Bunce C, Tufail A. A randomised, double-masked phase III/IV study of the efficacy and safety of Avastin(R) (Bevacizumab) intravitreal injections compared to standard therapy in subjects with choroidal neovascularisation secondary to age-related macular degeneration: clinical trial design. Trials. 2008;9:56.

[54] Tufail A, Patel PJ, Egan C, Hykin P, da Cruz L, Gregor Z, et al. Bevacizumab for neovascular age related macular degeneration (ABC Trial): multicentre randomised double masked study. BMJ. 2010;340:c2459.

[55] Dejneka NS, Wan S, Bond OS, Kornbrust DJ, Reich SJ. Ocular biodistribution of bevasiranib following a single intravitreal injection to rabbit eyes. Mol Vis. 2008;14:997- 1005.

[56] Shen J, Samul R, Silva RL, Akiyama H, Liu H, Saishin Y, et al. Suppression of ocular neovascularization with siRNA targeting VEGF receptor 1. Gene Ther. 2006 Feb;13(3):225-34.

[57] Kleinman ME, Yamada K, Takeda A, Chandrasekaran V, Nozaki M, Baffi JZ, et al. Sequence- and target-independent angiogenesis suppression by siRNA via TLR3. Nature. 2008 Apr 3;452(7187):591-7.

[58] Shoshani T, Faerman A, Mett I, Zelin E, Tenne T, Gorodin S, et al. Identification of a novel hypoxia-inducible factor 1-responsive gene, RTP801, involved in apoptosis. Mol Cell Biol. 2002 Apr;22(7):2283-93.

[59] Lee DU, Huang W, Rittenhouse KD, Jessen B. Retina Expression and Cross-Species Validation of Gene Silencing by PF-655, a Small Interfering RNA Against RTP801 for the Treatment of Ocular Disease. J Ocul Pharmacol Ther. 2012 Feb 3.

[60] Resnikoff S, Pascolini D, Etya'ale D, Kocur I, Pararajasegaram R, Pokharel GP, et al. Global data on visual impairment in the year 2002. Bull World Health Organ. 2004 Nov;82(11):844-51.

[61] Yau JW, Rogers SL, Kawasaki R, Lamoureux EL, Kowalski JW, Bek T, et al. Global prevalence and major risk factors of diabetic retinopathy. Diabetes Care. 2012 Mar;35(3):556-64.

[62] Qian H, Ripps H. Neurovascular interaction and the pathophysiology of diabetic retinopathy. Exp Diabetes Res. 2012;2011:693426.

[63] Willard AL, Herman IM. Vascular complications and diabetes: current therapies and future challenges. J Ophthalmol. 2012;2012:209538.

[64] Photocoagulation treatment of proliferative diabetic retinopathy. Clinical application of Diabetic Retinopathy Study (DRS) findings, DRS Report Number 8. The Diabetic Retinopathy Study Research Group. Ophthalmology. 1981 Jul;88(7):583-600.

[65] http://www.antisense.com.au/product-pipeline/atl1103-for-growth-sight-disorders/. [cited]; Available from.

[66] Gayton JL. Etiology, prevalence, and treatment of dry eye disease. Clin Ophthalmol.
2009;3:405-12.

[67] Qazi Y, Wong G, Monson B, Stringham J, Ambati BK. Corneal transparency: genesis, maintenance and dysfunction. Brain Res Bull. 2010 Feb 15;81(2-3):198-210.

[68] Seta F, Patil K, Bellner L, Mezentsev A, Kemp R, Dunn MW, et al. Inhibition of VEGF expression and corneal neovascularization by siRNA targeting cytochrome P450 4B1. Prostaglandins Other Lipid Mediat. 2007 Nov;84(3-4):116-27.

[69] Panda A, Vanathi M, Kumar A, Dash Y, Priya S. Corneal graft rejection. Surv Ophthalmol. 2007 Jul-Aug;52(4):375-96.

[70] Murthy RC, McFarland TJ, Yoken J, Chen S, Barone C, Burke D, et al. Corneal

transduction to inhibit angiogenesis and graft failure. Invest Ophthalmol Vis Sci. 2003 May;44(5):1837-42.
[71] Cursiefen C, Chen L, Dana MR, Streilein JW. Corneal lymphangiogenesis: evidence, mechanisms, and implications for corneal transplant immunology. Cornea. 2003 Apr;22(3):273-81.
[72] Bachmann BO, Bock F, Wiegand SJ, Maruyama K, Dana MR, Kruse FE, et al. Promotion of graft survival by vascular endothelial growth factor a neutralization after high-risk corneal transplantation. Arch Ophthalmol. 2008 Jan;126(1):71-7.
[73] Gerten G. Bevacizumab (avastin) and argon laser to treat neovascularization in corneal transplant surgery. Cornea. 2008 Dec;27(10):1195-9.
[74] Hos D, Saban DR, Bock F, Regenfuss B, Onderka J, Masli S, et al. Suppression of inflammatory corneal lymphangiogenesis by application of topical corticosteroids. Arch Ophthalmol. 2011 Apr;129(4):445-52.
[75] Miele C, Rochford JJ, Filippa N, Giorgetti-Peraldi S, Van Obberghen E. Insulin and insulin-like growth factor-I induce vascular endothelial growth factor mRNA expression via different signaling pathways. J Biol Chem. 2000 Jul 14;275(28):21695-702.
[76] Vuori K, Ruoslahti E. Association of insulin receptor substrate-1 with integrins. Science. 1994 Dec 2;266(5190):1576-8.
[77] Dietrich T, Onderka J, Bock F, Kruse FE, Vossmeyer D, Stragies R, et al. Inhibition of inflammatory lymphangiogenesis by integrin alpha5 blockade. Am J Pathol. 2007 Jul;171(1):361-72.
[78] Al-Mahmood S, Colin S, Farhat N, Thorin E, Steverlynck C, Chemtob S. Potent in vivo antiangiogenic effects of GS-101 (5′-TATCCGGAGGGCTCGCCATGCTGCT-3′), an antisense oligonucleotide preventing the expression of insulin receptor substrate-1. J Pharmacol Exp Ther. 2009 May;329(2):496-504.
[79] Andrieu-Soler C, Berdugo M, Doat M, Courtois Y, BenEzra D, Behar-Cohen F. Downregulation of IRS-1 expression causes inhibition of corneal angiogenesis. Invest Ophthalmol Vis Sci. 2005 Nov;46(11):4072-8.
[80] http://www.genesignal.com/index.php?id=23.
[81] Jabs DA, Griffiths PD. Fomivirsen for the treatment of cytomegalovirus retinitis. Am J Ophthalmol. 2002 Apr;133(4):552-6.
[82] Kuppermann BD. Therapeutic options for resistant cytomegalovirus retinitis. J Acquir Immune Defic Syndr Hum Retrovirol. 1997;14 Suppl 1:S13-21.
[83] Chou S, Miner RC, Drew WL. A deletion mutation in region V of the cytomegalovirus DNA polymerase sequence confers multidrug resistance. J Infect Dis. 2000 Dec;182(6):1765-8.
[84] Jabs DA. Ocular manifestations of HIV infection. Trans Am Ophthalmol Soc. 1995;93:623-83.
[85] Orr RM. Technology evaluation: fomivirsen, Isis Pharmaceuticals Inc/CIBA vision. Curr Opin Mol Ther. 2001 Jun;3(3):288-94.

[86] Silverstein BE, Conrad D, Margolis TP, Wong IG. Cytomegalovirus-associated acute retinal necrosis syndrome. Am J Ophthalmol. 1997 Feb;123(2):257-8.

[87] Atherton SS. Acute retinal necrosis: insights into pathogenesis from the mouse model.

Herpes. 2001 Nov;8(3):69-73.

[88] Ganatra JB, Chandler D, Santos C, Kuppermann B, Margolis TP. Viral causes of the acute retinal necrosis syndrome. Am J Ophthalmol. 2000 Feb;129(2):166-72.

[89] Mei H, Xing Y, Yang J, Wang A, Xu Y, Heiligenhaus A. Influence of antisense oligonucleotides targeting tumor necrosis factor-alpha on experimental herpetic- induced chorioretinitis of mouse eye. Pathobiology. 2009;76(1):45-50.

[90] Moerdyk-Schauwecker M, Stein DA, Eide K, Blouch RE, Bildfell R, Iversen P, et al. Inhibition of HSV-1 ocular infection with morpholino oligomers targeting ICP0 and ICP27. Antiviral Res. 2009 Nov;84(2):131-41.

[91] Grajewski RS, Li J, Wasmuth S, Hennig M, Bauer D, Heiligenhaus A. Intravitreal treatment with antisense oligonucleotides targeting tumor necrosis factor-alpha in murine herpes simplex virus type 1 retinitis. Graefes Arch Clin Exp Ophthalmol. 2011 Feb;250(2):231-8.

[92] Li J, Wasmuth S, Bauer D, Baehler H, Hennig M, Heiligenhaus A. Subconjunctival antisense oligonucleotides targeting TNF-alpha influence immunopathology and viral replication in murine HSV-1 retinitis. Graefes Arch Clin Exp Ophthalmol. 2008 Sep;246(9):1265-73.

[93] Zheng M, Atherton SS. Cytokine profiles and inflammatory cells during HSV-1-induced acute retinal necrosis. Invest Ophthalmol Vis Sci. 2005 Apr;46(4):1356-63.

[94] Zheng M, Qian H, Joshi RM, Nechtman J, Atherton SS. DNA microarray analysis of the uninoculated eye following anterior chamber inoculation of HSV-1. Ocul Immunol Inflamm. 2003 Sep;11(3):187-95.

[95] Streilein JW, Ksander BR, Taylor AW. Immune deviation in relation to ocular immune privilege. J Immunol. 1997 Apr 15;158(8):3557-60.

[96] Kim B, Tang Q, Biswas PS, Xu J, Schiffelers RM, Xie FY, et al. Inhibition of ocular angiogenesis by siRNA targeting vascular endothelial growth factor pathway genes: therapeutic strategy for herpetic stromal keratitis. Am J Pathol. 2004 Dec;165(6):2177-85.

[97] Tang Q, Chen W, Hendricks RL. Proinflammatory functions of IL-2 in herpes simplex virus corneal infection. J Immunol. 1997 Feb 1;158(3):1275-83.

[98] Thomas J, Gangappa S, Kanangat S, Rouse BT. On the essential involvement of neutrophils in the immunopathologic disease: herpetic stromal keratitis. J Immunol. 1997 Feb 1;158(3):1383-91.

[99] Inoue T, Inoue Y, Kosaki R, Nishida K, Shimomura Y, Tano Y, et al. Immunohistological study of infiltrated cells and cytokines in murine herpetic keratitis. Acta Ophthalmol Scand. 2001 Oct;79(5):484-7.

[100] Wasmuth S, Bauer D, Yang Y, Steuhl KP, Heiligenhaus A. Topical treatment with antisense oligonucleotides targeting tumor necrosis factor-alpha in herpetic stromal keratitis. Invest Ophthalmol Vis Sci. 2003 Dec;44(12):5228-34.

[101] Wasmuth S, Bauer D, Steuhl KP, Heiligenhaus A. Topical antisense-oligonucleotides targeting IFN-gamma mRNA improve incidence and severity of herpetic stromal keratitis by cytokine specific and sequence unspecific effects. Graefes Arch Clin Exp Ophthalmol. 2008 Mar;246(3):443-51.

[102] Zheng M, Deshpande S, Lee S, Ferrara N, Rouse BT. Contribution of vascular endothelial growth factor in the neovascularization process during the pathogenesis of herpetic stromal keratitis. J Virol. 2001 Oct;75(20):9828-35.

[103] Jun EJ, Won MA, Ahn J, Ko A, Moon H, Tchah H, et al. An antiviral small-interfering RNA simultaneously effective against the most prevalent enteroviruses causing acute hemorrhagic conjunctivitis. Invest Ophthalmol Vis Sci. 2011 Jan;52(1):58-63.

[104] Tan EL, Marcus KF, Poh CL. Development of RNA interference (RNAi) as potential antiviral strategy against enterovirus 70. J Med Virol. 2008 Jun;80(6):1025-32.

[105] Hayreh SS. Ischemic optic neuropathy. Prog Retin Eye Res. 2009 Jan;28(1):34-62.

[106] Hayreh SS. Management of ischemic optic neuropathies. Indian J Ophthalmol. 2011 Mar-Apr;59(2):123-36.

[107] Danesh-Meyer HV, Huang R, Nicholson LF, Green CR. Connexin43 antisense oligodeoxynucleotide treatment down-regulates the inflammatory response in an in vitro interphase organotypic culture model of optic nerve ischaemia. J Clin Neurosci. 2008 Nov;15(11):1253-63.

[108] Ferrari S, Di Iorio E, Barbaro V, Ponzin D, Sorrentino FS, Parmeggiani F. Retinitis pigmentosa: genes and disease mechanisms. Curr Genomics. 2011 Jun;12(4):238-49.

[109] Farrar GJ, Kenna PF, Humphries P. On the genetics of retinitis pigmentosa and on mutation-independent approaches to therapeutic intervention. EMBO J. 2002 Mar 1;21(5):857-64.

[110] O'Reilly M, Palfi A, Chadderton N, Millington-Ward S, Ader M, Cronin T, et al. RNA interference-mediated suppression and replacement of human rhodopsin in vivo. Am J Hum Genet. 2007 Jul;81(1):127-35.

[111] Maguire AM, Simonelli F, Pierce EA, Pugh EN, Jr., Mingozzi F, Bennicelli J, et al. Safety and efficacy of gene transfer for Leber's congenital amaurosis. N Engl J Med. 2008 May 22;358(21):2240-8.

[112] Gorbatyuk M, Justilien V, Liu J, Hauswirth WW, Lewin AS. Suppression of mouse rhodopsin expression in vivo by AAV mediated siRNA delivery. Vision Res. 2007 Apr;47(9):1202-8.

[113] Wang JJ, Zeng ZW, Xiao RZ, Xie T, Zhou GL, Zhan XR, et al. Recent advances of chitosan nanoparticles as drug carriers. Int J Nanomedicine. 2011;6:765-74.

[114] Tam LC, Kiang AS, Kennan A, Kenna PF, Chadderton N, Ader M, et al. Therapeutic benefit derived from RNAi-mediated ablation of IMPDH1 transcripts in a murine model of autosomal dominant retinitis pigmentosa (RP10). Hum Mol Genet. 2008 Jul 15;17(14):2084-100.

[115] Pearson RA, Barber AC, West EL, MacLaren RE, Duran Y, Bainbridge JW, et al. Targeted disruption of outer limiting membrane junctional proteins (Crb1 and ZO-1) increases integration of transplanted photoreceptor precursors into the adult wild-type and degenerating retina. Cell Transplant. 2010;19(4):487-503.

[116] Vetrini F, Tammaro R, Bondanza S, Surace EM, Auricchio A, De Luca M, et al. Aberrant splicing in the ocular albinism type 1 gene (OA1/GPR143) is corrected in vitro by morpholino antisense oligonucleotides. Hum Mutat. 2006 May;27(5):420-6.

[117] Alexopoulou L, Holt AC, Medzhitov R, Flavell RA. Recognition of double-stranded RNA and activation of NF-kappaB by Toll-like receptor 3. Nature. 2001 Oct 18;413(6857):732-8.

[118] Heil F, Hemmi H, Hochrein H, Ampenberger F, Kirschning C, Akira S, et al. Species- specific recognition of single-stranded RNA via toll-like receptor 7 and 8. Science. 2004 Mar 5;303(5663):1526-9.

[119] Krug A, Towarowski A, Britsch S, Rothenfusser S, Hornung V, Bals R, et al. Toll-like receptor expression reveals CpG DNA as a unique microbial stimulus for plasmacytoid dendritic cells which synergizes with CD40 ligand to induce high amounts of IL-12. Eur J Immunol. 2001 Oct;31(10):3026-37.

[120] Gil J, Esteban M. Induction of apoptosis by the dsRNA-dependent protein kinase (PKR): mechanism of action. Apoptosis. 2000 Apr;5(2):107-14.

[121] Samuel CE. Antiviral actions of interferons. Clin Microbiol Rev. 2001 Oct;14(4):778-809, table of contents.

[122] Yoneyama M, Fujita T. RNA recognition and signal transduction by RIG-I-like receptors. Immunol Rev. 2009 Jan;227(1):54-65.

[123] Kato H, Takeuchi O, Sato S, Yoneyama M, Yamamoto M, Matsui K, et al. Differential roles of MDA5 and RIG-I helicases in the recognition of RNA viruses. Nature. 2006 May 4;441(7089):101-5.

[124] Sioud M. Single-stranded small interfering RNA are more immunostimulatory than their double-stranded counterparts: a central role for 2'-hydroxyl uridines in immune responses. Eur J Immunol. 2006 May;36(5):1222-30.

[125] Sioud M. RNA interference and innate immunity. Adv Drug Deliv Rev. 2007 Mar 30;59(2-3):153-63.

[126] Song E, Zhu P, Lee SK, Chowdhury D, Kussman S, Dykxhoorn DM, et al. Antibody mediated in vivo delivery of small interfering RNAs via cell-surface receptors. Nat Biotechnol. 2005 Jun;23(6):709-17.

[127] Stein-Streilein J. Immune regulation and the eye. Trends Immunol. 2008 Nov;29(11):548-54.

[128] Jackson AL, Linsley PS. Recognizing and avoiding siRNA off-target effects for

target identification and therapeutic application. Nat Rev Drug Discov. 2009 Jan;9(1):57-67.

[129] Ui-Tei K, Naito Y, Takahashi F, Haraguchi T, Ohki-Hamazaki H, Juni A, et al. Guidelines for the selection of highly effective siRNA sequences for mammalian and chick RNA interference. Nucleic Acids Res. 2004;32(3):936-48.

[130] Yuan B, Latek R, Hossbach M, Tuschl T, Lewitter F. siRNA Selection Server: an automated siRNA oligonucleotide prediction server. Nucleic Acids Res. 2004 Jul 1;32(Web Server issue):W130-4.

[131] Bramsen JB, Kjems J. Chemical modification of small interfering RNA. Methods Mol Biol. 2011;721:77-103.

[132] Jackson AL, Burchard J, Leake D, Reynolds A, Schelter J, Guo J, et al. Position-specific chemical modification of siRNAs reduces "off-target" transcript silencing. Rna. 2006 Jul;12(7):1197-205.

[133] Bertrand JR, Pottier M, Vekris A, Opolon P, Maksimenko A, Malvy C. Comparison of antisense oligonucleotides and siRNAs in cell culture and in vivo. Biochem Biophys Res Commun. 2002 Aug 30;296(4):1000-4.

[134] Levin AA. A review of the issues in the pharmacokinetics and toxicology of phosphorothioate antisense oligonucleotides. Biochim Biophys Acta. 1999 Dec 10;1489(1):69-84.

[135] Watts JK, Corey DR. Silencing disease genes in the laboratory and the clinic. J Pathol. 2012 Jan;226(2):365-79.

[136] Haussecker D. The business of RNAi therapeutics. Hum Gene Ther. 2008 May;19(5):451-62.

8

Clinical Application of Photodisruptors in Ophthalmology

Emina Alimanović Halilović

1. Introduction

In ophthalmology today, laser photodisruptors are used besides laser photocoagulators. Photocoagulators transform light energy into heat energy, causing microcauterisation of tissue. Photodisruptors act non-thermally by controlled cutting of the unwanted tissue, causing microexplosions. The most frequently used photodisruptors are Neodymium YAG, Holmium YAG and Erbium YAG lasers. They differ by type of the active crystal. The laser beam of these lasers is highly coherent, low-divergent, which enables it a high precision. It is used as a microscalpel to cut optical membranes and tissues.

Meyer-Schwickerath was the first to describe the laser beam transmission through optical media. Photodisruptors such as Nd-YAG laser work by principles of the optical "breakdown". Laser beam energy is brought to as small focal point as possible, thus achieving a high energy density with a strong destructive effect. In the focal point there occurs a microexplosion with disruption of electrons from their nuclear orbits. This free floater is known as electronic plasma. The electronic plasma is able to absorb any further energy entering the eye in the same focal point. This significant feature of the protective plasma prevents damage to the eye structures beyond the protective plasma formation, i.e., conduction of the destructive effect outside the focus. Inside the protective plasma, the temperature is 15,000 ºC with a high pressure, so the plasma expands in concentric waves, "shock waves". In about 150ns after the "optical breakdown", it is possible to biomicroscopically see air bubbles as a sign of collapse and pressure equalisation inside the wave with atmospheric pressure. The "shock wave" is accompanied by an acoustic wave that is sometimes audible.

Two methods are used in the Nd-YAG laser beam production: "Q-switched" and "mode-locked". The former compresses energy in a single „nanosecond" pulse, and the latter produces a series of "picosecund" pulses. In the "mode-locked" method, we have a low energy power of single pulsations, while in the "Q-switched" method, pulse energy is higher at the same energy level. The "Q-switched" technology produces chiefly pulses whose main effect is mechanical – buckling. This is photodisruption, i.e., tearing of atoms with energy shocks. The effect of this method is creation of energy in the pipe being let through in short impulses, and during the still interval energy is kept, accumulated and enhanced, so that each impulse has a very high performing power.

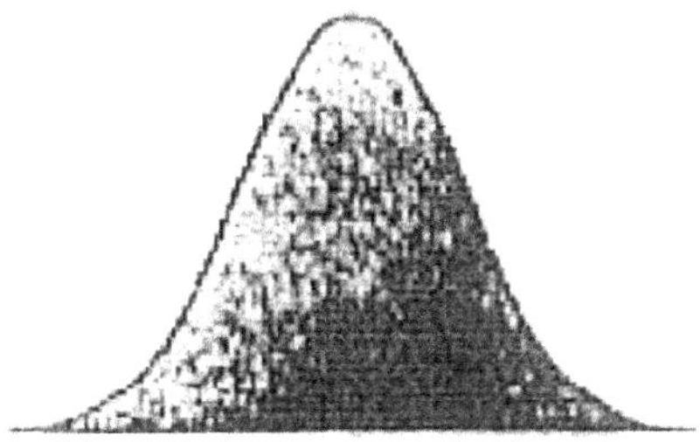

Figure 1. Q-switched pulse;

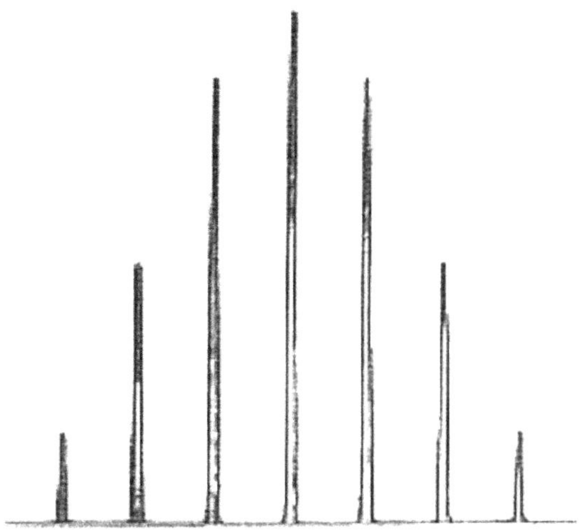

Figure 2. Mode-locked pulse train

The Nd-YAG laser beam causes damage to the tissue in the form of craters in the fields of vaporisation. The crater edges are carbonised, then towards the edges there follows the coagulation necrosis area, and at the far periphery the oedema area.

Erbium-YAG laser has found a broad application in aesthetic plastic microsurgery of eyelids, in blepharochalasis, ectropium, and phthisis. Multifocal Erbium-YAG laser systems have a multiple use in ophthalmology, in the cataract phaco surgery, vitrectomy and sclerectomy.

It is also used in dermatology for dermoabrasion for the skin rejuvenation.

2. Nd-Yag laser in ophthalmology

Modern cataract microsurgery with implantation of intraocular lenses is inseparable from the Nd-YAG laser microsurgery. The microsurgery of glaucoma and problems of the posterior segment also imply the use of Nd-YAG laser. Application of Nd-YAG laser:

with cataract in	
	anterior capsulotomy
	posterior capsulotomy
	removal of pigment from the anterior surface of IOL
	discission of secondary cataract and membrane
	synechiolysis
	cutting of corneal sutures after the cataract surgery or cheratoplastica
with corneal diseases	
	dendritic ulcers
	microabscesses
with glaucoma	
	transscleral cycolophotocoagulation
	iridectomy
	sphinteroctomy
with the vitreous body	
	anterior vitreoruption
	cutting of intravitreal
	vitreoretinal tractions and membranes

Table 1. Clinical application of Nd-YAG laser in ophthalmology

2.1. Nd-Yag laser posterior capsulotomy

The most frequent practical application of Nd-YAG laser is in posterior capsulotomy and discission of secondary membranes in aphakic (conditions after the cataract surgery), and pseudophakic (conditions after the cataract surgery with implantation of intraocular lens into the anterior or posterior eye chamber) of the eyes.

The surgical technique of intraocular lens placement is important for the development of posterior capsular opacity. The intraocular lens placement itself, manipulation with the iris, and lens contact with the posterior capsule may be a cause of accumulation of pigment on the lens anterior surface and development of opacity. Also, the lens implant size, its shape and the type of material of which it is made have a significant impact on the development of secondary cataract. Posterior lens capsular opacity develops through the migration of epithelium from the remaining parts of the anterior lens capsule, proliferation of the remaining epithelial cells of the anterior pole of lens and lens fibres. Through their metaplasia, myofibroblasts are developed, forming folds, reticles, uneven membranes which are difficult to see biomicroscopically; they do not significantly affect visual acuity. If epithelial cells accumulate in the form of round, uneven, pearl-shaped opacity - Elschnig's pearls - then such opacity reduces significantly vision. There may be also some other causes of opacity of the posterior lens capsule: remaining parts of the lens cortex intraoperatively and after incomplete aspiration. Masses can incorporate between the implanted lens and posterior capsule. Also, the remaining parts of the lens nucleus, blood cells in hyphema, pigment cells of the iris and ciliary body may accumulate on the lens or posterior capsule. Low-virulent, slow-growing, still bacterial colonies such as Propionibacterium acnes may settle in the posterior capsule field and look like ordinary opacity. If we mistake them for normal capsular opacity and perform the laser capsulotomy, we have opened a path for bacteria into the vitreous body, which can result in the occurrence of endophthalmitis.

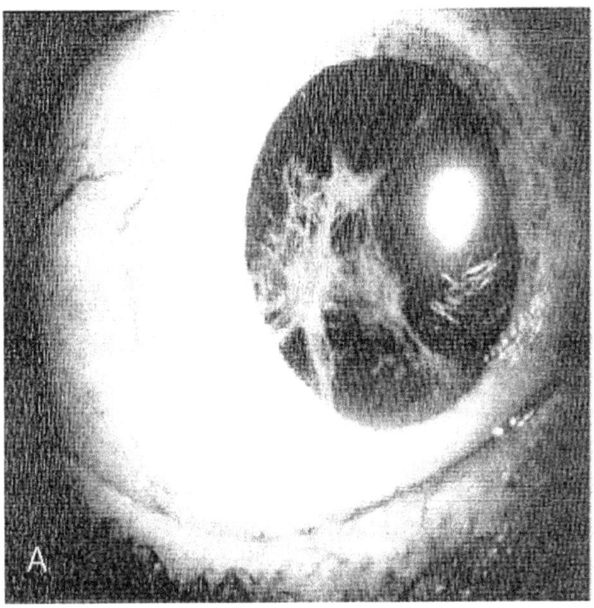

Figure 3. Posterior capsular opacification

Postoperative posterior capsular opacity leads to a fall of visual acuity. Patients complain of blurred images, they see things as if through "gauze or a sieve". In the first postoperative year, opacity occurs in 83% patients and from the second to the fifth years in 50% cases. The Nd-YAG laser posterior capsulotomy is a routine technique with which we resolve the problem. With the laser beam we make the "fenestra" opening on the posterior capsule through which light beams reach the retina without obstruction and form a clear image of an object.

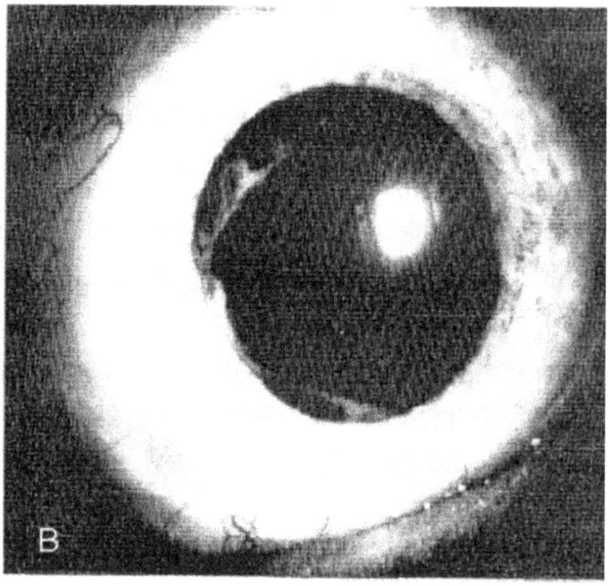

Figure 4. After Nd-YAG capsulotomy

Prior to the intervention itself, it is necessary to examine the patient's visual acuity, take intraocular pressure, examine biomicroscopically capsular opacity, direct and through the procedure of retroillumination of the capsule itself and the retrolental space. Opacity of the posterior lens capsule may be measured echographically, and the quantitative measuring "in vivo" with the Scheimpflug photographic computer system. The intervention is performed on the pupil dilated to the maximum, in the darkroom, with the surgeon's prior adaptation to the dark, with optimal enlargement on the biomicroscope, with the optimal light intensity, on the dilated pupil. The patient has to cooperate with the surgeon, keep still on the apparatus and follow the instructions from the surgeon in moving the eyes. The procedure is performed under local anaesthesia, by means of condensing Abraham or Peyman YAG planconvex contact lens for the posterior capsulotomy. Such lenses concentrate the laser beam to the smallest possible focus. At the same time, they immobilise the eye in restless patients. The angle of the incoming convergent laser beam depends on technical possibilities of the apparatus and it is selected by the surgeon. According to Eisner's discussions, the widest incoming angle, with the smallest focal point (mark), and clear focusing produce the clean beam, with the highest energy concentration in the focus and the smallest energy dispersion in the cornea or retina. The most frequently used capsulotomy techniques are Seaman's, which imply the knowledge of quality and thickness of opacity:

a. the „vertical opening" technique from 12 o'clock position to 6 o'clock position is applied in posterior capsular opacity;
b. the „cross-shaped" technique when horizontal cutting is performed by vertical opening from 9 o'clock position to 6 o'clock position;

c. the „concentric spreading" technique from the periphery to the centre, in abundant secondary;
d. the „fragmentation" technique with the widening of opening edges in fibrous membranes.

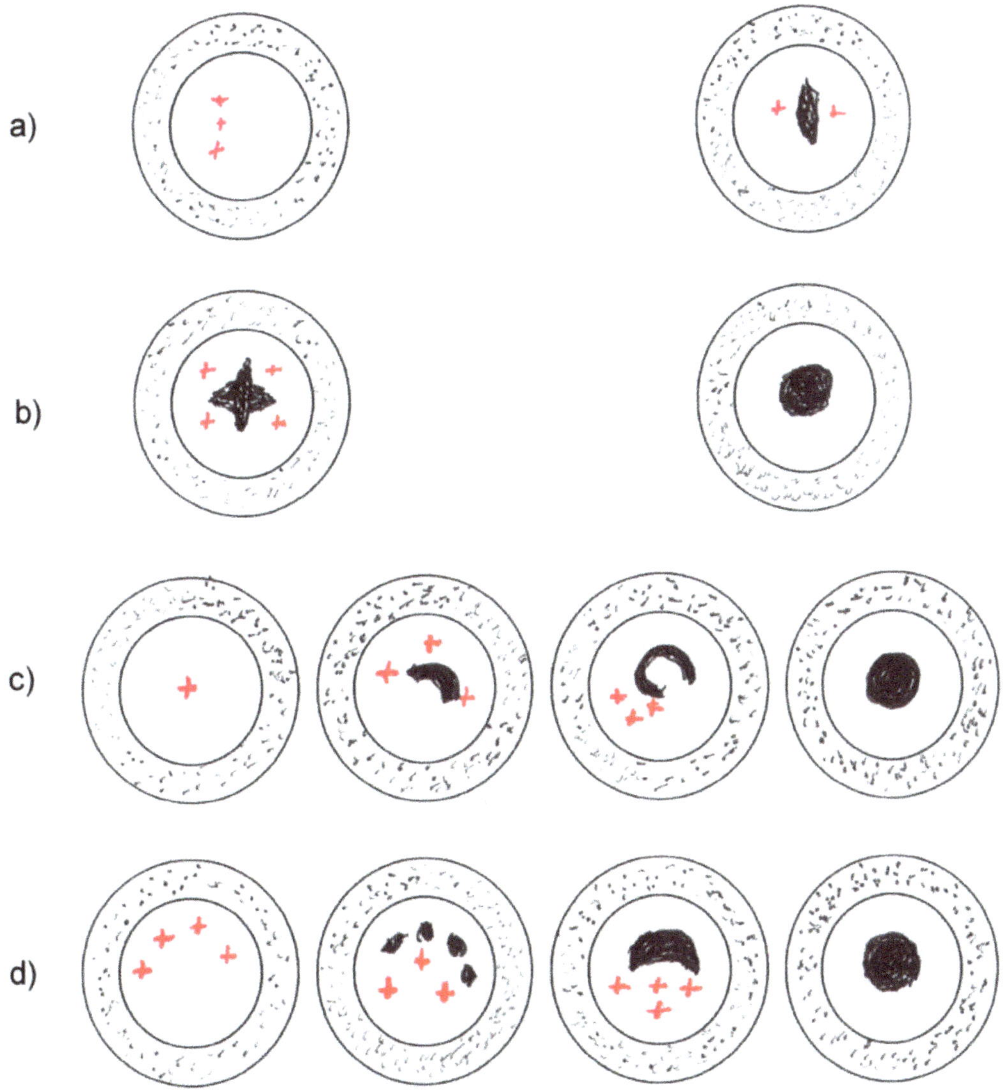

Figure 5. „Seaman's" capsulotomy techniques

Although the Nd-YAG laser capsulotomy is a non-invasive technique, efficient, painless, practical, easily-applicable, cost-effective, with fast recovery, today the method of choice, it is necessary that the laser surgery be performed by a well-trained, educated and experienced ophthalmologist. Only with the expertise and ethics of the laser surgeon can complications be avoided and reduced. All complications are a result of correlation of the laser action, methodological errors in performance and the condition of the eye. Use of the

Nd-YAG laser beam can lead to certain unwanted complications on the anterior and posterior poles of the eye.

On the anterior segment, we usually have: damage to the corneal epithelium, corneal perforation, damage to the intraocular lens, dislocation of the intraocular lens, changes of intraocular pressure, development of iritis, and hemorrhage into the anterior chamber.

On the posterior eye segment, the following complications can develop: rupture of the anterior hyaloid membrane, prolapse of the vitreous body into the anterior chamber, retinal rupture, cystic macular oedema, retinal detachment, retinal bleeding, macular fibrosis, macular rupture, and rarely endophthalmitis.

2.2. A jump of intraocular pressure

We have transient increase in IOP in 50-97% laser-treated patients after the posterior capsulotomy. Numerous investigations have shown that the highest jump takes place in the first four hours, and in the first 24-48 hours it returns to normal, stays increased by 5 mmHg respectively in the first week. In some cases, the increased IOP may stay on for two or three months. The IOP maximal values after the laser capsulotomy are 50-60 mmHg. Transient IOP increase after the Nd-YAG laser posterior capsulotomy is explained by the mechanical obstruction of the trabecular exhaust system with the posterior capsular residual particles, inflammatory cells, and high-molecular soluble proteins of the lens. An increased secretion of the ciliary epithelium is considered to be a cause of extended intraocular hypertension as a consequence of the "shock" wave effect. Also, according to Terry AC's opinion, there is a significant effect of prostglandins on the blood-aqueous barrier, which results in increased production of ocular water. The IOP jump is more frequent in the aphakic eye than in the pseudophakic eye. A higher IOP jump was proved in the lens implant into the anterior chamber compared to the eyes with the lens in the posterior chamber, or fixed to the iris. Glaucoma patients have a higher IOP jump compared to non-glaucoma patients.

2.3. Corneal damage

The laser beam, going through the cornea, may cause corneal oedema or perforation, usually unintentionally, due to the bad focusing or use of too much energy. The cornea absorbs 6% Nd-YAG laser energy, lens 15%, the vitreous body 36%. Capsulotomy causes a loss of endothelial cells of the cornea from 0 to 7%, but this loss does not decompensate the cornea.

Corneal damages are a consequence of the mechanical destruction and a heat effect of the linearly and non-linearly absorbed laser energy. Corneal epithelisation is completed in the first 24 hours. Corneal oedema may occur as secondary due to the increased IOP, or may be caused by exacerbation of inflammatory processes of the anterior segment after the YAG laser.

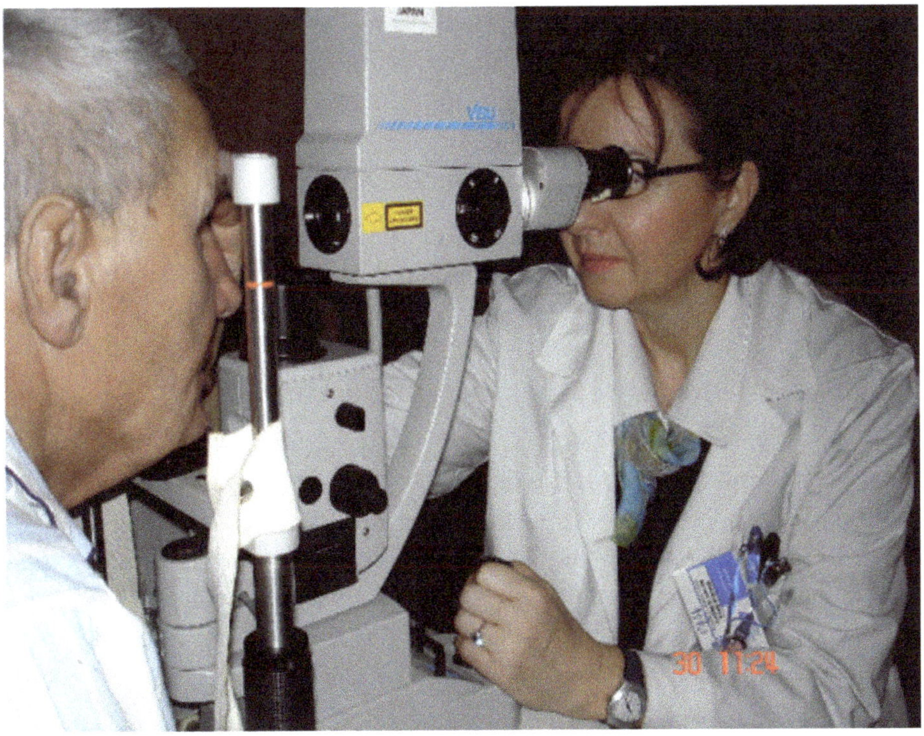

Figure 6. The Nd YAG laser procedure

2.4. Iris haemorrhage

As a consequence of damage to the delicate iris blood vessel by the laser beam during posterior capsulotomy, we can have bleeding in the anterior chamber with a slight pain. Incidence of this complication ranges from 1% to 3%. A slight pressure of the contact lens onto the cornea usually stops bleeding.

2.5. Damage to the intraocular lens

During posterior laser capsulotomy, damage to the intraocular lens may occur in 5% to 40% cases. They are usually recesses, fissures, cracks, lattice, and bursts of stellar shape. These damages affect visual acuity, especially if centrally located. They produce various visual effects, usually in the form of blinding glare, which affects the normal vision. The lens damage depends on individually and totally used energy, impulse duration, number of impulses, and the kind of the IOL material. Polymethylmethacrylat (PMMA) lenses may endure bigger energy without damages, and they are crater-shaped. Silicon lenses have damages in the form of smooth stratification.

2.6. Dislocation of the intraocular lens

Upon the Nd-YAG laser posterior capsulotomy, the IOL shifts to the vitreous body. The implanted lens shifting is monitored by measuring the depth of the anterior chamber with ultrasound biometry. It is a dislocation of 25μm (from 9 to 55 μm) with SD 13. It is difficult to prove the effect of dislocation on visual acuity as capsulotomy is followed by improvement of visual acuity.

2.7. Rupture of the anterior hyaloid membrane

Rupture of the anterior hyaloids membrane occurs as a complication after the Nd-YAG laser capsulotomy in 19% cases, which enables a prolapse of the vitreous body into the anterior chamber.

2.8. Prolapse of the vitreous body into the anterior chamber

We usually notice this complication three weeks after capsulotomy within the scope from 1.5% to 16%. Herniation of the vitreous body may cause an increased intraocular pressure. There are reports by the authors who, within a four-year period after intervention, do not find an increased IOP. Shifting of the vitreous body forward increases a danger of occurrence of macular oedema, retinal ruptures, and retinal detachment.

2.9. Retinal ruptures

After the laser posterior retinal capsulotomy, the number of retinal ruptures increases. The number, type and location of retinal ruptures are characteristic. They are asymptomatic, round, atrophic retinal ruptures observable usually a month upon capsulotomy, with incidence of 2.3%. The possibility of rupture occurrence is twice as big in laser-treated compared to non-laser treated eyes. Atrophic round retinal ruptures are more numerous than u-shaped ones. They occur in all meridians, including the macula, too. They may be isolated or within peripheral degenerations. They are chiefly localised in the upper temporal and nasal quadrants.

2.10. Retinal detachment

Occurrence of retinal detachment and retinal ruptures is statistically significantly more frequent in the eyes on which laser posterior capsulotomy was performed. Retinal detachment incidence after laser capsulotomy varies from 0.08% to 3.6% or 13% respectively, depending on the sample. Multiple studies have shown that post-laser retinal detachments occur more frequently in younger males. Risk factors, such as myopia, lattice degeneration, anamnesis of existence of retinal detachment on the other eye, and complicated surgeries, demonstrably increase the number of retinal detachments after capsulotomy. Retinal ablation development is influenced by tissue ionization and formation of gaseous "plasma", which then expands accompanied with the "shock and acoustic" wave. After the laser incision of tissue, we have a condition of a latent stress which further disintegrates the structures. All the three mechanisms act simultaneously, and the extent of destruction of the tissue around the optimal "breakdown" area depends on the laser pulse total energy, time of occurrence, and duration of electronic plasma, and the "shock" wave action. It is believed that the passage of the laser beam through the vitreous body and its "shock" and "acoustic" wave cause significant biochemical changes in the vitreous body. Animal experiments prove penetration of the physiological barrier, processes of depolymerisation of hyaluronic acid, liquefaction and separation of the vitreous body, and all this activates processes of vitreoretinal proliferation; as a consequence we have the occurrence of retinal ruptures and retinal detachment.

2.11. Cystoid macular oedema

Cystoid macular oedema incidence after the Nd-YAG laser capsulotomy varies in different authors from 0.5% to 4.9%. Oedema develops in first six months after the laser capsulotomy. Occurrence of cystoid macular oedema is related to the hyaloid membrane rupture, intraocular lens damage and a short time interval between the cataract surgery and laser intervention. Diagnosis is usually established on the basis of ophthalmoscopic finding and an unexpected fall of vision. Fluorescein angiography shows the flow of the contrast into the macular area. Fine and Brucker proved that cystoid macular oedema is a liquid which from perifoveolar capillaries pours via the damaged endothelium and accumulates in the plexiform, Henle's layer. The laser beam passing through optical tissues releases prostaglandin and leukotriene from the iris, which triggers a change of permeability of parafoveolar capillaries.

2.12. Macular rupture

After the Nd-YAG laser capsulotomy, we can have macular ruptures as a consequence. They are observable as early as 24 hours upon capsulotomy, and in the period from 10 to 21 days. They occur unilaterally more frequently, but there have been reports about bilateral occurrence as well. Macular rupture is almost always associated with other complications such as: a jump of intraocular pressure, prolapse of the vitreous body into the anterior chamber, macular haemorrhage, and occurrence of cystoid macular oedema. It manifests with a sudden fall of vision, appearance of central black spots and paracentral scotoma. They may create difficulties with recognition of colours.

Post-capsulotomy macular rupture occurs as a consequence of several mechanisms: thermal damages, mechanical disruptions, "optical breakdown" which leads to blood vessel bursts of the retina and chorioidea, thus causing subretinal, intraretinal, and vitreal bleeding. The third mechanism is the "shock wave" responsible for the occurrence of a series of changes in the vitreous body leading to the separation and ablation of the vitreous body. As a secondary effect, there occurs contraction of the perifoveolar vitreous body creating tangent tractions. They are considered to be a cause of macular rupture occurrence.

In most cases the macular rupture closes spontaneously within a period from three weeks to six months, and visual acuity improves significantly. Recently third-degree Gass macular ruptures are resolved surgically by vitrectomy with interior tamponade. After vitrectomy the macular rupture closes and visual acuity improves.

2.13. Macular fibrosis

After the Nd-YAG laser capsulotomy, macula bleeding may follow. Blood resorption is accompanied with formation of preretinal and retinal fibrogliosis bands and membranes which can be filled with abnormal blood vessels. Occurrence of macular fibrosis, after the Nd-YAG laser capsulotomy, is statistically significant. Macular fibrosis significantly reduces visual acuity and it is followed with metamorphopsia. It is confirmed by ophthalmological examination, fluorescein angiography, and fundus microphotography. Histologically, macular fibrosis is made up of: cells of retinal pigment epithelium 51%, astocytes 29%, fibrocytes 14%, and myofibroblasts 7%. With the epiretinal peeling technique within vitrectomy, preretinal membranes are removed. This technique requires the surgeon's enormous experience, and it gives significant results in the sphere of central visual functions.

2.14. Other photomacular damages

After the Nd-YAG laser capsulotomy, photomacular damages have incidence from 7% to 20%. Most photomacular damages appear asymptomatically or with a minimal symptomatology due to their frequent extrafoveolar location. They may manifest as macular haemorrhage, subretinal, intraretinal, and preretinal bleeding, or as semi-ruptures. Sometimes bleeding may occur in the vitreous body, which significantly reduces vision transiently. Despite big, visible, semi-ruptured macular changes, the condition may be almost fully repaired after the Nd-YAG laser capsulotomy.

2.15. Endophthalmitis

After the Nd-YAG laser capsulotomy, there may develop endophthalmitis. It develops from the fifth day to the sixth week after intervention. Proved causative agents are Propionibacterium acnes and Staphylococcus epidermis all-present, saprophyte bacteria with a low degree of pathogenicity. They are found in the normal conjunctival flora. Propionibacterium acnes is gram-positive, anaerobic, producing lipolytic enzyme which serves as a trigger of inflammatory processes. During the extra-capsular cataract extraction with lens implantation, bacteria are brought into the eye. The Nd-YAG laser capsulotomy is an activating factor, a trigger for the development of the anterior uveitis, which then spreads into panuveitis, endophthalmitis respectively. Formation of the fenestra on the posterior capsule, often on the anterior hyloid membrane as well, opens the path for bacteria from the anterior to the posterior ocular chamber, i.e., into the middle and posterior parts of the vitreous body. Diagnosis is confirmed by the characteristic ophthalmological picture, i.e., positive cultures of ocular water and vitreous body. The ocular water culture grows in nine days, while the vitreous body culture is earlier and more frequently positive.

Research has shown that the most common complication is a jump of ocular pressure, then damage to the intraocular lens, anterior hyaloid membrane rupture, bleeding in the anterior chamber, retinal rupture, and macular fibrosis.

Development of complications is significantly affected by a total of applied energy, number of pulsations, individual pulse energy, and opening diameter made during capsulotomy.

To prevent complications, the suggested optimal pulse energy is up to 2.0 mJ, total applied energy of 200-300 mJ. The optimal size of the opening made on the posterior capsule is 4 mm.

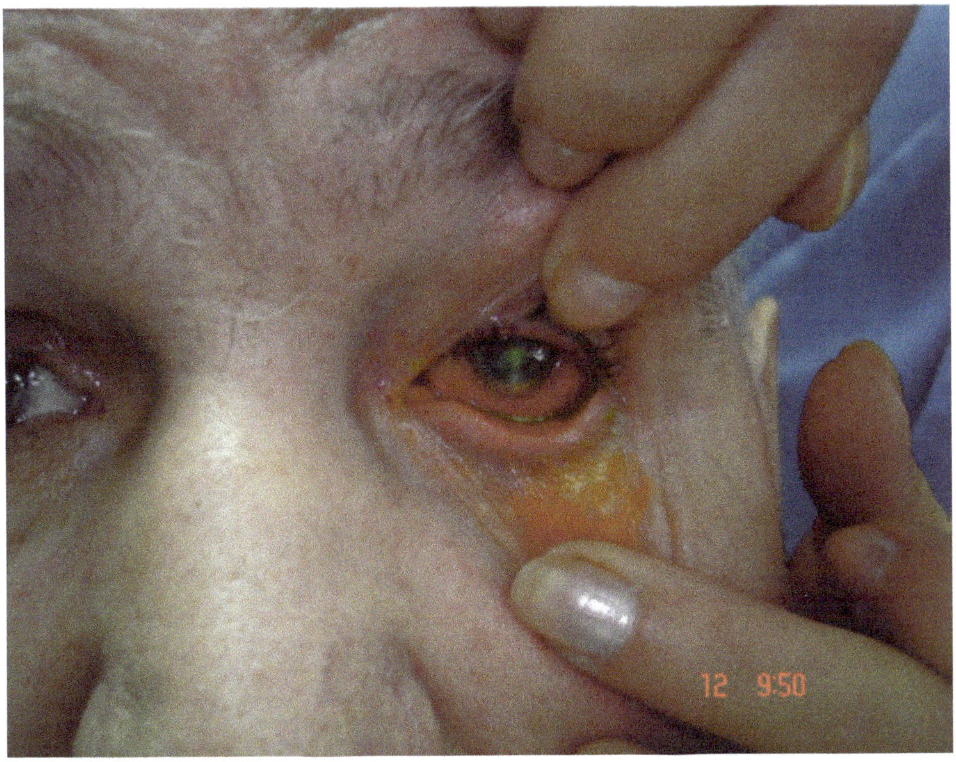

Figure 7. Endophthalmitis after Nd-YAG laser capsulotomy

3. Neodymium Yag laser iridectomy

Nd-YAG laser is used as an alternative treatment to the classic iridectomy in primary glaucoma of the closed angle, puppilary block, and secondary glaucoma of various mechanisms of origin.

Intervention is performed under local anaesthesia, in artificial myosis provoked by 2-4% pilocarpine. Abraham or Goldmann lenses are used. A total to be applied is from 1 to 12 mJ, usually from 3 to 5 mJ through 1-10 applications. The most common location is the central part of the iris on the basis of the iris crypts in the upper nasal quadrant in the 10:30 meridian, or the upper temporal quadrant in the 1:30 meridian. Studies carried out on a larger sample point to a successful iridectomy in 99% cases. After 1-2 hours intraocular pressure falls. The use of corticosteroid drops is suggested in the postoperative period. Upon the Nd-YAG laser iridectomy, there may occur complications described earlier in the chapter on posterior capsulotomy.

4. Nd-Yag laser on the posterior segment

Within diabetic retinopathy, the Valsalva retinopathy, or a sudden rupture of arterial retinal aneurysm, premacular haemorrhage may develop with a sudden loss of vision. According to the accepted opinions, such condition could be observed, waiting for spontaneous haemorrhage resorption. Vitrectomy with premacular haemorrhage aspiration is certainly a more effective method. Today membranectomy with the double-frequency Nd-YAG laser is offered a as an alternative therapy.

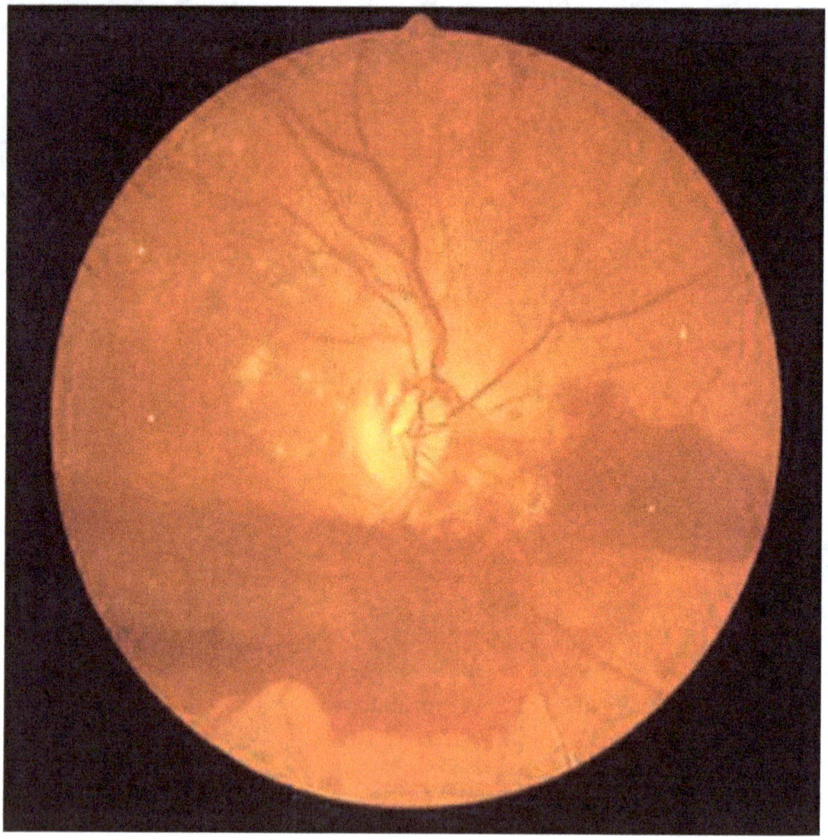

Figure 8. Preretinal haemorrhage

By this intervention, we drain haemorrhage and speed up blood resorption. Immediately upon the laser intervention, vision improves significantly. So today the Nd-YAG laser membranectomy, in premacular haemorrhage, occurs as a non-invasive alternative method to vitrectomy, due to the good results it achieves. Within proliferative diabetic retinopathy with vitreoretinal proliferation, Neodymium-YAG laser may be used to cut adhesions located in the central and posterior vitreous. Prior to that, bases of such proliferations may be ensured by placing argon laser barriers. We can have adhesions in the anterior vitreous body as well; we see them after cataract operations complicated with the vitreous body prolapse and development of iridicyclitis. In these interventions, special Peyman lenses are used for the middle and posterior vitreous.

5. Erbium-Yag laser

Erbium-YAG laser has also found its application in ophthalmology in phaco surgeries. Micropulse laser waves break up blurred lenses, which is followed with aspiration of the broken up and fragmented masses. The laser beam, in this surgery, is an alternative to the ultrasound wave. Erbium-YAG laser, which is introduced by means of special endo-probes into the bulbus, is used in sclerectomy and vitrectomy.

Author details

Emina Alimanović Halilović
University Clinical Center Sarajevo, Sarajevo, Bosnia and Herzegovina

References

[1] Alimanović-Halilović E. Complications after Neodymium-YAG laser capsulotomy in Phakic and Pseudophakic Eyes : PhD thesis. Sarajevo: Faculty of Medicine, 2001:5-20;78-105.
[2] Alward WLM. Laser Iridotomy. In: Weingeist TA. Laser Surgery in Ophthalmology Practical Applications. San Mateo California USA: Appleton & Lange, 1992:139-147.
[3] Aron-Rose DS et al. Rhegmtogenous retinal Detachment After Neodymium-YAG. Laser capsulotomy in Phakic and Pseudophakic Eyes. In Richard R et al. Use of apulsed picosecond Nd-YAG laser. Am J of Ophthalmology 1986;(101):81-9.
[4] Blacharski AP, Newsome AD. Bilateral macular holes after Nd-YAG laser posterior capsulotomy. American Journal of Ophthalmology 1988:417-8.
[5] Carstocea B, Pascu RA. Yttrium Aluminium Garnet Crystal (I).Oftalmologia 2005;49(3): 3-9.
[6] Cinal A. Intraocular lens position after capsulotomy. J Cataract Refract Surg 2000;26:5- 6.
[7] Collins JF, Donnenfeld ED. Opthalmic Desk Reference. New York: Raven Press, 1991: 456-7.
[8] Farvadin M, Mehryar M, Maghaddasi H, Farvadin M. Neodymium-YAG laser treatment for macular hemorrhages. Arch Indian Med 2005; 8(1):8-13.
[9] Georg E. Learning to be a YAG Surgeon. In: March FW. Ophthalmic Laser. 1990; 119-29.
[10] Glacet-Bernard, Brahim R, Mokhtari et al. Retinal detachment following Nd-YAG capsulotomy. A retrospective study of 144 capsulotomies. J Fr Ophthalmol 1993;16(2):87-94.
[11] Holweger R, Marefat B. Intraocular pressure change after neodymium-YAG capsulotomy. Journal of Cataract & Refractive Surgery 1997; 23(7):1095-102.

[12] Hal DB, Wayne FM, James HL. Use of the YAG Laser in Posterior Capsulotomies. In: Wayne FM. Ophthalmic Laser 1990:131-9.

[13] Hayashi K, Hayashi H, Nakao F, Hayash F. In vivo quantitative measurement of posterior capsule opacification after extracapsular catarac surgery. Am J of Ophthalmology 1998;125:837-43.

[14] Isola V, Spinelli G, Misefari W. Transpupillary retinopexy of chorioretinal lesions predisposing to retinal detachment with the use of diode (810 nm) microlaser. Retina 2001;21(5):453-9.

[15] Javitt et.al In: Ninn-Pedersen K, Bauer B. Cataract patients in a defined Swedish population 1986-1990. Nd-YAG laser capsulotomies in relation to preoperative and surgical conditions. Act Ophthal Scandinavica 1996;114:382-86

[16] Lerman S, Thrasher B, Moran M. Vitreus changes after Neodymium-YAG laser irradiation of the posterior lens capsule or midvitreus. Am J of Ophthalmology 1997;470-5.

[17] Mackool JR. Antiinflammatory regimen for cystoid macular edem after cataract surgery. J Cataract Refract Surg 2000;26:474.

[18] Meisler et al. In: Tetz MR, Apple JD et al. A newly described complication of Nd-YAG laser capsulotomy: Exacerbation of an intraocular infection. Arch Ophthalmology 1987;105:1324 5.

[19] Ranta P, Kivela T. Retinal detachement in pseudophakic eyes with and without Nd-YAG laser posterior capsulotomy. Ophthalmology 1998;105(11):2127-33.

[20] Rennie CA, Newman DK, Snead MP, Flanagan DW. Nd:YAG laser treatment for premacular subhyaloid haemorrhage. Eye 2001;15(Pt 4):519-24.

[21] Rakofsky S, Koch D. et al. Levobunolol 0,5% and Timolol 0,5% to prevent intraocular pressure elevation after Neodymium-YAG laser posterior capsulotomy. J of Cataract & Refractive Surgery 1997;23(7):1075-80.

[22] Sefić S, Firdus H, Alimanović E, Ljaljević S, Sefić M. Oštećenja oka kod pomraèenja sunca. Med Arch 2000;54(1):41-4.

[23] Sefić M. Bolesnik sa kataraktom pita: Da li se može poboljšati vid laserom? Sarajevo: KCU, 1999: 10.

[24] Smith RT, Moscoso WE, Trokel S, Auran J. The barrier function in Neodymium-YAG laser capsulotomy. Arch Ophthalmol 1995;113:645-52.

[25] Stilma JS, Boen-Tan TN. Timolol and intraocular pressure elevation following Neodymium-YAG laser surgery. Documenta Ophthalmologica 1986; 64:59-67.

[26] Sheidow T, Gonder RJ, Merchea MM. Macular hole following Nd-YAG capsulotomy. Br J of Ophthalmology 1999;83(6):755.

[27] Thach AB, Lopez PF, Snady-Mc Coy LC. et al. Accidental Nd-YAG laser injuries to the macula. Am J of Ophthalmology 1995; 119(6):767-773.

[28] Zeyen P, Zeyen T. The long term effect of YAG laser posterior capsulotomy on intraocular pressure after combined glaucoma and cataract surgery. Belge d Ophthalmologie 1999; 271:99-103.

[29] Bhargava R, Kumar P, Prakash A, Chaudhary KP. Estimation of mean ND: Yag laser capsulotomy energy levels for membranous and fibrous posterior capsular opacification. Nepal J Ophthalmol. 2012;4(7):108-13.

[30] Larrañaga-Osuna G, Garza-Cantú D. Intraocular pressure in patients undergoing capsulotomy Nd: YAG laser Rev Med Inst Mex Seguro Soc. 2011;49(3):259-66.

[31] Giocanti-Aurégan A, Tilleul J, Rohart C, Touati-Lefloc'h M, Grenet T, Fajnkuchen F, Chaîne G. OCT measurement of the impact of Nd:YAG laser capsulotomy on foveal thickness. J Fr Ophtalmol. 2011;34(9):641-6.

9

Nontuberculous Mycobacterial Keratitis

Ana Lilia Pérez-Balbuena,
David Arturo Ancona-Lezama,
Lorena Gutiérrez-Sánchez and
Virginia Vanzzini-Zago

1. Introduction

Mycobacterium species that are considered typical are the tuberculosis species such as *M.tuberculosis, M.bovis, M.africarium* and *M.leprae*. These species have only human or animal reservoirs and are not transmitted by water. In contrast, the species Non-Tuberculosis or "atypical", naturally are ubiquitous in soil and water and have been found as normal flora of skin, sputum, and gastric contents. These bacteria are resistant to common, disinfectants, chlorine, formaldehyde and glutaraldehyde.

NTM can cause infections on all adnexal and ocular tissues including the cornea, iris, lens, retina, choroid and optic nerve. Most NTM infections are caused by *M.chelonae* and *M. fortuitum*, that as we will discuss later, belong to the rapid growers group.

In this chapter, we will focus on keratitis caused by atypical mycobacterium, since a great number of recent clinical reports of NTM ocular infections are of keratitis. In common general ophthalmology procedures like refractive surgery, for example laser in situ keratomileusis (LASIK), Laser epithelial keratomileusis (LASEK), photorefractive keratectomy (PRK), and other specialized procedures such as penetrating keratoplasty (PKP), a transgression to natural barriers occurs, this constitutes a risk factor for infection by these organisms. In addition, LASIK is one of the most commonly performed procedures in ophthalmology practice.

Several factors may contribute to the development of mycobacterial keratitis following LASIK, making it difficult to determine the true origin of the infection in most cases. This procedure is often performed utilizing aseptic, but non sterile techniques. *Mycobacterium chelonei, M. abscessus, M. fortuitum, M. szulgai,* and *M. mucogenicum* have been reported as the result of improper asepsis.

Atypical Mycobacteria corneal infections are rare, but devastating complications. Although rare, are a diagnostic and therapeutic challenge. Mycobacterium have been involved in several isolated cases as well as in outbreaks.[4-12]

2. Microbiological and laboratory profile

Mycobacterium species that are considered typical are the tuberculosis specie; *M.tuberculosis*. Many species enclosed in genus *Mycobacteriaceae* are true human pathogens as *Mycobacterium tuberculosis* complex, that include *M tuberculosis, M bovis,* non pathogenic *M bovis* BCG, *M africanum, M caprae, M microti,* and *M pinnipedii* are characterized by different phenotypes and mammalian host ranges, displays the most extreme genetic homogeneity with 0.01 to 0.03% nucleotides variation only. Growth rate in this group is 6 to 12 weeks. *M leprae* is the only non cultivable in vitro specie and has some genetic variations in relation to *M tuberculosis complex*.

The only genus of the *Mycobacteriaceae* family is the *Mycobacterium*, the *Mycobacteriaceae* belongs to the order *Actinomycetales*. Mycobacteria is an unusual ocular pathogen that has the following characteristics: intracellular bacilli, slow growing organisms, obligate aerobic, non-motile, non-capsulated, non-sporing, present a large amounts of lipids and true waxes in their cell walls, and are considered gram-positive and acid-fast.

Other places where NTM have been isolated are: contaminated tap water, saline solutions, disinfectant solutions, and hemodialyzers. Mycobacteria influences a number of ocular structures, including the cornea,iris, lens,retina, choroid and optic nerve.

Clinical manifestations of the typical mycobacteria are : lupus vulgaris on eyelid, phlyctenule, scleritis, lacrimal gland involvement, orbital periostitis, granulomatous panuveitis, secondary glaucoma and cataract, chorioretinal plaque or nodule, nerve palsies.

The incidence of tuberculosis has increased due to the growth in homelessness, the upsurge of intravenous drug abuse, neglect of tuberculosis programs, acquired immunodeficiency syndrome.

Runyon classified nontuberculous mycobacteria into four groups, described in [Table 1]. Runyon Classification of tuberculous and non-tuberculous *Mycobacterium* is based, on the growth rate, and pigment production. Groups I to III are slow growers that require approximately 2 to 3 or more weeks to form visible colonies in culture at 27°C. Group IV organisms are rapid growers, forming non-pigmented colonies in culture in one week.[1,14,15]

Out of the more than 130 actually validated species of non-tuberculousmycobacteria, 60 are slowly growingmycobacteria, that shows in solid culture media growth rates of 2 to 4 weeks, the most clinically significance and most frequently in isolated human samples are *M avium, M intracellulare, M kansasii, M marinum, M xenopi, M malmoense and M ulcerans*. In the rapidly growing mycobacteria group with 7 -10 days of growing rate on solid culture media, there are three major clinically important species responsible for 80% of diseases in humans *M chelonae, M abscessus* and *M fortuitum,* that are too frequently located in tap water and have been related with sepsis in bone marrow transplant, post-traumatic, surgical ocular and other surgical wound infections.

SlowGrowers			**Rapid Growers**
Group I	**Group II**	**Group III**	**Group IV**
(photochromogens) *6-12 weeks*	*(scotochromogens)* *2-4 weeks*	*(nonchromogens)* *2-4 weeks*	*(nonchromogens)* *7-10 days*
M. marinum	M. scrofulaceum	M. avium	M. fortuitum group
M. kansasii	M. szulgai	M. intracellulare	*M. fortuitum*
M. simiae	M. gordonae	M. haemophilum	*M. peregrinum*
M. asiaticum	M. xenopi	M. paratuberculosis	*M. mucogenicum*
	M. flavescens	M. gastri	*M. Senegalese*
		M. malmoense	*M. septicum*
		M. nonchromogenicum	*M. mageritense*
		M. terrae	M. chelonae-abscessus group
		M. triviale	*M. chelonae*
			M. abscessus
			M. immunogenum
			M. smegmatis group
			M. smegmatis
			M. goodii
			M. wolinskyi

Problem statement: To describe the experience in México (Asociación Para Evitar La Ceguera I.A.P. "Hospital Dr. Luis Sánchez Bulnes" [APEC]) in the management of keratitis caused by nontuberculous mycobacteria.

Application area: Cornea and Refractive Service and Mycrobiology Service

Research course: To describe of atypical *Mycobacterium* keratitiscases diagnosed and attended in the Cornea Service of our Hospital in the last 10 years.

Methods: This is a descriptive retrospective case series of five patients treated in our service.

Table 1. Runyon's Classification of Nontuberculous Mycobacterium

3. Laboratory diagnosis and bacteriology

In ophthalmological infections traumatic or post-surgical in origin, are frequently involved in non-tuberculous or atypical fast growing *Mycobacteria,* the species *M. chelonae, M. chelonae /abscesus, M. fortuitum* have been isolated in many cases. These rapidly growing *Mycobacteria* share the cellular characteristics of *Mycobacterium* genus,like mycolic acids esters in its cell wall, long straight or curved rods with irregular Gram staining [Figure 1], and specific red-magenta staining characteristic with Ziehl-Neelsen or Kinyoun cold techniques.[Figure 2] They are aerobic and capable of growing in 5 -10% CO_2 atmosphere and in blood agar media.[Figure 3] In addition, these microorganisms are arylsulfatase positive, catalase positive and niacin negative. [Figure 4]

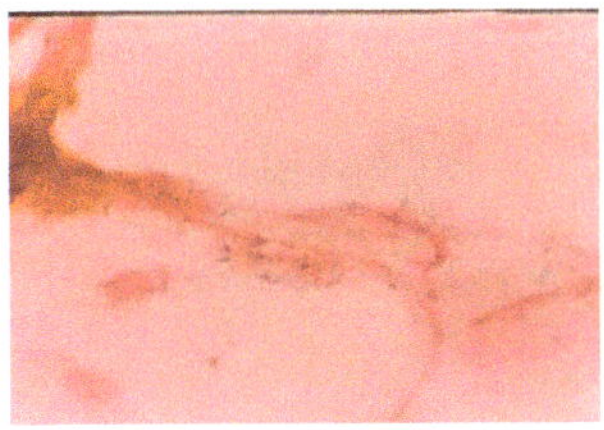

Figure 1. Gram positive and irregular stain and forms of *Mycobacterium chelonae*

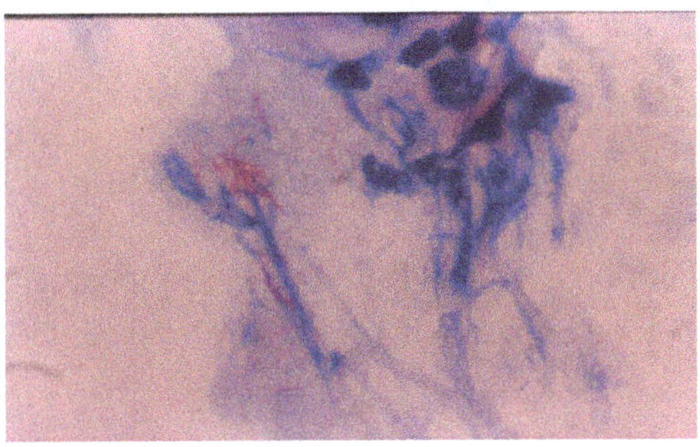

Figure 2. Red-magenta rods of *M. chelonae* in a corneal smear of patient with keratitis.

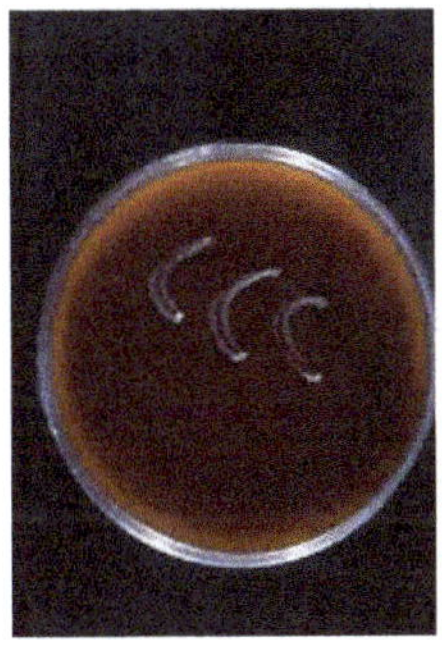

Figure 3. Colonies of *M. chelonae* in agar blood with Brain Heart Infusion (BHI) agar base after 7 days of incubation at 27°C and 5% CO_2 atmosphere.

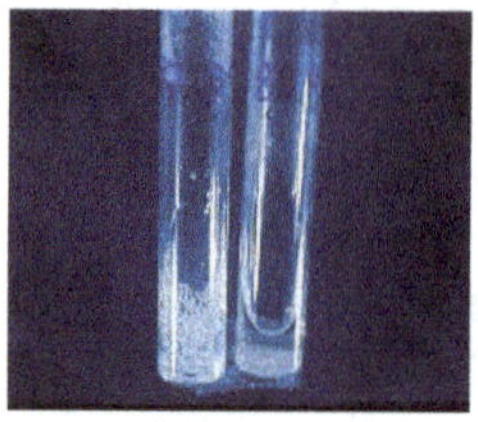

Figure 4. Catalase 65°C positive test (O_2 bubbles) for *Mycobacterium chelonae*.

To identify the microorganism, its phenotypic characteristics were used, such as pigmentation of colonies growing in the darkness (presented in Table 1) on Lowenstein-Jensen media.

The most common species of rapidly growing *Mycobacteria* belong to group IV of Runyon's classification, also known as colorless or nonchromatogens.[Figure 5]

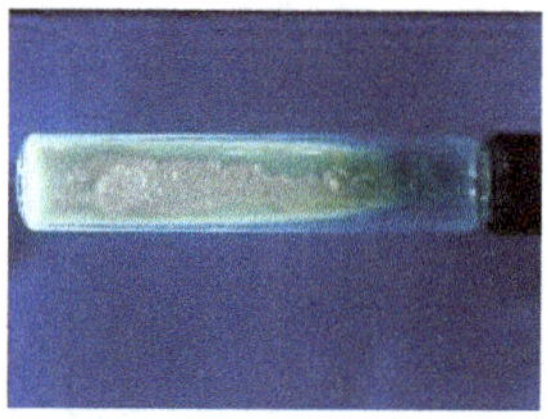

Figure 5. *Mycobacterium chelonae* colonies in Lowenstein-Jensen medium after 7 days of incubation at 27°C.

For genotypic characterization, the 16Sr RNA gene sequencing, high performance liquid chromatography and polymerase chain reaction has been used.

4. Clinical features

Nontuberculous Mycobacteria can cause infections of all adnexal and ocular tissues. Most atypical Mycobacteria infections are caused by *M. chelonae*, and *M. fortuitum*.

Dacryocystitis and Canaliculitis: Present as epiphora and erythematous swelling in the medial canthal area, purulent material can be expressed with massage of the lacrimal sac.

Orbital Infections: Present with a gradual development of periorbital edema, without a significant proptosis and a superficial skin lesion may be present. The visual acuity will depend on the involvement of the optic nerve. [18,19]

Conjuntivitis and Scleritis: Present as conjunctival or as scleral injection and tenderness accompanied with chronic redness, irritation, discharge and pain. Sometimes, marked scleral thinning may develop. Scleral abscesses manifest late in the course of the disease as subconjunctival nodules. [20,21]

Endoftalmitis: Present with severe pain, decreased vision, and redness and discharge, may exist hypopyon, and variable amounts of granulomatous keratitic precipitates. Moderate vitreous inflammation is present in most cases.

Keratitis: The greatest number of recent clinical reports of nontuberculous Mycobacteria ocular infections are of keratitis, as seen in our hospital (Asociación Para Evitar La Ceguera en México "Dr. Luis Sánchez Bulnes" I.A.P. [APEC]). Keratitis most commonly follows trauma or surgery and has been associated with penetrating keratoplasty and refractive surgery.

Nontuberculous Mycobacteria keratitis is characterized by a delayed onset of symptoms that range typically from 1 to 3 weeks following the exposing event. There is decreased vision and an indolent course and some cases various degrees of pain, ranging from indolent to severe.

Presenting symptoms can include any of the following: pain, redness, photophobia, decreased vision, foreign body sensation and/or mild irritation. Presenting clinical signs include infiltrates in the corneal interface that can either be multiple white granular opacities <0.5mm in diameter with well defined borders or radiating projections, or a single white round lesion (0.1-2 mm in diameter) which may progress to satellite lesions. These infiltrates spread subsequently into the corneal stroma posteriorly and anteriorly and can result in perforation though the flap to surface. [Table 2].A hypopyon is often found in untreated or poorly treated cases. [25,26]

Lazar and colleagues first described the presence of a "cracked windshield" appearance to the cornea around the edge of the central area of ulceration and infiltrate, seen transiently early in the course of the infection. [25,27,28] This sign consist of radiating lines from the central infiltrate in the middle third of the corneal stroma. It is important to mention that NTM keratitis has also been noted in the abscence of epithelial defect with deep stromal keratitis. The corneal infiltrate may show irregular margins.

Signs	Symptoms
Single or multiple white granular opacities with well	Pain (mild)
defined borders or radiating projections	Redness
Satellite infiltrates	Photophobia
Hypopyon	Tearing
Mild or absent anterior chamber reaction	Foreign body sensation
"Cracked windshield" appearance	Decreased visual acuity

Table 2. Signs and symptoms of keratitis caused by mycobacterias

5. Predisposing factors

Nontuberculous Mycobacteria are opportunistic pathogens that require an alteration in the ocular barriers to produce infection. In nearly all reports, a previous history of minor to severe trauma is the common denominator.Men and women are equally affected among NTM keratitis patients who have had LASIK, in contrast to a 70% male preponderance among patients who have not had LASIK, the result of a higher prevalence of trauma in males. [Table 3] [5,29]

Risk factors associated with NTM keratitis
Trauma
Surgical trauma
Refractive surgeries
Laser in situ keratomileusis (LASIK)
Laser epithelial keratomileusis (LASEK)
Corneal transplantation
Radial keratotomy
Photorefractive keratectomy (PRK)
Penetrating keratoplasty (PKP)
Other ophthalmologic surgeries
Extracapsular cataract extraction
Small incision corneal cataract surgery
Suture removal
Contact lens wear
Corticosteroid use
Improper aseptic technique or sterilization of surgical instrumentation

Table 3. Risk factors for the development of nontuberculous mycobacterial keratitis.

Post-LASIK NTM keratitis: Laser in situ keratomileusis (LASIK) is the most commonly performed refractive surgical procedure, since it offers rapid visual rehabilitation, decreased stromal scarring, less postoperative pain, and the ability to treat a wider range of refractive disorders. LASIK preserves the integrity of Bowman's membrane and the overlying epithelium, thus decreasing the risk for microbial keratitis. Several studies have reported an incidence of bacterial infection following LASIK procedures varying between 0% to 1.5%. [29,31,32] Solomon et. al published the first survey that provides information about post-LASIK infectious keratitis. The most common organisms cultured were nontuberculous mycobacteria (48%) and staphylococci (33%).. These findings are consistent with Chang's research, where he found that nearly 47% of infectious keratitis cases after LASIK appear to be caused by NTM; 32% being caused by *Mycobacterium chelonei* alone. In contrast to the acute or subacute onset of symptoms generally seen postoperatively in bacterial and fungal keratitis, rapid growing atypical mycobacteria may present with a slower onset of clinical disease, from 3 to 14 weeks (3.5 weeks in average) after the procedure. It is important to keep in mind that this is not a rule, and more rapidly growing NTM such as the *Mycobacterium chelonae-abscessus* group may present as soon as 10 days posterior to the refractive surgery. [1,33,34]

Innoculation of NTM to the flap-stromal interface probably takes place at the time of surgery, therefore, it is infrequent to find an epithelial defect, being present in less than half of cases. Corneal infiltrates appear to be entirely within the lamellar flap or at the flap interface and may be either multiple, tiny, white, granular opacities less than 0.5mm in diameter or a single white lesion ranging between 0.1-0.2mm in diameter. Anterior extension of infiltrate with ulceration or anterior perforation of the corneal flap or posterior extension into the stroma is a rare finding and is usually associated with a delay in diagnosis and the beginning of therapy. Anterior chamber reaction is not a common finding, occurring in only 20% of cases.[1,29]

6. Differential diagnosis

NTM keratitis can often be mistaken with other bacterial infections that cause nonsuppurative keratitis. Several authors suggest to keep in mind other causative organisms that may present, in the course of disease, similar clinical features such as fungal keratitis, infectious crystalline keratopathy, Nocardia keratitis, herpes simplex virus, and rarely Acanthamoeba keratitis. In our experience at APEC, the principal differential diagnosis must be made between fungal and Nocardia keratitis.

Fungal keratitis: Often preceded by history of trauma involving plants or foreign bodies. Like NTM, mycotic keratitis may worsen with the use of topical corticosteroids. These keratitis often do not respond to topical antibiotics, as seen with NTM keratitis. Multiple corneal fungal abscesses may emulate the multifocal presentation of NTM keratitis. Sabouraud's agar is essential for the identification of the causative fungus. [Figure 6]

Infectious Crystalline Keratopathy (ICK): "Cracked windshield" corneal appearance may be also seen in this keratitis caused most commonly by Streptococcus species, but unlike this entity, NTM keratitis presents with this sign transiently early in the course. Gorovoy et al first described Infectious crystalline keratopathy in 1984, describing it as a unique corneal infection characterized by and indolent, progressive course: a paucity of inflammation; and

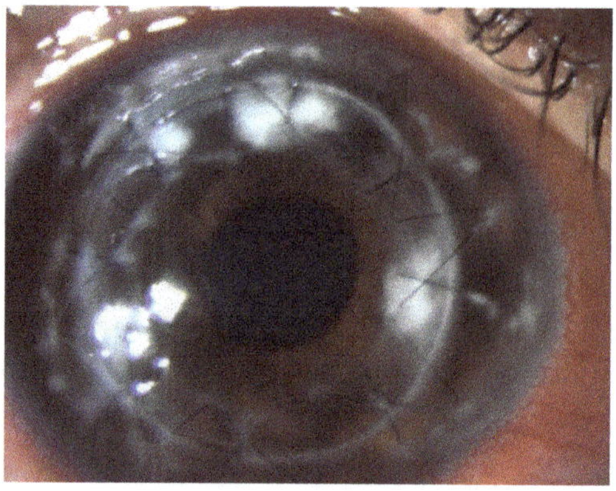

Figure 6. Candida keratitis after penetrating keratoplasty for keratoconus.

the formation of sharply demarcated, gray-white, branching, round, stellate, or needle-like opacities in the corneal stroma. Although the duration of the relatively recalcitrant course of the infectious crystalline keratopathy may mimic NTM keratitis, the crystalline appearance persists in ICK but is transient in NTM keratitis. Among post-LASIK patients, crystalline NTM keratitis occurs rarely (less than 10%).

Nocardiaasteroides infection: should also be considered, since it is an acid-fast microorganism capable of producing bacterial keratitis. The best way to differentiate Nocardia infection from NTM keratitis is with a Gram stain. Nocardia keratitis is more fulminant than NTM keratitis.[Figure 7]

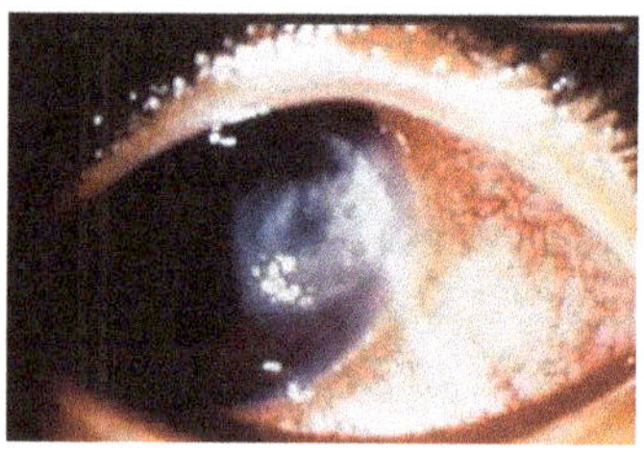

Figure 7. Nocardial keratitis as a differential diagnosis of NTM keratitis.

Deep lamellar keratitis can be confused with post-LASIK NTM keratitis. It usually presents within the first 7 days post-LASIK, and unlike NTM keratitis, it clears with topical corticosteroids. If the wrong diagnosis is made, the improper use of such medications contribute to the delay in diagnosis of post-LASIK NTM keratitis.

Acanthamoeba keratitis generally presents with out-of-proportion pain in comparison to the clinical findings. It is common to see ring ulcers in Acanthamoeba keratitis. This agent responds, unlike NTM, to topical biguanides and diamidines, and topical corticosteroids may be of some benefit.

Herpetic keratitis. In necrotizing stromal keratitis, herpetic keratitis can cause dense white stromal infiltrates that may be confused with NTM keratitis. Special features that are more typically found in herpetic keratitis are decreased corneal sensation and previous or concomitant history of herpes labialis lesions. NTM keratitis may simulate a non-suppurative herpetic keratitis, especially in cases caused by Mycobacterium marinum. There may also be a dendritic or geographic epithelial defect with minimal stromal infiltration, misleading the clinician and prompting treatment with antivirals. This can lead to the development of a severe, wide corneal infiltrate.

7. Our experience

Keratitis caused by atypical *Mycobacteria* is characterized by an indolent course and poor response to antibiotics. The diagnosis requires a high index of suspicion and their treatment is usually very difficult. The early diagnosis of nontuberculous mycobacterial keratitis following LASIK is not easy, because the overlying, noninvolved stroma hinders the collection of sufficient material for culture. In addition, such organisms are only detectable by culture in special media, such as Lowenstein-Jensen, and special stains like Ziehl-Neelsen, which may not be included among routine cultures in the microbiology service.

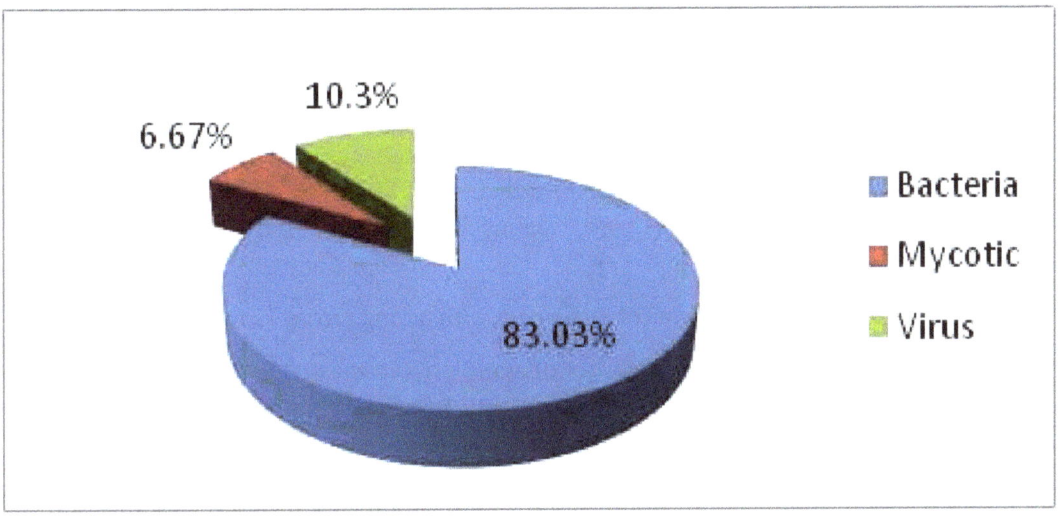

Table 4. Profile of microorganisms causing infectious keratitis; 2025 cases, during 10 years (2000-2010). Data of Asociación Para Evitar La Ceguera en México "Dr. Luis Sánchez Bulnes" I.A.P.

In our hospital, our service found an incidence of 2025 cases of infectious keratitis in the last 10 years (2000-2010). We found that 83.03% corresponded to infections caused by bacteria, 6.67% mycotic, and 10.3% originated by virus. [Table 4] Out of this percentage of bacterial keratitis, we report a frequency of 73.57% caused by gram positive, 9.22% caused by gram negative and 0.24% originated by nontuberculous mycobacteria. [Table 5]

In 100% of cases, the causative agent was *Mycobacterium chelonae,* correlating with the reported in literature.

Several authors reported an incidence between 0% and 1.5% of mycobacterial keratitis post-LASIK, our results (0.24%) correlate with these values. [29,31,32]

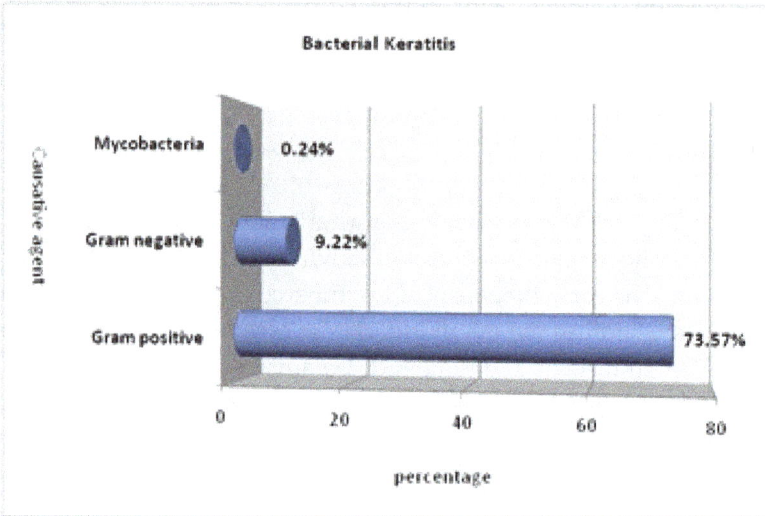

Table 5. The spectrum of bacterial agents causing keratitis. Data of Asociación Para Evitar La Ceguera en México "Dr. Luis Sánchez Bulnes" I.A.P

Almost all our cases (4 out of 6) of nontuberculous mycobacterial keratitis had as common background, a previous history of surgical trauma, specifically speaking of LASIK and PKP. We report one case of a contact lens user. A clinical summary of all cases reported in APEC to date, has been compiled in [Table 6,7]

The average age in our patients was of 36.6 years with a range from 12 to 58 years.

The average time that took from the onset of symptoms to the stabishment of correct diagnosis in patients that underwent previous surgical therapy was 4.25 weeks, which results similar to the average of weeks reported in literature (3.5 weeks). [1,33,34]

In our hospital 15,028 LASIK surgeries were performed from 2001-2011. We report in our service a total of 4 cases ok infectious keratitis following a LASIK procedure, which resembles an incidence of 1 infection every 3,757 procedures (0.026%). 2 cases (50%) correspond to post-LASIK keratitis caused by *Mycobacterium chelonae, a*nd the remaining 2 cases (50%) by gram positive bacteria (*Streptococcus pneumoniae*). These findings correlate with the reported by Solomon et al. (year 2003)of 1 infection for every 2919 procedures (0.034%), Donnenfeld et al. (year 2005) who reported an incidence of 1 in every 2131 (0.04%) LASIK procedures and LLovet et al. (year 2010) with an incidence of 1 in every 2841 cases (0.035%). The study also mentions that 65.5% (76 cases) of the infections reported, presented in the first week postoperatively. 6.03% (7 cases) presented in the second week, 14.65% (17 cases) presented between the second and fourth week and lastly 13.79% (16 cases) presented after 1 month. 2 of our cases, the ones caused by *Streptococcus pneumoniae,* presented in the first week postoperatively. 1 nontuberculous mycobacterial case presented between the second and fourth week (3 weeks), and lastly the remaining NTM keratitis case presented presented after 1 month (7 weeks). Speaking of ethiological factors, Solomon et al. reported that the most common microorganisms involved in post-LASIK keratitis are mycobacteria (48%) and coccus (33%), we found similar data in our retrospective analysis; Mycobacterial keratitis 50% and Streptococcus 50%.[30,39,40]

Case	Age/Sex	Eye	Delay in diagnosis	History	Infiltrates /localization	Initial VA	Previous Eye therapy	Causative organism	Medical therapy
1	57/F	OS	7 weeks	Unilateral redness, photophobia and tearing 6 weeks after bilateral LASIK associated with flap ulcer.	A central epithelial defect measuring 5.0 x 3.0 mm associated with stromal infiltrates involving area of flap. Hypopyon of 1mm.	*CF 50cm*	*Multitreated with Moxifloxacin, Dexamethasone Natamycin and Aciclovir*	*M. chelonae*	Amikacin 3.3% Gatifloxacin 0.3% Topical Rifampin Clarithromycin PO BID
2	58/M	OS	3 weeks	DM. Uneventful bilateral PKP as treatment for keratoglobus. 14 years later unilateral corneal trauma with graft dehiscense and endothelial rejection. Second graft evolved with redness, photophobia, pain and diminished VA, 3 weeks later.	Paracentral lesion 3.0 x 2.0 mm at the graft-host junction, infiltrate with irregular edges, satellite lesion.	*CF 2m*	*Multitreated with Neomycin, Polymixin and Dexamethasone phosphate*	*M. chelonae*	Amikacin 3.3% Gatifloxacin 0.3% Clarithromycin PO BID Fluorometholone
3	27/M	OS	4 weeks	PKP for herpetic leucoma, 4 months later presented with loose suture and ulcer at the site.	Ulcer in graft-host junction.	CF 1m	Multitreated with Prednisolone, Ciprofloxacin, Vancomycin, Fluorometholone	*M. chelonae*	Gatifloxacin 0.3% Ciprofloxacin PO BID Lubricant eye drops
4	43/F	OS	6 weeks	Redness, photophobia and tearing. Contact lens user.	Paracentral infiltrate with satellite lesion.	CF 2m	Multitreated with Vancomycin, Tobramycin, Ofloxacin	*M. chelonae*	Amikacin c/3hrs. Gatifloxacin 0.3% Clarithromycin PO BID
5	23/M	OD	3 weeks	Bilateral LASIK. post surgery unilateral hyperemia, photophobia and tearing.	3.5 mm intralamellar central infiltrate	20/400	Multitreated with Ofloxacin, Vancomycin, Moxifloxacin	*M. chelonae*	Amikacin c/3hrs. Gatifloxacin 0.3% Clarithromycin PO BID

F=female, M=male, CF=count fingers, OS=left eye, OD=right eye, PO=per oral, BID=twice daily, DM=Diabetes Mellitus, VA= visual acuity, PKP=penetrating keratoplasty, LASIK=laser in situ keratomileusis

Table 6. Nontuberculousmycobacterialkeratitis in patients of Asociación Para Evitar La Ceguera en México "Dr. Luis Sánchez Bulnes" I.A.P.

Velotta reported that nearly 90% of NTM keratitis after LASIK cases are unilateral, all of our cases presented in just one eye.

Infectious keratitis after penetrating keratoplasty (PKP) is not a frequent complication with an incidence ranging from 1.8% to 11.0%; however, this infection has a high risk of loss of corneal clarity. In our present analysis, the remaining 2 patients that underwent surgical procedures, developed nontuberculous mycobacterial keratitis posterior to penetrating keratoplasty. Both cases were promptly diagnosed after onset of symptoms, resulting in satisfactory outcomes and good final visual acuity [Table 7] [Figure 8,9]

Case	Surgical Treatment	Follow up	Outcome	Final Visual Acuity	Refraction
1	Flap amputation + scraping + irrigation with gatifloxacin 0.3% First PKP (*with recurrence*) Second PKP + Ahmed valve implant + ECCE & IOL	30 months	resolved	*20/70*	*+8.00=-4.00x140°*
2	None	18 months	resolved	*20/30*	*Contact lens +3.50 D*
3	None	10 months	resolved	20/30	*Contact lens* 8.30 Power -7.00, Diameter 9.6
4	None	3 months	resolved	20/20	-4:00=-3:00 X180°
5	None	3 months	resolved	20/60	-2.00=-1.00x45°

PKP=penetrating keratoplasty, ECCE=extracapsular, IOL=intraocular lens.

Table 7. Surgical treatment and outcome in nontuberculousmycobacterial keratitis in patients of Asociación Para Evitar La Ceguera en México "Dr. Luis Sánchez Bulnes" I.A.P.

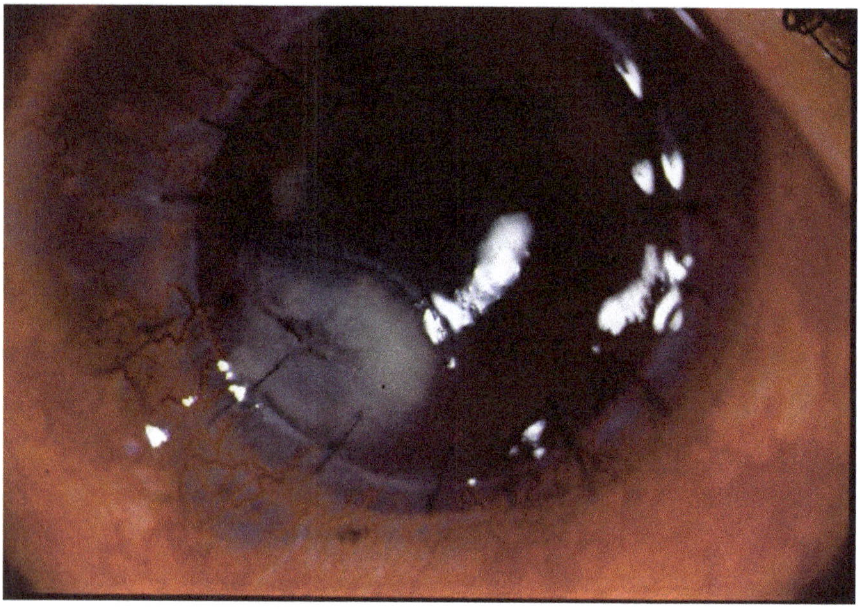

Figure 8. Patient 2, clinical examination 4 weeks after penetrating keratoplasty with conjunctival hyperemia and corneal infiltrate (3.0 x 2.0 mm) in graft-host junction caused by *Mycobacterium chelonae.*

8. Treatment

Management of this type of infectious keratitis often traduces in a medical challenge. In cases of identified NTM corneal infection, there is considerable benefit from the use of combined antibiotics, since atypical mycobacteria have a slower growth rate compared to other bacteria and may become resistant to a single antibiotic class during the course of extended treatment.

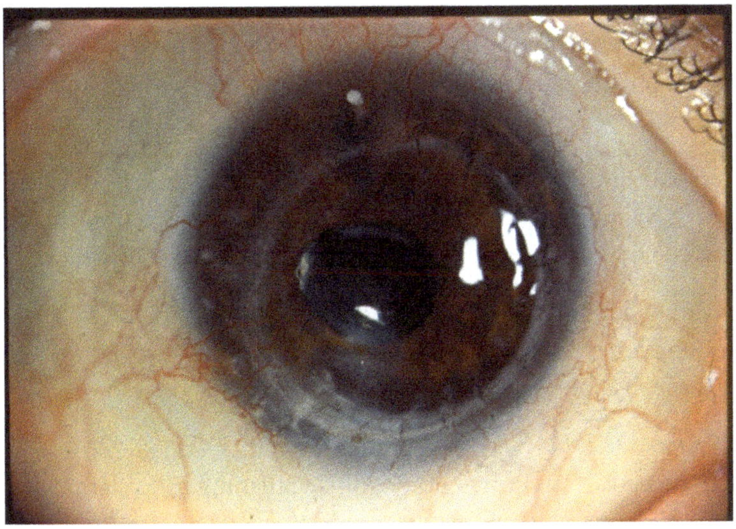

Figure 9. Patient 2, eighteen months after therapy discontinuation. Corneal graft is infection-free and clear in the visual axis; best-corrected vision of 20/30 was attained with a +3.50-D contact lens.

The base of treatment consists of a double approach; appropriate antibiotic and judicious surgical intervention. Such antimicrobial choice becomes complicated since a poor correlation exists between *in vitro* susceptibility profiles and the final clinical response. We recommend surgical debridement, depending on the case, to facilitate drug penetration to the interlamellar space. In some cases, flap amputation may be necessary, the rationale for this procedure is to lower the bacterial load, remove necrotic as well as infected tissue, and permit better antibiotic penetration. We recommend this surgical procedures in recalcitrant post-LASIK NTM keratitis to maintain the infection under control.

De La Cruz et al. suggest initial combined antibiotic therapy that includes at least 2 of the 3 most susceptible agents (clarithromycin, amikacin, and fourth-generation fluoroquinolones) for rapidly growing mycobacteria specially if known resistance has been documented. The initial therapy recommended for many years has been the use of topical Amikacin sulfate 20-40mg/mL.This antibiotic is the most frequently used agent in the treatment of NTM keratitis. In our institution we use amikacin sulfate (Amikin® 500mg injectable solution. Bristol-Myers Squibb de México S. de R.L. de C.V.)diluted to a concentration of 20mg/mL, one drop every hour and dose-response. Even though this antibiotic constitutes the first line of treatment against atypical mycobacterial keratitis, only a success rate of 30-40% has been reported. This therapeutic agent has also been associated with high epithelium toxicity when it is applied for a prolonged course.

We recommend the addition of two additional antibiotics to the drug scheme, such as a macrolide like clarithromycin and a fourth-generation fluoroquinolone like gatifloxacin.[Table 6] In our hospital we employ oral clarithromycin Klaricid H.P.® 500mg (Abbott Laboratories de México S.A. de C.V. México, D.F.) twice daily, and Zymar® (gatifloxacin 0.3% Allergan Labs, Irvine, CA).

Fluoroquinolone antibiotics are concentration-dependent killers. Therefore, they require a minimum inhibitory concentration (MIC) to be reached in order to be effective. In vitro studies have shown that fourth-generation fluoroquinolones are effective against atypical mycobacteria, inhibiting 90% of isolates after reaching its proper concentration.[23,43]

The fourth-generation fluoroquinolones have significant advantages over earlier generation fluoroquinolones in treating mycobacterial infections, including superior bactericidal activity, higher corneal concentrations, and decreased risk for bacterial resistance.

The reason for adding a fourth-generation fluoroquinolone to the therapeutic scheme is that 8-metoxy-fluoroquinolones such as gatifloxacin and moxifloxacin has shown better in vitro activity against these organisms, in comparison to second-generation fluoroquinolones like ciprofloxacin.

Furthermore, the molecular structures of moxifloxacin and gatifloxacin have a greater binding affinity for 2 of the enzymes necessary for bacterial DNA synthesis (deoxyribonucleic acid gyrase [also called topoisomerase II] and tipoisomerase IV) in both gram-negative and gram-positive microorganisms. By inhibiting such enzymes, these bacteria require to undergo two genetic mutations in order to create resistance. Older fluoroquinolones adequately inhibit tipoisomerase II in gram-negative microorganisms but are not as effective in inhibiting topoisomerase IV in gram-positive organisms.

The great effectiveness of fourth-generation fluoroquinolones rely due to their superior bactericidal activity, the ability to reach higher corneal concentration, and better resistance pattern.In a rabbit model, fourth-generation fluoroquinolones were found to be synergistic to our first-line drug options, amikacin and clarithromycin against *M. chelonae.* Lastly, considering antibiotic resistance as an emerging problem; Ford et al. reported in their study that more than 60% of atypical mycobacteria are unresponsive to second-generation fluoroquinolones. [5,34]

Lazar et al reported a torpid answer to the use of Rifampin in nontuberculous mycobacteria ocular infections. In our experience, we required to add a new antibiotic drug in patient 1 (Table 6), when we reached the three antibiotics suggested by diverse authors in literature (Amikacin, Clarythromicin and Gatifloxacin). We added topical rifampin to the scheme obtaining positive outcomes. We prepared a topical solution of Rifampin at our hospital by dissolving 300mg of Rifampin (Rifadin®) (SANOFI-AVENTIS de México, S.A. de C.V.) with 10mL of Sodium Hyaluronate (Lagricel® SOPHIA, S.A. de C.V., Laboratorios. Guadalajara, México) indicating a drop every hour and dose-response.

Management of mycobacterial keratitis usually requires a prolonged and intensive therapy consisting of topical and systemic medication. In our experience, medical treatment of NTM keratitis can prolong as long as 30 months. Shih et al have reported full months of therapy even when the appropriate antibiotic, chosen by drug sensitivity test results, is used. In [Table 8]we summarize our suggested treatment for the proper management of nontuberculous Mycobacterial keratitis.

Suggested treatment		
Triple Antibiotic Therapy	*Topical*	1. Amikacin 20 mg/mL 2. Fourth-generation fluoroquinolone (gatifloxacin)
	Systemic	3. Clarithromycin 500mg PO BID
		* *In case of resistance addition of Rifampin 30mg/mL.*
SurgicalTherapy		1. Flap lift and irrigation 2. Flap amputation in post-LASIK 3. Biopsy and culture 4. Penetrating keratoplasty

Table 8. We suggest a triple antibiotic treatment combined if needed with surgical therapy.

9. Modification to initial therapy

The medical response of mycobacterial keratitis to antibiotic therapy can be achieved by constant clinical observance. This can be difficult to appreciate in the first days of treatment due to increase in inflammation and local reaction to topical agents. The clinical response varies depending on the microorganism and pathogenicity of the mycobacteria, duration of the infection, risk factors involved and the patient's individual response (immunosuppresion).

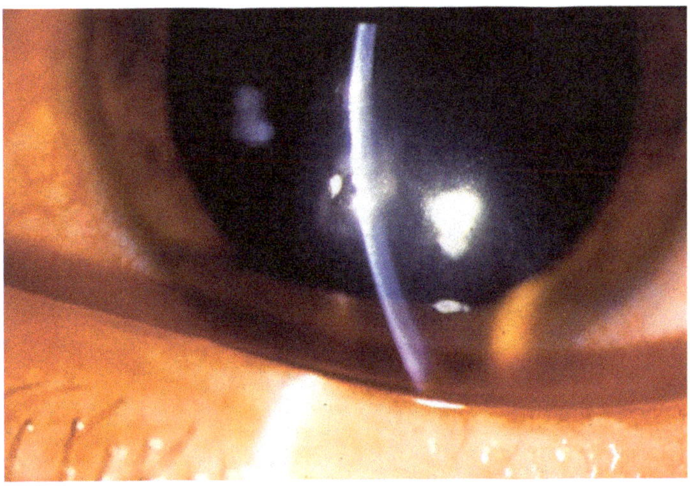

Figure 10. Patient 4 presented in the first clinical examination a paracentral infiltrate caused by *Mycobacteria chelonae*. Previous to initiation of proper antibiotic treatment. At this moment visual acuity was count fingers 2 meters.

If the chosen therapy is effective, some response should manifest within the first of 24 to 72 hours of appropriate treatment. [Figure 10,11]. Said response manifests with the decrease of stromal infiltrates and less anterior chamber inflammation in case it exists. [Figure 12, 13]

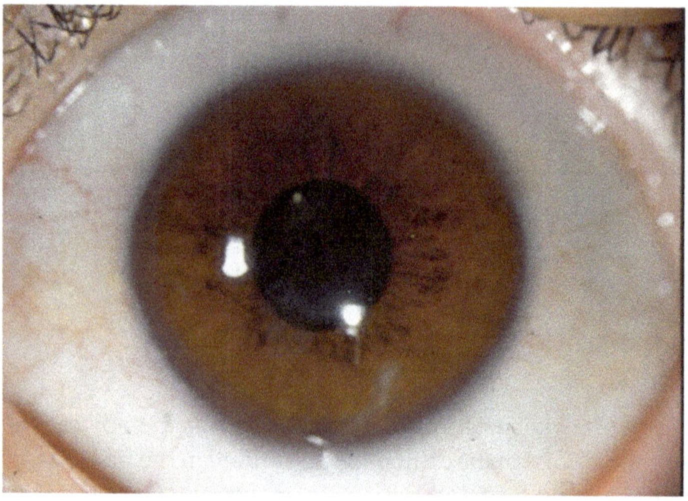

Figure 11. Patient 4 at 3 months follow-up after proper antibiotic treatment was applied. Final visual acuity was 20/30.

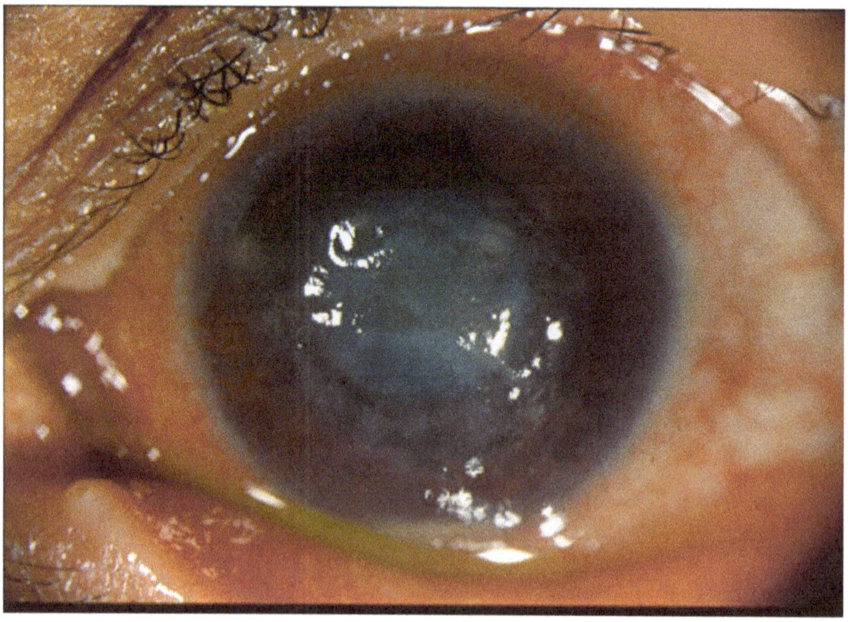

Figure 12. Patient 1 with preceding hypopyon (black arrow) and anterior chamber reaction who underwent a therapeutic flap amputation procedure.

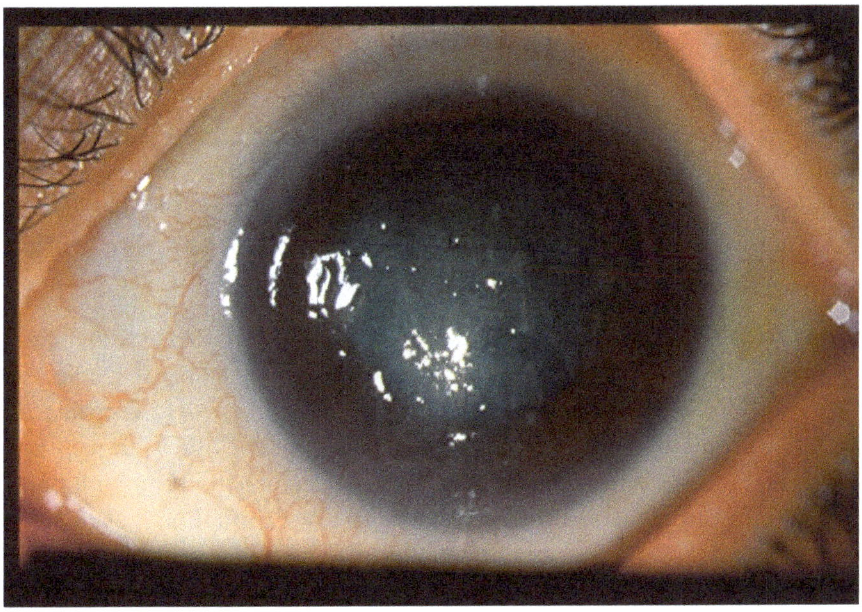

Figure 13. Absence of ahypopyon seen in Patient 1 as a manifestation of positive response to antibiotic treatment.

If clinical improvement exists at 48 hours of initiation of treatment, we encourage to continue the same pharmacological agents, reducing the administration time to 1 drop every 2 hours until completion of 5 days with night rest. After the 5 days, if further improvement exists, antibiotic doses should be decreased progressively in function of clinical response, drug tolerance and sensitivity tests results. Antibiotic with the best sensitivity should be the one chosen to continue the treatment for 2-3 more weeks.

Special caution should be kept when therapy is suspended, as some microorganisms may remain in corneal tissue. In this case, a prolonged treatment may be required.

If lesion progression occurs after 48 hours of initiation of treatment, manifested by evident increase in size, stromal thinning or incomplete resolution of symptoms, the ophthalmologist should consider a lack of sensitivity to the chosen treatment or a failure in the patient's attachment to the therapy. Culture results should be rechecked as well as sensitivity test results, as an addition of a different antimicrobial agent might be needed.[Table 9]

Positive clinical response parameters	Negative clinical response parameters
Peripheral corneal clearance of infiltrates and density reduction.	Increase in size or depth.
Decrease in stromal edema.	Stromal thinning.
Less anterior chamber inflammation.	Partial resolution of symptoms.
Corneal epithelial regeneration.	

Table 9. Response parameters associated with antibiotic therapy

10. Complementary therapy

Pain management: The cornea is a highly innervated tissue. Despite most of the times, these lesions tend to have an indolent course, on occasions, patients can refer any degree of pain, ranging from mild to severe. The clinician should administer a cyclopegic agent to ease the symptoms caused by ciliary spasms and to prevent the formation of sinequiae. We recommend the employment of cyclopentolate 1% eye drops or Atropine 1% collyrium every 12 hours.

Topical corticosteroids: Its role and appropriate moment of use is a controversial topic. Corticosteroids are applied to diminish the host's inflammatory response, capable of producing tissue destruction. Its use is also aimed to decrease the subsequent corneal cicatrization. Nevertheless, some potential adverse effects of these agents include bacterial growth stimulation by local immunosuppression, decrease in phagocytic activity, inhibition of collagen synthesis, drug-induced glaucoma and secondary cataract formation. Several experimental studies have shown a lack of harmful effects associated by addition of steroids to the preexistent bactericidal regime in keratitis. However, other studies documented an increase in bacterial growth with the addition of topical steroids to previous therapy. Due to the uncertain role of these agents in keratitis caused by nontuberculous mycobacteria, we recommend the use of low doses of steroids like fluorometholone (Flumetol® SOPHIA, S.A. de C.V., Laboratorios. Guadalajara, México) if it is considered appropriate, only when certainty exists of the infectious process being under control or in an inactive phase.

Alternate medical treatment: Authors have recommended the use of Azithromycin 2mg/mL or 1%, prepared Clarithromycin eye drops 10mg/mL, imipenem, tobramycin and systemic doxyciclin. We do not have experience with these drugs. [1,5]

Surgical treatment Conjunctival flap: Its purpose is aimed to provide blood vessels to the infected area, thus promoting curation. It is indicated in uncontrolled progression of the corneal lesion or infiltrates, limbal compromise with imminent scleritis or elevated risk of corneal perforation.

Therapeutic penetrating keratoplasty: It is difficult to perform in the initial stages of mycobacterium keratitis, furthermore it involves a higher incidence of complications and an inferior graft survival rate in comparison to optical PKP in an inactive process. We recommend to avoid this surgical option when possible. The indications for urgent therapeutic PKP are:

- Uncontrolled progression of the infection.
- Imminent risk of corneal perforation
- Confirmed cornealperforation.

We recommend maximal antibiotic therapy for 48 hours prior to surgery to decrease the number of bacterial colonies as much as possible and consequently the diminish the risk of endophthalmitis. Additional to topical antibiotics, we suggest the use of systemic antimicrobial and antiinflammatory agents in the preoperative period. The trepan employed on the recipient's cornea should be of enough size to extract the entire infected area, and the donor's corneal graft should be 0.5mm bigger than the measurement made on the recipient's cornea. It is advisable to obtain cultures from one half of the obtained cornea tissue (including stains and special culture media), and the other half should be sent for histopathological study. Sutures should be placed separately due to intense inflammatory reaction. In the postoperative period, corticosteroid therapy should be continued as well as specific antibiotics. Systemic therapy should continue. Posterior to the complete resolution of corneal infection, an optical PKP is an option of treatment to seek visual rehabilitation, as seen in out patient that appears on [Table 7]. As a consequence of the long term infectious process caused by mycobacterium keratitis, secondary cataract formation can be induced by the production of toxins, iridocyclitis, treatment toxicity and corticosteroid usage. For this complication, and optic PKP combined with a cataract extraction and Ahmed valve implantation can be considered as a treatment option, as seen in patient 1 who developed glaucoma.[Table 6,7]

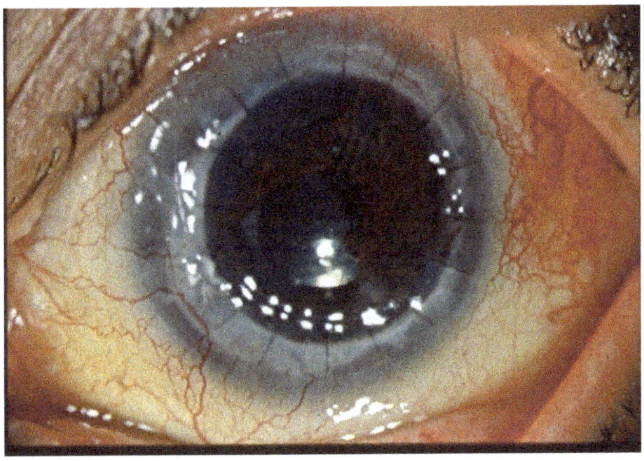

Figure 14. Patient 1 treated with optic PKP combined with Ahmed valve implantation and cataract extraction with colocation of intraocular lens posterior to the resolution of nontuberculous mycobacterial keratitis.

11. Conclusion

We describe our experience in patients who developed keratitis caused by nontuberculous mycobacteria. As the most common cause of post-LASIK keratitis is NTM, a greater degree of suspicion, recognition of typical clinical course and presentation, and knowledge of similar cluster of NTM keratitis prompts rapid institution of appropriate antibiotic therapy, granting this cases with a better prognosis in comparison with those of late diagnosis. Antibiotic resistance continues to be an emerging problem, thus a limitation in the coverage of this pharmacological agents exists. We emphasize the need for vigilance in the follow-up of patients. Appropriate adjustment of antimicrobial therapy may be required based on cultures and sensitivity tests when atypical mycobacteria are responsible for corneal infection.

We believe that fourth-fluoroquinolones adequately combined with first-line antibiotics constitute the best option so far to treat keratitis caused by atypical mycobacteria.

Acknowledgements

We express our gratitude to the cornea service and pathology service at Asociación Para Evitar La Ceguera en México "Hospital Dr. Luís Sánchez Bulnes" for their valuable contribution with images that helped making this chapter possible. Also to Miss. Elia Portugal for her assistance in the translation of this work.

Author details

Ana Lilia Pérez-Balbuena[1], David Arturo Ancona-Lezama[1], Lorena Gutiérrez-Sánchez[1] and Virginia Vanzzini-Zago[2]

1 Cornea Service. Asociación para Evitar la Ceguera en México I.A.P. "Hospital. Dr. Luis Sánchez Bulnes". Vicente García Torres,México D.F., México

2 Laboratory of Microbiology. Asociación para Evitar la Ceguera en México I.A.P. "Hospital. Dr. Luis Sánchez Bulnes". Vicente García Torres, México D.F., México

References

[1] Moorthy RS, Valluri S, Rao NA. Major Review; Nontuberculous Mycobacterial Ocular and Adnexal Infections.SurvOphthalmol 2012;57:202-235.

[2] Pallikaris IG, Papatzanaki ME, Stathi EZ, et al. Laser in situ keratomileusis. Lasers Surg Med 1990;10:463-468.

[3] Krachmer JH, Mannis MJ, Holland EJ. Cornea, Chapter 82. Nontuberculous Mycobacteria Keratitis. 3rd edition. ElSevier Mosby.

[4] Chandra NS, Torres MF, Winthrop KL, Bruckner DA, Heidemann DG, Calvet HM, Yakrus M, Mondino BJ, Holland GN. Cluster of Mycobacterium chelonae keratitis cases following laser in-situ keratomileusis. Am J Ophthalmol. 2001:132(6):819-830.

[5] Ford JG, Huang AJ, Pflugfelder SC, Alfonso EC, Forster RK, Miller D. Nontuberculous mycobacterial keratitis in south Florida. Ophthalmology. 1998:105(9):1652-1658.

[6] Freitas D, Alvarenga L, Sampaio J, Mannis M, Sato E, Sousa L, Vieira L, Yu MC, Martins MC, Hoffling-Lima A, Belfort R Jr. An outbreak of Mycobacterium chelonae infection after LASIK. Ophthalmology. 2003:110(2):276-285.

[7] Garg P, Bansal AK, Sharma S, Vemuganti GK. Bilateral infectious keratitis after laser in situ keratomileusis: a case report and review of the literature. Ophthalmology. 2001;108(1):121-125.

[8] Kouyoumdjian GA, Forstot SL, Durairaj VD, Damiano RE. Infectious keratitis after laser refractive surgery. Ophthalmology. 2001 Jul;108(7):1266-1268.

[9] Maloney RK. Cluster of Mycobacterium chelonae keratitis cases following laser in situ keratomileusis. Am J Ophthalmol. 2002:134(2):298-299.

[10] Solomon A, Karp CL, Miller D, Dubovy SR, Huang AJ, Culbertson WW. Mycobacterium interface keratitis after laser in situ keratomileusis. Ophthalmology. 2001:108(12):2201-2208.

[11] Sossi N, Feldman RM, Feldman ST, Frueh BE, McGuiere G, Davis C. Mycobacterium gordonae keratitis after penetrating keratoplasty Arch. Ophthalmol. 1991:109(8): 1064-1065.

[12] Winthrop KL, Steinberg EB, Holmes G, Kainer MA, Werner SB, Winquist A, Vugia DJ. Epidemic and sporadic cases of nontuberculous mycobacterial keratitis associated with laser in situ keratomileusis. Am J Ophthalmol. 2003;135(2):223-224.

[13] Pfyffer GE, Palicova F. Mycobacterium: General characteristics, laboratory detection, and staining procedures. In Versalovic J, Carrol KC, Funke G, Jorgensen JH, Landry ML, Warnock DW. Manual of Clinical Microbiology 10th ed. ASM press. Washington DC. 472-502.

[14] Runyon EH. Identification of mycobacterial pathogens using colony characteristics. Am J ClinPathol. 1970;54:578-586.

[15] Vincent V, Brown-Elliot BA, Jost KC Jr, et al. Mycobacterium: Phenotypic and Genotypic Identification, in Murray PR, Baron EJ, Jorgensen JH, Pfaller MA, Yolken RH (eds) Manual of Clinical Microbiology. Vol. 1. Washington, DC, ASM Press, 2003, 8th ed, pp 560-658.

[16] Broadway DC, Kerr-Muir MG, Eykyn SJ, Pambakian H. Mycobacterium chelonei keratitis: a case report and review of previously reported cases. Eye 1994; 8: 134-142.

[17] Fowler AM, Dutton JJ, Fowler WC, et al. Mycobacterium chelonaecanaliculitis associated with SmartPlug use. Ophthal Plast ReconstrSurg. 2008;24:241-243.

[18] Chang WJ, Tse DT, Rosa RH Jr, et al. Periocular atypical mycobacterial infections. [see comment]. Ophthalmology. 1999;106:86-90.

[19] Mauriello JA Jr. Atypical Mycobacterial Study G. Atypical mycobacterial infection of the periocular region after periocular and facial surgery. OphthalPlastReconstr Surg. 2003;19:182-188

[20] Margo CE, Pavan PR. Mycobacterium chelonae conjunctivitis and scleritis following vitrectomy. Arch Ophthalmol. 2000;118:1125—1128.

[21] Nash KA, Zhang Y, Brown-Elliott BA, et al. Molecular basis of intrinsic macrolide resistance in clinical isolates of Mycobacterium fortuitum. J AntimicrobChemother. 2005; 55:170-177.

[22] Benz MS, Murray TG, Dubovy SR, et al. Endophthalmitis caused by Mycobacterium chelonaeabscessus after intravitreal injection of triamcinolone. Arch Ophthalmol. 2003;121:271-273.

[23] Velotta JT. Nontuberculous (atypical) mycobacterial keratitis after LASIK: current status and clinical implications. Cornea. 2005;24:245-255

[24] Rola NH, Baha N, Hayham IS,Randa H, Johnny MK. Recalcitrant post-LASIK Mycobacterium chelonae Keratitis Eradicates after the Use of Fourtn–Generation Fluoroquinolone .Ophthalmology 2006;113:950-954.

[25] Lazar M, Nemet P, Bracha R, et al. Mycobacterium fortuitum keratitis. Am J Ophthalmol 1974;78:530-532.

[26] Reviglio V, Rodriguez ML, Picotti GS, et al. Mycobacterium Chelonae Keratitis Following Laser in situ Keratomileusis. J Refract Surg 1998;14:357-360.

[27] Mirate D, Hull D, Steel J, et al. Mycobacterium chelonei keratitis: a case report. Br J Ophthalmol 1983;67:324-327.

[28] Zabel R, Mintsioulis G, MacDonald I. Mycobacterium keratitis in a soft contact lens wearer. Can J Ophthalmol. 1988;23:315-317.

[29] Chang MA, Jain S, Azar DT. Infections following laser in situ keratomileusis: an integration of the published literature. SurvOphthalmol. 2004;49:269-280.

[30] Solomon R, Donnenfeld ED, Azar DT. Infectious keratitis after laser in situ keratomileusis: Results of an ASCRS survey. J Cataract Refract Surg 2003;29:2001-2006

[31] Lin RT, Maloney RK- Flap complications associated with lamellar refractive surgery. Am J Ophthalmol 1999;127(2):129-136.

[32] Machat J. LASIK complications and their management. In Machat J, editor: Excimer laser refractive surgery: practice and principles, Thorofare, NJ 1996, Slacc 359-400.

[33] Alvarenga L, Fretias D, Hofling-Lima AL, et al. Infectious post-LASIK crystalline keratopathy caused by nontuberculous mycobacteria. Cornea. 2002;21:426-429.

[34] De La Cruz J, Behlau I, Pineda R. Atypical mycobacteria keratitis after laser in situ keratomileusis unresponsive to fourth-generation fluoroquinolone therapy. J Cataract ReractSurg 2007;33:1318-1321.

[35] Shukla PK, Kumar M, Keshava GBS. Mycotic keratitis: an overview of diagnosis and therapy. Mycoses. 2008;51:183-199.

[36] Dart JKG, Saw VPJ, Kilvington S. Acanthamoeba keratitis: diagnosis and treatment update 2009. Am J Ophthalmol. 2009;148:487-499.

[37] Knickelbein JE, Hendricks RL, Charukamnoetkanok P. Management of herpes simplex virus stromal keratitis: An evidence-based review. SurvOphthalmol. 2009;54:226-234.

[38] Schonherr U, Naumann GO, Lang GK, et al. Sclerokeratitis caused by Mycobacterium marinum. Am J Ophthalmol. 1989;108:607-608

[39] Donnenfeld ED, Kim TK, Holland EJ Azar DT, Palmon FR, Rubenstein JB, Daya S, Yoo SH. American Society of Cataract and Refractive Sugery Cornea Clinical Committee. ASCRS White Paper. Management of infectious keratitis following laser in situ keratomileusis. J Cataract Refract Surg 2005;31:2008-2011.

[40] Llovet F, de Rojas V, Interlandi E, Martín C, Cobo-Soriano R, Ortega-Usobiaga J, Baviera J. Infectiouskeratitia in 204586 LASIK procedures. Ophthalmology 2010;117:232-238.

[41] Pérez-Balbuena AL, Vanzzini-Zago V, Garza M, Cuevas-Cancino D. Atypical Mycobacterium Keratitis Associated With Penetrating Keratoplasty: Case Report of Successful Therapy With Topical Gatifloxacin 0.3%. Cornea 2010;29:468-470.

[42] Bullington RH Jr, Lanier JD, Font RL. Nontuberculous mycobacteria keratitis; report of two cases and review of the literature. Arch Ophthalmol 1992;110:519-524.

[43] Hu F-R, Luh K-T. Topical ciprofloxacin for treating nontuberculous mycobacterial keratitis. Ophthalmology 1998;105:269-272.

[44] Schlech BA, Alfonso E. Overview of the potency of moxifloxacin ophthalmic solution 0.5% (VIGAMOX®). SurvOphthalmol 2005;50(suppl):S7-S15.

[45] Hamam RN, Noureddin B, Salti H, et al. Recalcitrant post-LASIK Mycobacterium chelonae keratitis eradicated after the use of fourth-generation fluoroquinolones. Ophthalmology 2006;113:950-954.

[46] Hyon JY, Joo MJ, Hose S, et al comparative efficacy of topical gatifloxacin with ciprofloxacin, amikacin, and clarithromycin in the treatment of experimental Mycobacterium chelonae keratitis. Arch Ophthalmol 2004,122:1166-1169.

[47] Shih et al have reported full months of therapy even when the appropriate antibiotic, chosen by drug sensitivity test results, is used. (Shih MH, Huang FC. Effects of Photodynamic Therapy on Rapidly Growing Nontuberculous Mycobacteria Keratitis. Invest Ophthalmol Vis Sci. 2011; 52:223-229.

[48] Banoch PR, Hay GJ, McDonellPJ, et al. A rat model of bacterial keratitis :effects of antibiotics and corticosteroids. Arch Ophthalmol 1980,98:718-20.

[49] Leibowitz HM, Kupferman A. Topically administered corticosteroids: effect with antibiotic treated bacterial keratitis. Arch opthalmol 1980, 98: 1287-1290.

[50] Pérez-Balbuena AL, Santander-García D, Vanzzini-Zago V. Therapeutic Keratoplasty for Microbial Keratitis. In: MoscaL. Keratoplasties. Surgical Techinques and Complications. Rijeka: InTech; 2011.

10

Genetics and Environmental Stress Factor Contributions to Anterior Segment Malformations and Glaucoma

Yoko A. Ito and Michael A. Walter

1. Introduction

Glaucoma is one of the leading causes of irreversible blindness worldwide [1]. A gradual loss of retinal ganglion cells (RGCs) result in degeneration of the optic nerve head and visual field loss. Glaucoma is an age-related disease with a strong genetic basis. The risk of developing glaucoma significantly increases after age 40 [2,3]. An estimated 79.6 million people worldwide will have glaucoma by 2020 [1]. Patients with mutations in glaucoma-associated genes are more likely to develop juvenile-onset and early adult-onset glaucoma. In any case, early detection of glaucoma is essential to effectively manage the progression of the disease by preventing further loss of RGCs. Despite many years of research in this field, the precise cause(s) of RGC death remain unknown. The pathophysiology of glaucoma is complicated as environmental, genetic, and even stochastic factors all contribute to the pathology of glaucoma. Also, both the posterior segment, where the RGCs are located, and the anterior segment of the eye play key roles in the disease.

Glaucoma can be classified as being primary, secondary, or congenital. These groups can then be further categorized to be open-angle or closed-angle, depending on the anterior chamber angle. In closed-angle glaucoma, the angle between the iris and the cornea is closed resulting in obstruction of aqueous humor flow. Primary glaucoma is non-syndromic and is not associated with any underlying condition. Primary congenital glaucoma is a rare form of glaucoma present at birth or within the first two years after birth. Glaucoma that develops as a result of an underlying ocular or systemic condition or eye injury is categorized as secondary glaucoma. Pseudoexfoliative glaucoma is an example of secondary glaucoma whereby fibrillar extracellular material deposits and accumulates in various ocular tissues, predisposing the patient to developing glaucoma.

Primary open angle glaucoma (POAG) is a common type of glaucoma where the iridocorneal angle is unobstructed. Although POAG can occur in patients with normal intraocular pressure (IOP), sometimes referred to as normal-tension glaucoma, elevated IOP is a major risk factor of developing POAG. IOP is dependent on proper flow of aqueous humor from the site of production in the posterior chamber to the site of drainage in the anterior chamber of the eye. The anterior chamber structures that function in regulating the drainage of aqueous humor from the eye are the trabecular meshwork (TM) and Schlemm's canal. Disruptions of the aqueous humor flow pathway are predicted to result in elevated IOP.

In this chapter, the recent advances in research regarding the contribution of the TM in maintaining proper IOP will be reviewed. An overview of the anterior chamber drainage structures, the TM and Schlemm's canal, and how these structures maintain the aqueous humor outflow pathway will be provided. Also, the changes that occur in the TM during the normal aging process and in the glaucoma phenotype will be compared. Then, the specific types of stresses that TM cells are exposed to, mainly mechanical, oxidative, and phagocytic stresses, and the effects these stresses have on gene expression will be examined. Recent advances in technology have enabled the analysis of global gene expression profiles. These analyses have revealed that signal transduction pathways play an important role in the cellular adaptive response to environmental stresses. Finally, the effect that environmental stresses have on glaucoma-associated genes will be considered.

2. Trabecular meshwork and aqueous humor outflow pathway

Aqueous humor is a colourless and transparent fluid that makes contact with various structures in both the anterior and posterior chambers of the eye including the lens, iris, and cornea. The lens and the cornea are clear and avascular, which enables light to be effectively transmitted to the photoreceptors in the back of the eye. Aqueous humor provides nutrients to the avascular lens and cornea and also removes metabolic waste products. The composition of aqueous humor has been of great interest due to the potential regulatory effects on all the structures to which it makes contact. For example, the presence of antioxidants such as glutathione and ascorbic acid [4,5] in the aqueous humor suggest that this fluid affects the ability of cells to respond and adapt to stress.

Aqueous humor flows from the site of production, which is the non-pigmented ciliary epithelial cells [6,7] in the posterior chamber, to the site of drainage, which is the TM and Schlemm's canal in the anterior chamber (Figure 1). Production and drainage of aqueous humor is a continuous and dynamic process. Diurnal variations in aqueous humor turnover rates occur ranging from 3.0μL/min in the morning to 1.5μL/min at night [8]. The balance between aqueous humor production and drainage is essential for maintaining a healthy IOP of approximately 15mmHg within the eye [9]. Abnormalities in aqueous humor drainage due to increased resistance at the TM are thought to result in elevated IOP, which is a major risk factor for developing glaucoma [10].

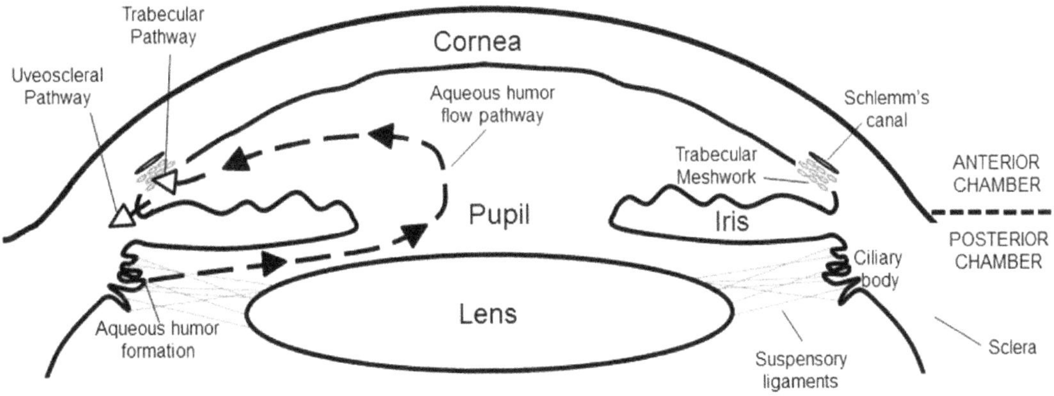

Figure 1. Schematic diagram of aqueous humor flow pathway. Aqueous humor is produced by the ciliary body in the posterior chamber and then flows into the anterior chamber. The majority of the aqueous humor will be drained from the eye via the trabecular pathway through the trabecular meshwork (TM) and Schlemm's canal. The rest of the aqueous humor is drained via the uveoscleral pathway. Increased resistance occurs when the TM and Schelmm's canal malfunctions. This disruption in aqueous humor outflow leads to increased intraocular pressure (IOP), which is a major risk factor for developing glaucoma.

Aqueous humor is drained from the eye by two distinct outflow pathways: the trabecular (aka conventional) pathway and the uveoscleral (aka unconventional) pathway. The uveoscleral pathway is an IOP-independent pathway in which the aqueous humor leaves the anterior chamber by passing through the ciliary muscle bundles into the supraciliary and suprachoroidal spaces and eventually into the sclera [11,12]. Direct measurement of the percentage of aqueous humor leaving the human eye via the uveoscleral pathway has proven to be difficult [13]. There appears to be great variation between individuals with values ranging from 36% to 54% in healthy young subjects [14,15]. The percentage of aqueous humor leaving the eye via the uveoscleral pathway decreases with age with values ranging from 4% to 46% in older subjects [15,16]. Thus, as aging progresses, a larger portion of aqueous humor is drained via the trabecular pathway.

Despite the individual variations, it is generally accepted that in humans, the majority of aqueous humor is transported through the TM via the trabecular pathway. Disruption of aqueous humor drainage through the trabecular pathway is thought to be the major contributing factor to alteration of IOP. The TM is a multi-layered tissue located in the anterior chamber angle. From the anterior chamber the aqueous humor passes through the multiple layers of the TM: the uveal meshwork, the corneoscleral meshwork, and the juxtacanalicular meshwork (also known as the cribriform plexus). Each layer consists of a central connective tissue (aka beam) surrounded by an outer endothelial layer. Connecting fibrils tightly connect the network of elastic fibres in the juxtacanalicular meshwork to the inner endothelial wall of Schlemm's canal [17-20]. As the aqueous humor passes through each layer of the TM, the intercellular space narrows resulting in increased resistance. Then, aqueous humor progresses through the inner endothelial cell layer of Schlemm's canal. The endothelial cells of Schlemm's canal express the tight junction protein Zona occludens-1 (ZO-1), which allows aqueous humor to be transported via the intercellular route [21]. The aqueous humor is also transported via the transcellular route through giant vacuoles [22-24]. Aqueous humor passes through Schlemm's canal and returns to the general circulation via the aqueous and episcleral veins [23,25]. IOP is affected by the episcleral venous pressure and the resistance to aqueous humor flow within the TM. Episcleral venous pressure directly affects IOP because aqueous humor must flow out of the eye against the pressure in the episcleral veins. The main source of resistance to aqueous humor flow is thought to be located in the intercellular (aka subendothelial) region of the juxtacanalicular network [26-29].

Extracellular matrix (ECM) occupies the intercellular space between the beams of TM cells. The ECM consists of glycosaminoglycans (GAGs), proteoglycans, laminin, various collagens, fibronectin, and vitronectin (reviewed in [30]). The constant turnover of this ECM has been proposed to play a role in maintaining proper aqueous humor resistance. The family of matrix metalloproteinases (MMPs) are secreted zinc proteinases that initiate ECM turnover [31,32]. MMP activity is inhibited by the family of tissue inhibitors of metalloproteinases (TIMPs). MMP activity is suggested to be important in regulating aqueous humor outflow facility by proteolytic alterations. Using perfused human anterior segment, Bradley *et al*. observed that increasing MMP activity increased the outflow rate while inhibiting MMP activity by the addition of TIMP decreased outflow rate [32]. MMP activity is suggested to have various functional consequences including degradation of ECM components, cleavage and modification of signaling molecules, and cleavage of intercellular junctions and basement membrane (reviewed in [33]).

Another factor that affects resistance is the ciliary muscle. The elastic anterior tendons of the ciliary muscle insert into the network of elastic fibres in the juxtacanalicular meshwork and corneoscleral meshwork [19,20,34]. The elastic fibres are surrounded by a collagen-based sheath [20]. Ciliary muscle contractions result in increased aqueous humor outflow facility [35]. Upon ciliary muscle contraction, the connecting fibres straighten. Since the ciliary muscle is connected to the TM and the inner wall of Schlemm's canal by the connecting fibrils, ciliary muscle contraction widens the intercellular space in the juxtacanalicular meshwork allowing aqueous humor to flow against less resistance [35]. In contrast, relaxation of the ciliary muscles results in the opposite effect where there is increased resistance to aqueous flow [36].

As outlined above, the aqueous humor flow pathway is a complex process regulated by structures in both the posterior and anterior chambers of the eye. The TM is a highly specialized tissue that is able to adapt to the dynamic nature of aqueous humor outflow. The ability to adapt is an essential characteristic of the TM, especially because these cells are located in an environment that is constantly changing (Figure 2).

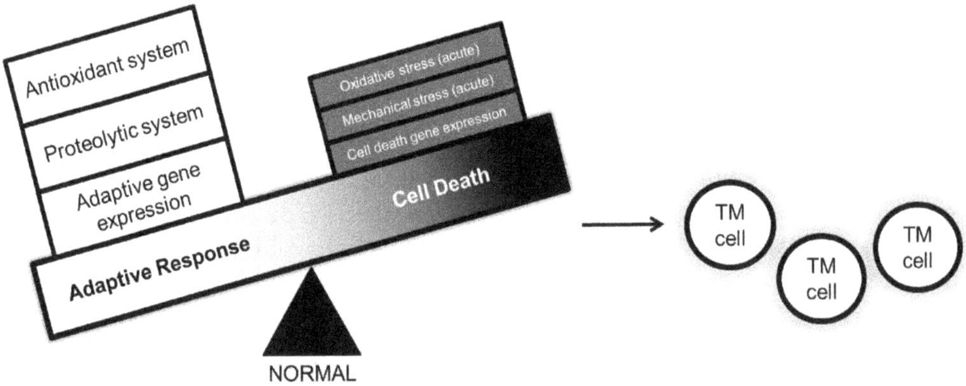

Figure 2. Trabecular meshwork under normal conditions. Even under normal conditions, the cells of the trabecular meshwork (TM) are constantly exposed to mechanical and oxidative stresses. TM cells have defense mechanisms including the antioxidant and proteolytic systems to protect the cells from these stresses. Also, specific changes in global gene expression occur in response to the specific stress, which enables TM cells to adapt to the environment and survive.

3. Change in trabecular meshwork during the normal aging process

Aging is a major risk factor for developing glaucoma. However, at the physiological level, minimal changes in aqueous humor flow dynamics occur in normal healthy subjects as aging progresses (reviewed in reference [37]). Using tonography, many studies have observed that aqueous humor outflow facility decreases with age [15,38-40]. The tonographic procedure measures outflow facility. IOP is first increased by applying force to the cornea using a tonometer probe. The subsequent decrease in IOP over the time of the test is used to determine aqueous humor outflow via the trabecular pathway. However, interpretation of results using the tonographic technique is limited because ocular rigidity is not taken into account. Since ocular rigidity increases with age [39,41], older subjects may appear to have a reduction in aqueous humor outflow facility because the stiffer eyes are less responsive to the tonographic technique, which involves applying force to the cornea. Also, the tonographic measurements do not take into account the change in pseudofacility, which refers to the probe-induced change in aqueous humor flow into the anterior chamber. In contrast to tonography, fluorophotometry is not affected by ocular rigidity and pseudofacility because no force is applied to the cornea. The outflow facility measured by fluorophotometry was 0.23±0.10μL/min/mmHg in 20-30 year old subjects (n=51) and 0.27±0.13μL/min/mmHg in subjects 60 years and older (n=53) [15]. Thus, fluorophotometric measurements indicate that there is in fact no difference in outflow facility as aging progresses [15]. Many studies using tonographic and fluorophotometric measurements have consistently shown that with age, aqueous humor production decreases [15,38,39,42-44]. Although outflow facility remains stable and aqueous humor production decreases, IOP remains stable in normal healthy subjects as aging progresses. Toris *et al.* have recently measured IOP to be 14.7±2.5mmHg in 20-30 year old subjects (n=51] and 14.3±2.6mmHg in subjects 60 years and older (n=53) [15]. A decrease in anterior chamber depth [15,45,46] with aging may account for the lack of change in IOP.

Interestingly, prominent changes at the structural and cellular levels occur with age. Connecting fibrils ensure that contact is maintained between the juxtacanalicular meshwork and the inner endothelial wall of Schlemm's canal [19,20]. The sheath surrounding these elastic fibres thickens with age [47]. The intercellular space narrows due to an increase in the amount of extracellular material from the thickened sheath, resulting in increased resistance [48,49]. Also, as aging progresses, the number of TM cells decrease [50,51]. Grierson and Howes estimate that at age 20, there are approximately 763 000 cells in the TM. By age 80, approximately 403 000 cells remain [51]]. The outer TM layers lose more TM cells while the least number of TM cells are lost from the inner juxtacanalicular layer [51,52]. This decline in TM cells appears to be a continuous and linear process with an estimated 0.58% loss of cells annually [50,52]. The linear decrease in TM cellularity is intriguing because the mechanism of cell loss may be different between the ages [52]. Age-related mechanisms such as accumulation of reactive oxygen species (ROS) and misfolded proteins are likely to contribute to cell loss in older subjects. However, other non-age-related mechanisms, such as exposure to mechanical stress, are likely responsible for cell death in the TM in younger subjects. Interestingly, Alvarado *et al.* noted that TM cells may have a reduced reparative capacity, which would further contribute to the decreased cellularity with age [52]. The loss of TM cells with age could have a more severe consequence in some individuals because there appears to be great variation in the absolute number of TM cells between individuals [53]. Therefore, individuals with less TM cells would be predicted to be less efficient in fulfilling the function of TM cells (Figure 3).

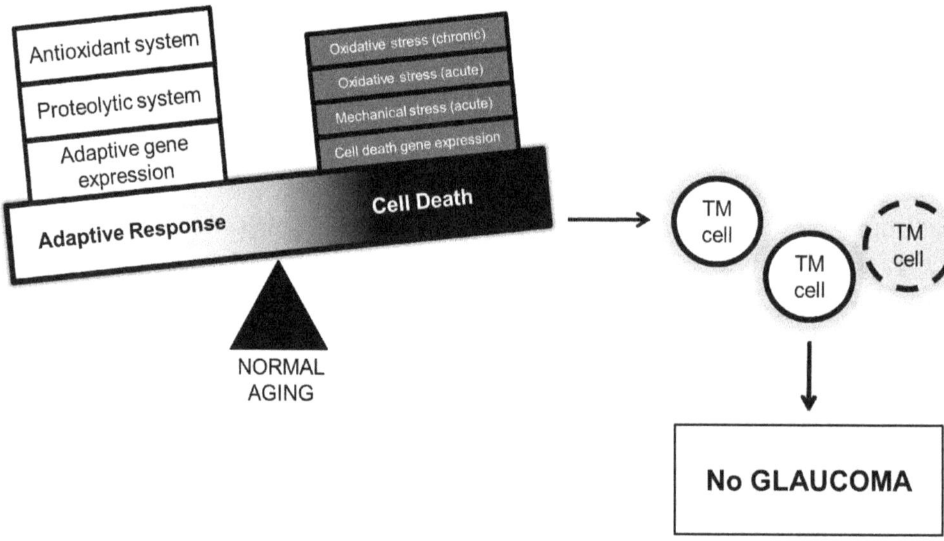

Figure 3. Trabecular meshwork during normal aging. During normal aging, the cellular defense mechanisms of the trabecular meshwork (TM) cells become less efficient. As in normal conditions (see Figure 2), the TM cells are exposed to a variety of stresses. However, the TM cells will also be exposed to other types of stresses such as chronic oxidative stress because there is an accumulation of reactive oxygen species (ROS) as aging progresses. Since the TM cells are no longer able to adapt to the environment, there will be increased TM cell death (dotted circle). However, the TM tissue still functions, preventing the onset of glaucoma.

Regardless of the individual variation in TM cell number, the consequence of losing TM cells in all aging individuals can be predicted. As avid phagocytes, TM cells are thought to clear debris from the aqueous humor outflow pathway [54-58]]. Although TM cells have the ability to ingest particulate matters rapidly, the phagocytic process may have detrimental effects on the overall health of the cell, even leading to necrosis [59]. Zhou *et al.* also showed that after phagocytosis, temporary alteration of TM cells occurred including rearrangement of the cytoskeleton and increased migratory activity [60]. These alterations, although temporary, have been speculated to be linked to the age-related loss of TM cells [60]. TM cells also maintain aqueous humor outflow by releasing factors that regulate permeability of the endothelial cells of Schlemm's canal [61]. TM cells release various enzymes and cytokines both in the presence and absence of stimulation such as mechanical stretching and exposure to pro-inflammatory cytokines [61,62]. TM endothelial cells constitutively secrete cytokines such as Interleukin 8 (IL8], Chemokine, CXC motif, ligand 6 (CXCL6), and Monocyte chemotactic protein 1 (MCP1], strengthening the notion that the release of cytokines is important in maintaining aqueous humor outflow [62].

4. Change in trabecular meshwork in glaucoma disease phenotype

Even with the age-related structural and cellular changes, the TM effectively functions to drain aqueous humor. However, in patients with glaucoma, the structural and cellular changes are more pronounced and as a result, TM function is disrupted. In glaucomataous eyes, there is more prominent and irregular thickening of the sheaths of the elastic fibers. Also, there is increased deposition of sheath-derived plaques compared with normal eyes [47,63]. This increase in extracellular material in the TM is predicted to block aqueous humor outflow [20] contributing to the development of disease. As in normal aging, there is a linear decrease in cellularity as aging progresses in the TM of POAG patients. Moreover, Alvarado *et al.* observed fewer cells in the glaucomatous TM compared with the non-glaucomatous TM over a wide range of ages [50].

The risk of developing glaucoma significantly increases after age 40. Despite the fact that glaucoma is an age-related disease, aging in most people does not result in this disease (Figure 3). The changes that occur in the TM during the normal aging process may make the tissue more susceptible to malfunction. However, other unknown factors and even stochastic factors must be present for the TM to fail to a point that the glaucoma phenotype develops (Figure 4).

5. Exposure of trabecular meshwork to mechanical stress

In order to survive, TM cells must be able to constantly adapt to their continuously changing environment. Similar to any other cell in the body, TM cells are exposed to a variety of environmental stresses. Due to the location of cells of the TM, one of the major types of stress these cells are exposed to is mechanical stress. IOP continuously fluctuates throughout the day with a higher IOP occurring during the nocturnal period. The fluctuation in IOP is part of a normal physiological process and is unavoidable. Fluctuations in IOP occur with blinking, eye

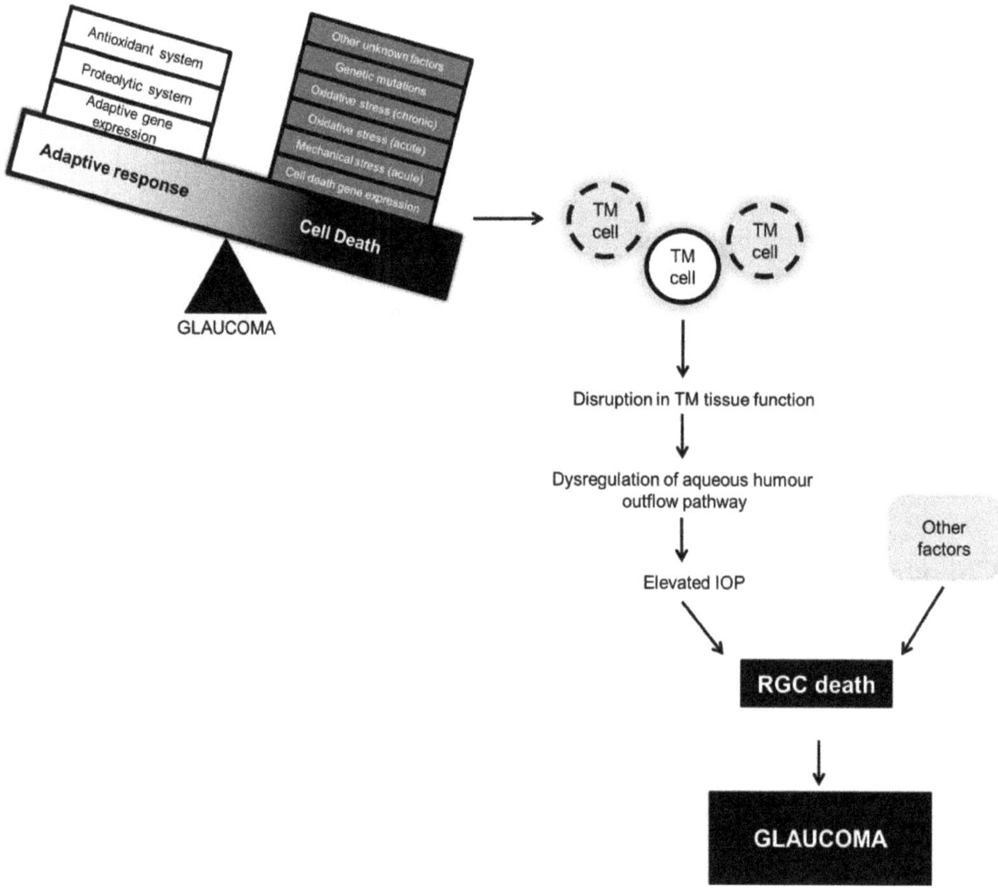

Figure 4. Trabecular meshwork of glaucoma phenotype. Similar to normal non-aging and aging conditions, trabecular meshwork (TM) cells are exposed to a variety of stresses. However, other unknown factors are present to initiate the cascade of events that lead to the development of glaucoma. Also, genetic mutations could compromise normal TM cell function. All of these factors are predicted to result in TM cell death (dotted circles) to the extent that the TM tissue is no longer able to function properly. Consequently, there will be dysregulation of aqueous humor drainage resulting in increased intraocular pressure (IOP), which would ultimately lead to retinal ganglion cell (RGC) death and glaucoma.

movements, and even with a change in body position. A supine body position has been shown to result in higher IOP compared with an upright body position [64,65]. The temporary fluctuation in IOP can vary up to 10mmHg [66]. This change in IOP results in distortions (including stretching and compression) of the cells and is sensed by the cells of the TM as mechanical stress.

6. Exposure of trabecular meshwork to oxidative stress

Another type of environmental stress that TM cells are exposed to is oxidative stress. Cells are constantly exposed to free radicals that are the by-products of normal cellular metabolism. In addition, the aqueous humor is itself a source of free radicals. Hydrogen peroxide (H_2O_2) is normally present in the aqueous humor and is suggested to be the key source of oxidative stress for the TM [67]. Initially, the concentration of H_2O_2, a reactive oxygen species (ROS), was reported to be between 25-60 μM in the aqueous humor using the dichloropheno-indopheno (DCPIP) assay [5,68-70]. However, technical issues with the DCPIP method, including the interference of ascorbic acid with the assay [70] and the spontaneous auto-oxidization of DCPIP in the presence of oxygen [71], has resulted in the re-examination of H_2O_2 in the aqueous humor. Different methods have indicated that H_2O_2 is present in the aqueous humor, but at much lower concentrations than previously thought [70,71]. An accurate concentration of H_2O_2 is still difficult to obtain and may vary greatly between individuals. Since cells of the TM are in direct contact with aqueous humor, these cells are exposed both intracellularly and extracellularly to oxidative stress.

Free radicals at lower concentrations are beneficial to the cell (reviewed in [72,73]). Low concentrations of ROS act as second messengers for signal transduction and gene regulation. For example, low concentrations of ROS activate the Nuclear factor kappa-B (NF-κB) transcription factor, which plays a key role in many cellular processes including inflammation, cell proliferation, and apoptosis (reviewed in [74]) However, higher concentrations of free radicals can have negative effects on the cell (Figure 5). Free radicals can damage proteins and DNA, promote lipid peroxidation, disrupt mitochondrial function, and trigger cell death (reviewed in [73]). Cells have an antioxidant defense mechanism to counter the deleterious effects of ROS. For example, superoxide dismutase (SOD) is an antioxidant enzyme that converts superoxide free radical anion (O_2^-) into H_2O_2 and molecular oxygen (O_2) [75]. H_2O_2 must then be converted into H_2O by two other antioxidant enzymes: peroxisomal catalases and the family of glutathione peroxidases (GPx). In the event that H_2O_2 is not converted, then it may split into the hydroxyl radical (OH•), which can be dangerous because it can react with almost any macromolecule within a short diffusion distance. Cells, through the activity of nitric oxide synthase, are able to produce the free radical nitric oxide (NO). NO itself is hardly toxic and is in fact important in regulating various cellular functions. In fact NO has been suggested to increase aqueous humor outflow by relaxing the ciliary smooth muscles [76,77]. However, NO becomes dangerous when it spontaneously reacts with superoxide O_2^- , forming the powerful oxidant peroxynitrite (ONOO-) [78]. Peroxynitrite is highly reactive and can damage biological molecules resulting in cell death (reviewed in [79]). In this way, the antioxidant defense mechanism also functions in minimizing the deleterious effects of reactive nitrogen species (RNS).

Chronic oxidative stress is recognized to be a major contributor to the aging process and various diseases including neurodegenerative diseases such as Parkinson's [80,81] and Alzheimer [82-84], cancer [72,85], and cardiovascular diseases [86]. Since POAG is an age-related disease, chronic oxidative stress is also suggested to have a role in the pathophysiology of this disease (reviewed in [87]). In POAG, both the RGCs and the anterior segment structures such as the TM are exposed to chronic oxidative stress conditions. TM cells are exposed to acute oxidative stress under normal physiological conditions [67]. The presence of cellular defense mechanisms in TM cells enables TM cells to quickly and effectively respond and adapt to their environment (Figure 2). Two cellular defense mechanisms present in TM cells are the antioxidant system, which defends against ROS, and the proteolytic system, which removes unwanted biomaterials from the cell, many of which are products of oxidative stress-related damage. However, as aging progresses, the normal cellular defense mechanisms become less effective and the cell is less able to remove potential toxic materials such as ROS and misfolded proteins (Figure 3). The gradual accumulation of toxic materials will lead to an environment where the cells are exposed to chronic oxidative stress. We hypothesize that the cellular defense mechanisms, already compromised due to the aging process, become completely overwhelmed under such chronic oxidative stress conditions. Cell death will occur when the cells are no longer able to adapt to the environment. Since accumulation of ROS occurs with age, the loss of TM cells during the aging process may also be in part due to exposure of TM cells to chronic oxidative stress conditions. The presence of fewer TM cells as aging progresses could also be detrimental to the TM tissue as there are fewer cells to protect against ROS in the aqueous humor. Although it remains a likely possibility, evidence that chronic oxidative stress directly contributes to the loss of TM cells with age is currently lacking.

In comparison to non-glaucomatous individuals, the TM cells of glaucoma patients appear to have more oxidative stress-related damages, including the accumulation of oxidatively damaged DNA[88,89], proteins[90], and organelles, as well as lipid peroxidation products [91,92] (Figure 5). Oxidative stress can damage DNA, resulting in the formation of 8-hy-

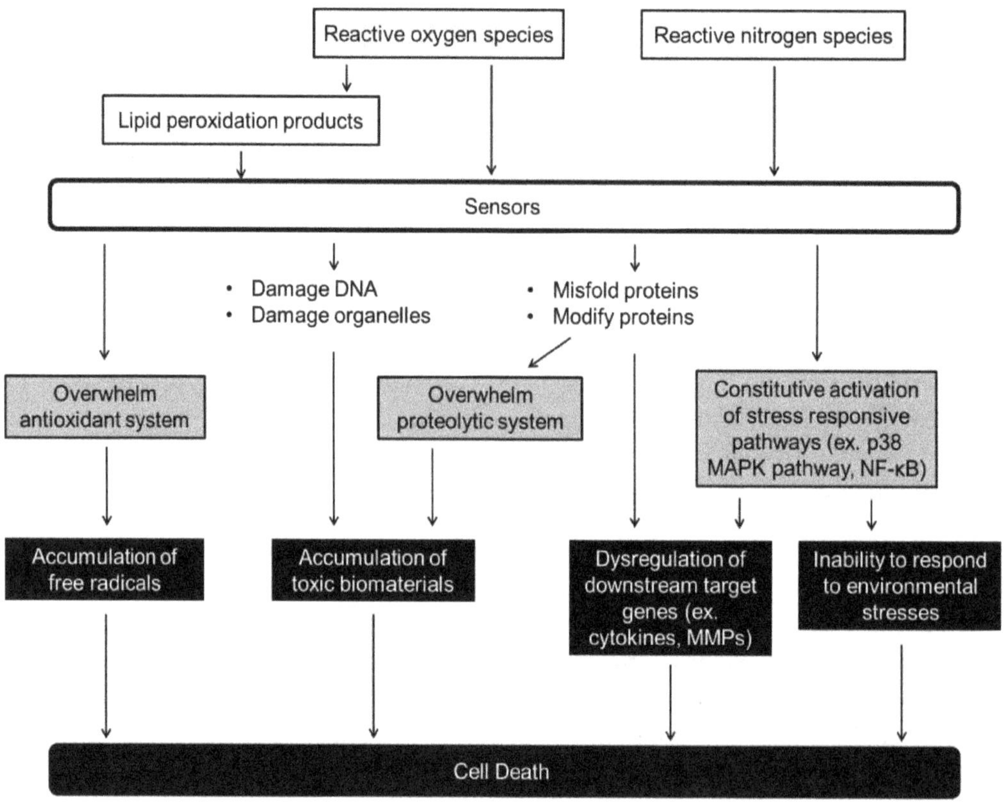

Figure 5. Overview of various oxidative stress-related effects on the cell, which would contribute to cell death.

droxy-2`-deoxyguanosine (8-OHdG). The levels of 8-OHdG were increased in DNA extracts from glaucomatous TM cells compared with healthy controls [88,89]. Also, aqueous humor and serum levels of 8-OHdG were significantly higher in glaucoma patients (n=28] compared with the age-matched control group of senile cataract patients (n=27) [93].

Despite having more oxidative stress-related damages, TM cells of glaucoma patients appear to have increased activity of some components of the antioxidant defense mechanism. Increased levels of glutathione peroxidase (GPx) and superoxide dismutase (SOD) activities were measured in aqueous humor of glaucomatous patients compared with the control group of senile cataract patients [94,95]. However, no apparent change in catalase activity levels have been detected [94,95]. Thus, at least some components of the antioxidant defense mechanism are functioning to prevent TM cell death under glaucomatous conditions.

Aqueous humor is both a source of free radicals and a source of antioxidants. Since low concentrations of free radicals are necessary for normal cellular function, TM cells rely on the very high content of antioxidants in the aqueous humor to achieve a balance that maximizes cell survival. High aqueous humor concentration of the antioxidant ascorbic acid (aka Vitamin C), which is about 20 times higher than in plasma [70], suggests that this antioxidant may be a major protector against free radicals in the eye [96-98]. Ascorbic acid has also been suggested to protect cells against ultraviolet light [98,99]. In addition to being an antioxidant, ascorbic acid is suggested to also have a role regulating the ECM of the TM. TM cells synthesize many types of glycosaminoglycans (GAGs) into the ECM including hyaluronic acid [100]. Ascorbic acid can increase hyaluronic acid synthesis [100]. Since hyaluronic acid has been shown to increase the expression of several MMPs [101], altered levels of this GAG would affect ECM turnover. Interestingly, Knepper *et al.* has shown that there is significantly less hyaluronic acid in the TM of POAG patients compared with the TM of normal subjects [102,103]. Thus, ascorbic acid is predicted to affect the aqueous outflow pathway by acting as an antioxidant and by regulating the ECM components that are important in maintaining the aqueous humor outflow pathway. Although some groups observed no difference in aqueous ascorbic acid levels between POAG patients and senile cataract patients [104,105], Lee *et al.* observed greater levels of ascorbic acid in the aqueous humor of POAG patients [106]. The difference in observation may be due to the great individual variation in ascorbic acid levels [105]. Nevertheless, ascorbic acid appears to play a protective role for TM cells.

In addition to the antioxidant system, the proteolytic system is another cellular defense mechanism present in TM cells. The proteolytic system is essential for the removal of oxidatively damaged proteins and organelles. The 20S proteasome, 26S proteasome, and immunoproteasome are the main cellular systems in eukaryotic cells that eliminate damaged proteins. The 20S proteasome tends to degrade oxidized proteins while the 26S proteasome degrade ubiquitynated proteins. In many tissues, including the TM, there is a decline in proteasomal activity with age. Caballero *et al.* reported that primary cultures of human trabecular meshwork (HTM) cells from healthy older donors (ages 66, 70, and 73) had decreased proteasomal activity compared with healthy young donors (ages 9, 14, and 25) [90]. Since the overall proteasomal content did not change between the older and younger donors, the decrease in proteasomal activity is most likely due to oxidation of the proteasomal subunits and the overload of the proteasomal machinery with damaged proteins. Caballero *et al*. observed an increase in oxidized proteins in the older donors [90]. Accumulation of oxidized protein is not the only biomolecule detrimental to proteasomal function.

The accumulation of lipid peroxidation products in the TM is suggested to also contribute to proteasomal dysfunction [107]. Lipid peroxidation occurs when a ROS attacks a polyunsaturated fatty acid, thus initiating the lipid peroxidation chain reaction, which results in highly reactive aldehydes [108,109]. Lipid peroxidation products interact with protein, which results in modification to the protein structure and activity [109]. Accumulation of lipid peroxidation end products have been observed in many neurodegenerative diseases including Alzheimer's disease [110] and Parkinson's disease [111]. In glaucoma, an increase in lipid peroxidation end products, including diene and triene conjugates, and Schiff's bases, were observed in glaucomatous TM tissue (n=17) and aqueous humor (n=16) compared to age-matched controls (n=13 and n=17, respectively) [91]. In addition, Fernandez-Durango *et al.* measured increased levels of the lipid peroxidation mediator, malondialdehyde (MDA), in the aqueous humor of patients with terminal cases of POAG (n=38) compared to the cataract control group (n=48) [92]. Accumulation of lipid peroxidation products is predicted to have severe consequences on the TM by modifying proteins such as calpain-1. The calpains are a family of calcium-activated non-lysosomal cysteine proteases. In glaucomatous TM tissue, aggregated and degraded calpain-1 is present, but calpain-1 activity is lower compared with normal TM tissue [107]. In the TM of glaucomatous eyes, the lipid peroxidation products isolevuglandins, specifically iso[4]levuglandin E2, modifies calpain-1, thereby inhibiting calpain-1 activity. Although the physiological function of calpain-1 in the TM remains to be elucidated, calpain-1 modified by isolevuglandins is more prone to form larger aggregates. One of the major consequences of this modification is a disruption in the proteasomal machinery. This type of malfunction of the proteasomal machinery appears to be specific to the TM and does not occur in the posterior segment of the eye. Thus, accumulation of oxidative stress-related biomolecules along with a decrease in proteasomal activity with age perpetuates a vicious cycle that is postulated to greatly hinder cell survival.

7. Global change in gene expression in response to stress

As reviewed in the previous sections, cells of the TM are exposed to a variety of environmental stresses. The stresses can vary in form (mechanical, phagocytic, and oxidative), magnitude, and duration (acute or chronic). The antioxidant system and the proteolytic system are effective cellular defense mechanisms that protect cells. Recent advances in technology have shown that a change in the global gene expression profile is another major part of a cell's adaptive response to stress (reviewed in [112]. The change in gene expression profile in response to stress has revealed that signal transduction pathways are a necessary means of integrating complex signals and propagating these signals to effectors. In the next section, we will examine the specific sensors and signal transduction pathways that result in an appropriate response to stress in TM cells.

8. Sensors of TM cells

Cells have stress sensors that are highly specialized for survival in a particular environment. The specific mechanism of how TM cells sense various stimuli is largely unknown [48]. Mechanosensitive ion channels, specifically calcium-dependent maxi-K+ channels, are present in TM cells [113]. Stretch-activated channels located on the TM cell membrane are predicted to increase intracellular calcium levels. Another potential mechanism through which TM cells sense mechanical stress is the ECM. ECM receptors such as integrins are connected to the cytoskeleton, which is attached to the nuclear membrane. Thus, signals may be propagated from the extracellular environment where the mechanical stress occurs to the nucleus where gene expression can be altered in response to the stress [114]. Although the consequences of oxidative stress-related damages have been extensively studied, how the cell initially senses oxidative stress remains largely unknown [48,115]. In fact, the identification of oxidative stress sensors in any cell type has proven to be very difficult. In the future, identifying more sensors in TM cells will give insight into how TM cells achieve specificity in responding to specific stresses such as mechanical and oxidative stresses.

9. Global change in gene expression in response to mechanical stress

Exposure of TM cells to acute mechanical stress requires a quick and specific adaptive response to ensure maximal survival occurs. Recent studies examining the change in the global gene expression profile of TM cells has given insight into how TM cells are able to adapt and respond to the constant exposure to mechanical stress.

Several groups have examined the change in global gene expression profile of TM cells in response to mechanical stress [116-119]. Vittitow *et al.* and Vittal *et al.* both observed a change in expression of a large number of genes in response to mechanical stress. In TM from postmortem human donors, application of mechanical stress resulted in the upregulation of 40 genes and the downregulation of 14 genes [116]. Mechanical stretching of cultured porcine TM cells resulted in the upregulation of 126 genes and downregulation of 29 genes [117]. However, there was very little overlap in genes between the studies most likely due to the use of different experimental models as well of stochastic factors. Nevertheless, these studies reveal that TM cells appear to respond specifically to the *type* of stress. A large number of genes that changed expression levels were involved in ECM and cytoskeletal function, which is predicted to function in response to mechanical-stretch related changed to the cell and extracellular environment [117,118]. Several studies have shown that exposure of TM cells to mechanical stress results in increased levels of active MMPs, specifically MMP2 [120-123]. The MMP family of zinc proteases initiate ECM turnover, which has been predicted to regulate aqueous humor outflow facility by altering resistance. Furthermore, temporal variation of mechanical stretching resulted in a different gene expression profile indicating that TM cells are also able to respond specifically to the *magnitude* of mechanical stress.

Induction of stress response is thought to result in conditions that are detrimental to cell growth due in part to activation of cell cycle checkpoints [115,124]. Also, during stress response, the cell diverts energy to the adaptive response and as a result, less energy is available for cell growth-related functions [112,125]. Thus, there is a continuous balance between cell growth and stress response. In order to achieve this balance, stress responses must be transient and be temporally restricted. Consistent with this theory, exposure to mechanical stress resulted in a change in expression of a large number of stress-related genes while few growth-related genes were affected [117]. Another related characteristic of stress response is the highly reversible nature of the global change in gene expression. After removal of stress, inactivation of the stress-induced signal transduction pathway occurs, likely because constitutive activation of stress response would be detrimental to the overall health of the cell. Although the specific reversal of the gene expression profile in TM cells after the removal of mechanical stress has not been examined, TM cells appear to physiologically return to the pre-stress state after a period of time. Perfusion of anterior segment cultures is an effective experimental model for examining TM function [126].In this model, anterior segment explants are perfused with culture medium at a constant pressure, resulting in a stable and physiologically relevant flow rate [122,127]. Using perfused human anterior segment culture, Bradley *et al.* observed that doubling the flow rate resulted in immediate doubling of IOP [122]. However, after two days, TM cells lowered outflow resistance and thus, restored the IOP to pre-stress levels even under conditions where the flow rate remained doubled. In this study, the TM cells appear to reach a new homeostatic condition even when the stress is not removed.

Cells use multiple signal transduction pathways to integrate various input signals and coordinate an appropriate stress response. In TM cells, activation of signal transduction pathways appears to be important in mediating an appropriate stress response. Vittitow *et al.* observed that nearly 32% of genes altered in the global gene expression profile in response to mechanical stretch of TM cells functioned in various signal transduction pathways [116]. One particularly interesting signal transduction pathway is the stress-activated protein kinase (SAPK) pathways, a highly conserved signalling pathway in eukaryotes that are activated by many different environmental stresses. A rapid response to stress is essential to maximize cell survival. Thus, the SAPK pathway enables rapid phosphorylation of components of various signal transduction pathway so that a response occurs within minutes of initial exposure to the stress [128,129]. In mammals, the SAPKs are the p38 mitogen-activated protein kinases (MAPKs). There is evidence that the MAPK signal transduction pathway is involved in the TM cell response to mechanical stress [130]. In TM cells, the p38 MAPK pathway is suggested to modulate the regulation of stretch-induced cytokines such as TGF-β1 and IL-6 [131]. Thus, the p38 MAPK pathway functions in co-ordinating and regulating signal transduction pathways in response to stress. However, in primary glaucomatous TM cells, Zhang *et al.* demonstrated that the p38 MAPK pathway is unresponsive to exogenous manipulation, including the administration of Interleukin 1 (IL1), which has been shown to activate the p38 MAPK pathway in non-glaucomatous TM cells [132]. Although examination of the p38 MAPK pathway *in vivo* is required, this pathway may be unresponsive in glaucomatous TM cells because it is already maximally activated [132]. The cause of this constitutive activation remains unknown. Nevertheless, the constitutive activation of the stress-responsive MAPK pathway is predicted to have serious consequences as the TM cells will lose its ability to mediate the stress response through the stress-dependent activation of the p38 MAPK pathway.

10. Global change in gene expression in response to oxidative stress

Despite the evidence that TM cells are exposed to oxidative stress, not much is currently known about the change in global gene expression profile in TM cells in response to chronic oxidative stress. Examining the effects of chronic oxidative stress on TM cells is especially challenging because it is difficult to experimentally create an environment where TM cells are exposed to chronic oxidative stress.

Porter *et al.* examined the global gene expression profile of phagocytically challenged TM cells under normal and acute oxidative stress conditions [133]. As avid phagocytes, TM cells are predicted to keep the aqueous humor outflow pathway clear of debris [55]. When TM cells were phagocytically challenged to *E. coli* under normal conditions, 1190 genes were upregulated and 728 genes were downregulated [133]. When TM cells were phagocytically challenged to E. coli under oxidatively stressed conditions at 40% O_2, 976 genes were upregulated and 383 genes were downregulated. Although many of the altered genes were involved in immune response, cell adhesion, and regulation of ECM, there were only 6 genes that were altered in both the normal and oxidatively stressed conditions. TM cells therefore appear to have distinct gene expression profiles specific to the type of stress. Under experimental conditions, different types of stresses tend to be examined one at a time to elucidate the response of the cells to that particular stress. However, TM cells under physiological conditions are simultaneously exposed to different stresses. Studies in yeast have shown that cells are able to combine and integrate these different signals and produce an adaptive response [128]. Thus, analyzing a combination of stresses in TM cells will possibly reveal the role that cross-protection plays in these cells. Cross-protection refers to the ability of cells to become resistant to stress after first being exposed to a sub-lethal stress [134].

Transcription factors are essential regulators of signal transduction pathway components. NF-κB was identified as the transcription factor responsible for activation of many of the genes in the gene expression profile of phagocytically challenged TM cells including MMP1 and MMP3 [133]. The NF-κB transcription factor has also been shown to mediate the activation of endothelial leukocyte adhesion molecule (ELAM1) and the inflammatory cytokine IL1 [135]. ELAM1 is a cell adhesion molecule that is readily expressed in glaucomatous TM cells [135-137]. Activation of ELAM1 and IL1 by the NF-κB transcription factor in response to oxidative stress promotes cell survival. However, constitutive activation of NF-κB is predicted to be detrimental to cell survival and even contribute to the development of glaucoma [135]. The NF-κB transcription factor regulates the expression of numerous downstream target genes with varying functions including MMPs that regulate ECM turnover. Dysregulation of these downstream target genes is predicted to cause disruptions to TM cell function. In many situations, the altered gene expression returns to a steady-state level that is comparable to unstressed conditions even when the cells remain exposed to a particular stress [125]. As mentioned previously, activation of stress-related genes during a stress response diverts energy and resources from cell growth. Thus, situations where steady state levels are not achieved can pose a great risk to the overall health of the cell, ultimately affecting its ability to survive.

11. Unspecific gene expression response

Studying the change in the global gene expression profile of TM cells reveals that a large number of genes are either upregulated or downregulated in response to various environmental stresses. Many of the genes that have altered expression do not appear to have any relevant function in the adaptive response to the specific stress. Analysis of global gene expression profiles in other systems such as *S. cerevisiae* yield similar findings of an unspecific gene expression response [138-140]. Furthermore, studies in *E.coli* have revealed that when cells are exposed to an unknown stress that the cell would not encounter under normal biological conditions, an unspecific and stochastic gene expression response was triggered [141,142]. Since cells may not have specific sensors to detect multiple stresses simultaneously, the unspecific stress response has been suggested to protect cells under multiple stress conditions by changing the expression of a large number of genes, some of which function in promoting a general adaptive response [125]. Furthermore, this unspecific and stochastic gene expression response may be an important evolutionary mechanism, thereby allowing cells to adapt to an unpredictable challenge [125]. Even though cells of the TM are in a dynamic environment with a multitude of challenges, the unspecific gene expression response may enable these cells to quickly and effectively adapt to a new steady state. In the future, distinguishing between stress-essential genes (necessary for immediate response) and stress-induced genes (most likely necessary for unspecific or long-term response) in TM cells is critical in understanding how TM cells adapt to stress in the long-term and prepare for subsequent stresses. Finally, although examining a particular stress-induced gene is important in elucidating its role in aqueous humor regulation, examining the *network* of genes altered in response to stress will provide further insight into the complex nature of the adaptive response of TM cells.

12. Effect of environmental stress on glaucoma-associated genes

Exposure of anterior segment structures, specifically the TM, to environmental stresses disrupts the aqueous humor outflow pathway and contributes to the development of glaucoma. Glaucoma, however, has a complex etiology. In addition to the environmental stress factors, genetic factors contribute to the development of this disease. At least 14 chromosomal loci have been identified for POAG (GLC1A to GLC1N) [143]. Currently three genes from these loci have been associated with glaucoma: *myocilin* (*MYOC*), *optineurin* (*OPTN*), and *WD repeat domain 36* (*WDR36*). Mutations in these three genes account for less than 5% of POAG cases [144]. Glaucoma is also a major consequence for many anterior segment dysgenesis disorders including Axenfeld-Rieger Syndrome (ARS) and Peter's anomaly. Mutations in the transcription factor genes, *FOXC1* and *PITX2*, are associated with ARS [145-147]. How mutations in *FOXC1* and *PITX2* cause disease is not well understood. Recent findings have suggested that patients with these types of mutations may be more sensitive to environmental stresses [148,149]. The cells of the TM may be less tolerant when exposed to various stresses, resulting in dysregulation of aqueous humor outflow. In this section, we will take a closer look at the effects of environmental stresses on two genes, *MYOC*, which is associated with POAG, and *FOXC1*, which is associated with ARS.

MYOC was the first POAG gene to be reported [150-152]. Patients with *MYOC* mutations tend to present with juvenile and early adult-onset forms of POAG. However, the most commonly reported MYOC mutation, Q368X, is associated with later adult-onset POAG. MYOC is expressed in most ocular tissues [153] including the TM and is secreted into the aqueous humor [154,155]. The release of MYOC is associated with the release of exosomes. Signaling molecules within these exosomes is predicted to function in maintaining TM homeostasis [156]. Specific MYOC mutations appear to sensitize cells to oxidative stress. Joe *et al*. observed that Human Embryonic Kidney 293 (HEK293) cells stably transfected with the Y437H MYOC mutation have decreased expression of antioxidant genes and produced more ROS [156,157]. Also, more H_2O_2-induced cell death occurred in HEK293 cells overexpressing various *MYOC* mutations compared with wild type. The extent of cell death differed between mutants. Furthermore, 18 month old Y437H mutant mice had increased expression of ER stress markers and decreased levels of antioxidant proteins [157]. These findings suggest that patients with *MYOC* mutations are more sensitive to oxidative stress. The decreased ability to response to oxidative stress may contribute to the development of glaucoma earlier on in these patients' lives.

Anterior segment dysgenesis covers a wide spectrum of developmental anomalies that can affect the iris, cornea, lens, TM, and Schlemm's canal. We have already discussed the importance of the TM and Schlemm's canal in maintaining the aqueous humor outflow pathway. Disruptions in this pathway may result in increased IOP, which is a major risk factor of developing glaucoma. Glaucoma is estimated to develop in approximately 50% of patients with anterior segment dysgenesis [158-160]. Although the mechanism that leads to glaucoma may vary between different anterior segment dysgenesis disorders and even between individuals with the same disorder, recent findings suggest that environmental stresses affect the normal functioning of the disease-associated gene. Patients with ARS can present with a variety of ocular anomalies and systemic anomalies. Ocular anomalies include iris hypoplasia, corectopia, polycoria, and posterior embryotoxon while systemic anomalies include dental anomalies and redundant periumbilical skin. ARS patients with FOXC1 mutations have a 50-80% risk of developing earlier-onset glaucoma [161]. As a transcription factor, FOXC1 regulates the expression of a myriad of genes including genes that function in proteolysis, cell matrix adhesion, apoptosis, signal transduction, and stress response [148]. Berry *et al.* observed that FOXC1 plays a role in TM cell viability by directly regulating the transcription factor FOXO1A which is involved in the cellular stress response pathway and apoptosis. Decreasing the expression of FOXC1 increased the sensitivity of TM cells to oxidative stress. Tight regulation of the FOXC1 transcription factor is essential because both a high (FOXC1 duplications) and low FOXC1 (loss of function mutations) gene dose results in anterior segment dysgenesis phenotypes associated with glaucoma. Interestingly, FOXC1 itself appears to be responsive to stress as well (Y.A.I. and M.A.W. personal observations). Thus, the FOXC1 transcription factor appears to play an important role in responding to environmental stresses. Disruptions to normal FOXC1 function are predicted to disrupt the regulation of downstream target genes that are involved in executing a rapid and effective adaptive response. Therefore, ARS patients with FOXC1 mutations may have a compromised ability to respond to environmental stresses resulting in the early age of development of glaucoma. Thus, even in the case of anterior segment developmental disorders, oxidative stress appears to have an impact on the TM. Studying genes that are associated with both the primary and secondary glaucomas provide an invaluable tool to understanding the contribution of environmental stresses on the development of glaucoma.

13. Conclusion

The functional nature of the TM inevitably results in exposure of this tissue to a highly dynamic environment. Examining the functional roles of single genes have provided invaluable insight into how specific genes contribute to normal TM cell function and how these TM cells are able to respond to specific stresses. However, the recent analyses of global gene expression profiles have indicated that an extensive number of genes are involved in mediating the TM cell stress response. We are beginning to piece together how these singles genes function as part of a 'network' of genes. Individual components of this network of genes are potential therapeutic targets for promoting cell survival and maintaining TM cell function. However, future research needs to examine how these genes interact with each other and the environment in a more physiologically relevant context; as part of a TM stress-response network. Understanding the network of genes that are involved in executing the adaptive response is complicated, but essential to developing effective treatments for anterior segment malformations and glaucoma.

Acknowledgements

We would like to thank Dr. Fred Berry and Mr. Tim Footz for critically reviewing this manuscript. Y.A.I. is supported by the Sir Frederick Banting and Dr. Charles Best Canada Graduate Scholarship provided by the Canadian Institutes of Health Research.

Author details

Yoko A. Ito and Michael A. Walter*

*Address all correspondence to: mwalter@ualberta.ca

Department of Medical Genetics, University of Alberta, Edmonton, AB, Canada

References

[1] Quigley, H. A, & Broman, A. T. The number of people with glaucoma worldwide in 2010 and 2020. Br J Ophthalmol (2006). , 90, 262-267.

[2] Rudnicka, A. R, Mt-isa, S, Owen, C. G, Cook, D. G, & Ashby, D. Variations in primary open-angle glaucoma prevalence by age, gender, and race: a Bayesian meta-analysis. Invest Ophthalmol Vis Sci (2006). , 47, 4254-4261.

[3] Leske, M. C. Open-angle glaucoma-- an epidemiologic overview. Ophthalmic Epidemiol 200;, 14, 166-172.

[4] Giblin, F. J, Mccready, J. P, Kodama, T, & Reddy, V. N. A direct correlation between the levels of ascorbic acid and H2O2 in aqueous humor. Exp Eye Res (1984). , 38, 87-93.

[5] Bhuyan, K. C, & Bhuyan, D. K. Regulation of hydrogen peroxide in eye humors. Effect of 3-amino-1H-triazole on catalase and glutathione peroxidase of rabbit eye. Biochim Biophys Acta (1977). , 1(2), 4.

[6] Mark, H. H. Aqueous humor dynamics in historical perspective. Surv Ophthalmol (2010). , 55, 89-100.

[7] Goel, M, Picciani, R. G, Lee, R. K, & Bhattacharya, S. K. Aqueous humor dynamics: a review. Open Ophthalmol J (2010). , 4, 52-59.

[8] Brubaker, R. F. Measurement of Aqueous Flow By Fluorophotometry. The Glaucomas; (1989). , 337.

[9] Millar, C, & Kaufman, P. L. Aqueous humor: Secretion and dynamics. In: Jaeger EA, Tasman W, editors. DUANE'S FOUNDATIONS OF CLINICAL OPHTHALMOLOGY: Philadelphia: Lippincott; (1995). , 1.

[10] Hollows, F. C, & Graham, P. A. Intra-ocular pressure, glaucoma, and glaucoma suspects in a defined population. Br J Ophthalmol (1966t). , 50, 570-586.

[11] Bill, A. The aqueous humor drainage mechanism in the cynomolgus monkey (Macaca irus) with evidence for unconventional routes. Invest Ophthalmol (1965). , 4, 911-919.

[12] Bill, A, & Hellsing, K. Production and drainage of aqueous humor in the cynomolgus monkey (Macaca irus). Invest Ophthalmol (1965). , 4, 920-926.

[13] Fautsch, M. P, & Johnson, D. H. Aqueous humor outflow: what do we know? Where will it lead us? Invest Ophthalmol Vis Sci (2006). , 47, 4181-4187.

[14] Townsend, D. J, & Brubaker, R. F. Immediate effect of epinephrine on aqueous formation in the normal human eye as measured by fluorophotometry. Invest Ophthalmol Vis Sci (1980). , 19, 256-266.

[15] Toris, C. B, Yablonski, M. E, Wang, Y. L, & Camras, C. B. Aqueous humor dynamics in the aging human eye. Am J Ophthalmol (1999). , 127, 407-412.

[16] Bill, A, & Phillips, C. I. Uveoscleral drainage of aqueous humor in human eyes. Exp Eye Res (1971). , 12, 275-281.

[17] Fine, B. S. Observations on the Drainage Angle in Man and Rhesus Monkey: a Concept of the Pathogenesis of Chronic Simple Glaucoma. a Light and Electron Microscopic Study. Invest Ophthalmol (1964). , 3, 609-646.

[18] Fine, B. S. Structure of the trabecular meshwork and the canal of Schlemm. Trans Am Acad Ophthalmol Otolaryngol (1966). , 70, 777-790.

[19] Rohen, J. W, Futa, R, & Lutjen-drecoll, E. The fine structure of the cribriform meshwork in normal and glaucomatous eyes as seen in tangential sections. Invest Ophthalmol Vis Sci (1981). , 21, 574-585.

[20] Lutjen-drecoll, E, Futa, R, & Rohen, J. W. Ultrahistochemical studies on tangential sections of the trabecular meshwork in normal and glaucomatous eyes. Invest Ophthalmol Vis Sci (1981). , 21, 563-573.

[21] Underwood, J. L, Murphy, C. G, Chen, J, Franse-carman, L, Wood, I, Epstein, D. L, et al. Glucocorticoids regulate transendothelial fluid flow resistance and formation of intercellular junctions. Am J Physiol (1999). C, 330-42.

[22] Tripathi, R. Tracing the bulk outflow route of cerebrospinal fluid by transmission and scanning electron microscopy. Brain Res (1974). , 80, 503-506.

[23] Epstein, D. L, & Rohen, J. W. Morphology of the trabecular meshwork and inner-wall endothelium after cationized ferritin perfusion in the monkey eye. Invest Ophthalmol Vis Sci (1991). , 32, 160-171.

[24] Brilakis, H. S, & Johnson, D. H. Giant vacuole survival time and implications for aqueous humor outflow. J Glaucoma (2001). , 10, 277-283.

[25] Ascher, K. W. The aqueous veins: I. Physiologic importance of the visible elimination of intraocular fluid. Am J Ophthalmol. (1942). , 25, 1174-1209.

[26] Lutjen-drecoll, E. New findings on the functional structure of the region of the angle of the chamber and its changes after glaucoma surgery (author's transl). Klin Monbl Augenheilkd (1973). , 163, 410-419.

[27] Maepea, O, & Bill, A. Pressures in the juxtacanalicular tissue and Schlemm's canal in monkeys. Exp Eye Res (1992). , 54, 879-883.

[28] Ethier, C. R, Kamm, R. D, Palaszewski, B. A, Johnson, M. C, & Richardson, T. M. Calculations of flow resistance in the juxtacanalicular meshwork. Invest Ophthalmol Vis Sci (1986). , 27, 1741-1750.

[29] Seiler, T, & Wollensak, J. The resistance of the trabecular meshwork to aqueous humor outflow. Graefes Arch Clin Exp Ophthalmol (1985)., 223, 88-91.

[30] Acott, T. S, & Kelley, M. J. Extracellular matrix in the trabecular meshwork. Exp Eye Res (2008)., 86, 543-561.

[31] Woessner, J. F. Jr. Matrix metalloproteinases and their inhibitors in connective tissue remodeling. FASEB J (1991)., 5, 2145-2154.

[32] Bradley, J. M, Vranka, J, Colvis, C. M, Conger, D. M, Alexander, J. P, Fisk, A. S, et al. Effect of matrix metalloproteinases activity on outflow in perfused human organ culture. Invest Ophthalmol Vis Sci (1998)., 39, 2649-2658.

[33] Page-McCaw A., Ewald AJ, Werb Z.Matrix metalloproteinases and the regulation of tissue remodelling. Nat Rev Mol Cell Biol (2007)., 8, 221-233.

[34] Rohen, J. W, Lutjen, E, & Barany, E. The relation between the ciliary muscle and the trabecular meshwork and its importance for the effect of miotics on aqueous outflow resistance. A study in two contrasting monkey species, Macaca irus and Cercopithecus aethiops. Albrecht Von Graefes Arch Klin Exp Ophthalmol (1967)., 172, 23-47.

[35] Lutjen-drecoll, E, Wiendl, H, & Kaufman, P. L. Acute and chronic structural effects of pilocarpine on monkey outflow tissues. Trans Am Ophthalmol Soc (1998). , 96, 171-95.

[36] Barany, E. H. The mode of action of miotics on outflow resistance. A study of pilocarpine in the vervet monkey Cercopithecus ethiops. Trans Ophthalmol Soc U K (1966)., 86, 539-578.

[37] Gabelt, B. T, & Kaufman, P. L. Changes in aqueous humor dynamics with age and glaucoma. Prog Retin Eye Res (2005)., 24, 612-637.

[38] Becker, B. The decline in aqueous secretion and outflow facility with age. Am J Ophthalmol (1958)., 46, 731-736.

[39] Gaasterland, D, Kupfer, C, Milton, R, Ross, K, & Mccain, L. MacLellan H. Studies of aqueous humor dynamics in man. VI. Effect of age upon parameters of intraocular pressure in normal human eyes. Exp Eye Res (1978)., 26, 651-656.

[40] Croft, M. A, Oyen, M. J, Gange, S. J, Fisher, M. R, & Kaufman, P. L. Aging effects on accommodation and outflow facility responses to pilocarpine in humans. Arch Ophthalmol (1996)., 114, 586-592.

[41] Armaly, M. F. The consistency of the 1955 calibration for various tonometer weights. Am J Ophthalmol (1959)., 48, 602-611.

[42] Bloom, J. N, Levene, R. Z, Thomas, G, & Kimura, R. Fluorophotometry and the rate of aqueous flow in man. I. Instrumentation and normal values. Arch Ophthalmol (1976)., 94, 435-443.

[43] Brubaker, R. F, Nagataki, S, Townsend, D. J, Burns, R. R, Higgins, R. G, & Wentworth, W. The effect of age on aqueous humor formation in man. Ophthalmology (1981). , 88, 283-288.

[44] Kupfer, C. Clinical significance of pseudofacility. Sanford R. Gifford Memorial Lecture. Am J Ophthalmol (1973). , 75, 193-204.

[45] Foster, P. J, Alsbirk, P. H, Baasanhu, J, Munkhbayar, D, Uranchimeg, D, & Johnson, G. J. Anterior chamber depth in Mongolians: variation with age, sex, and method of measurement. Am J Ophthalmol (1997). , 124, 53-60.

[46] Rufer, F, Schroder, A, Klettner, A, Frimpong-boateng, A, Roider, J. B, & Erb, C. Anterior chamber depth and iridocorneal angle in healthy White subjects: effects of age, gender and refraction. Acta Ophthalmol (2010). , 88, 885-890.

[47] Lutjen-drecoll, E, Kaufman, P. L, & Eichhorn, M. Long-term timolol and epinephrine in monkeys. I. Functional morphology of the ciliary processes. Trans Ophthalmol Soc U K (1986). , 105, 180-195.

[48] Llobet, A, Gasull, X, & Gual, A. Understanding trabecular meshwork physiology: a key to the control of intraocular pressure? News Physiol Sci (2003). , 18, 205-209.

[49] Lutjen-drecoll, E. Morphological changes in glaucomatous eyes and the role of TGFbeta2 for the pathogenesis of the disease. Exp Eye Res (2005). , 81, 1-4.

[50] Alvarado, J, Murphy, C, & Juster, R. Trabecular meshwork cellularity in primary open-angle glaucoma and nonglaucomatous normals. Ophthalmology (1984). , 91, 564-579.

[51] Grierson, I, & Howes, R. C. Age-related depletion of the cell population in the human trabecular meshwork. Eye (Lond) (1987). , 1, 204-210.

[52] Alvarado, J, Murphy, C, Polansky, J, & Juster, R. Age-related changes in trabecular meshwork cellularity. Invest Ophthalmol Vis Sci (1981). , 21, 714-727.

[53] Tschumper, R. C, & Johnson, D. H. Trabecular meshwork cellularity. Differences between fellow eyes. Invest Ophthalmol Vis Sci (1990). , 31, 1327-1331.

[54] Buller, C, Johnson, D. H, & Tschumper, R. C. Human trabecular meshwork phagocytosis. Observations in an organ culture system. Invest Ophthalmol Vis Sci (1990). , 31, 2156-2163.

[55] Grierson, I, & Chisholm, I. A. Clearance of debris from the iris through the drainage angle of the rabbit's eye. Br J Ophthalmol (1978). , 62, 694-704.

[56] Grierson, I, & Lee, W. R. Erythrocyte phagocytosis in the human trabecular meshwork. Br J Ophthalmol (1973). , 57, 400-415.

[57] Johnson, D. H, Richardson, T. M, & Epstein, D. L. Trabecular meshwork recovery after phagocytic challenge. Curr Eye Res (1989). , 8, 1121-1130.

[58] Rohen, J. W, & Van Der Zypen, E. The phagocytic activity of the trabecularmeshwork endothelium. An electron-microscopic study of the vervet (Cercopithecus aethiops). Albrecht Von Graefes Arch Klin Exp Ophthalmol (1968). , 175, 143-160.

[59] Shirato, S, Murphy, C. G, Bloom, E, Franse-carman, L, Maglio, M. T, Polansky, J. R, et al. Kinetics of phagocytosis in trabecular meshwork cells. Flow cytometry and morphometry. Invest Ophthalmol Vis Sci (1989). , 30, 2499-2511.

[60] Zhou, L, Li, Y, & Yue, B. Y. Alteration of cytoskeletal structure, integrin distribution, and migratory activity by phagocytic challenge in cells from an ocular tissue--the trabecular meshwork. In Vitro Cell Dev Biol Anim (1999). , 35, 144-149.

[61] Alvarado, J. A, Alvarado, R. G, Yeh, R. F, Franse-carman, L, Marcellino, G. R, & Brownstein, M. J. A new insight into the cellular regulation of aqueous outflow: how trabecular meshwork endothelial cells drive a mechanism that regulates the permeability of Schlemm's canal endothelial cells. Br J Ophthalmol (2005). , 89, 1500-1505.

[62] Shifera, A. S, Trivedi, S, Chau, P, Bonnemaison, L. H, Iguchi, R, & Alvarado, J. A. Constitutive secretion of chemokines by cultured human trabecular meshwork cells. Exp Eye Res (2010). , 91, 42-47.

[63] Rohen, J. W, & Witmer, R. Electrn microscopic studies on the trabecular meshwork in glaucoma simplex. Albrecht Von Graefes Arch Klin Exp Ophthalmol (1972). , 183, 251-266.

[64] Liu, J. H, Zhang, X, Kripke, D. F, & Weinreb, R. N. Twenty-four-hour intraocular pressure pattern associated with early glaucomatous changes. Invest Ophthalmol Vis Sci (2003). , 44, 1586-1590.

[65] Liu, J. H, Bouligny, R. P, Kripke, D. F, & Weinreb, R. N. Nocturnal elevation of intraocular pressure is detectable in the sitting position. Invest Ophthalmol Vis Sci (2003). , 44, 4439-4442.

[66] Coleman, D. J, & Trokel, S. Direct-recorded intraocular pressure variations in a human subject. Arch Ophthalmol (1969). , 82, 637-640.

[67] Rose, R. C, Richer, S. P, & Bode, A. M. Ocular oxidants and antioxidant protection. Proc Soc Exp Biol Med (1998). , 217, 397-407.

[68] Spector, A, & Garner, W. H. Hydrogen peroxide and human cataract. Exp Eye Res (1981). , 33, 673-681.

[69] Garcia-castineiras, S, Velazquez, S, Martinez, P, & Torres, N. Aqueous humor hydrogen peroxide analysis with dichlorophenol-indophenol. Exp Eye Res (1992). , 55, 9-19.

[70] Bleau, G, Giasson, C, & Brunette, I. Measurement of hydrogen peroxide in biological samples containing high levels of ascorbic acid. Anal Biochem (1998). , 263, 13-17.

[71] García-castiñeiras, S. Hydrogen peroxide in the aqueous humor: 1992-1997. (1998). , 17, 335-343.

[72] Valko, M, Rhodes, C. J, Moncol, J, Izakovic, M, & Mazur, M. Free radicals, metals and antioxidants in oxidative stress-induced cancer. Chem Biol Interact (2006). , 160, 1-40.

[73] Valko, M, Leibfritz, D, Moncol, J, Cronin, M. T, Mazur, M, & Telser, J. Free radicals and antioxidants in normal physiological functions and human disease. Int J Biochem Cell Biol (2007). , 39, 44-84.

[74] Gloire, G, Legrand-poels, S, & Piette, J. NF-kappaB activation by reactive oxygen species: fifteen years later. Biochem Pharmacol (2006). , 72, 1493-1505.

[75] Mccord, J. M, & Fridovich, I. Superoxide dismutase. An enzymic function for erythrocuprein (hemocuprein). J Biol Chem (1969). , 244, 6049-6055.

[76] Wiederholt, M, Sturm, A, & Lepple-wienhues, A. Relaxation of trabecular meshwork and ciliary muscle by release of nitric oxide. Invest Ophthalmol Vis Sci (1994). , 35, 2515-2520.

[77] Kamikawatoko, S, Tokoro, T, Ishida, A, Masuda, H, Hamasaki, H, Sato, J, et al. Nitric oxide relaxes bovine ciliary muscle contracted by carbachol through elevation of cyclic GMP. Exp Eye Res (1998). , 66(1), 1-7.

[78] Huie, R. E, & Padmaja, S. The reaction of NO with superoxide. Free Rad. Res. Com. (1993). , 18, 195-199.

[79] Pacher, P, Beckman, J. S, & Liaudet, L. Nitric oxide and peroxynitrite in health and disease. Physiol Rev (2007). , 87, 315-424.

[80] Jenner, P. Oxidative stress in Parkinson's disease. Ann Neurol (2003). Suppl 3:Sdiscussion S36-8., 26-36.

[81] Zhou, C, Huang, Y, & Przedborski, S. Oxidative stress in Parkinson's disease: a mechanism of pathogenic and therapeutic significance. Ann N Y Acad Sci (2008). , 1147, 93-104.

[82] Nunomura, A, Perry, G, Aliev, G, Hirai, K, Takeda, A, Balraj, E. K, et al. Oxidative damage is the earliest event in Alzheimer disease. J Neuropathol Exp Neurol (2001). , 60, 759-767.

[83] Pratico, D, Uryu, K, Leight, S, Trojanoswki, J. Q, & Lee, V. M. Increased lipid peroxidation precedes amyloid plaque formation in an animal model of Alzheimer amyloidosis. J Neurosci (2001). , 21, 4183-4187.

[84] Reddy, P. H, Mcweeney, S, Park, B. S, Manczak, M, Gutala, R. V, Partovi, D, et al. Gene expression profiles of transcripts in amyloid precursor protein transgenic mice: up-regulation of mitochondrial metabolism and apoptotic genes is an early cellular change in Alzheimer's disease. Hum Mol Genet (2004). , 13, 1225-1240.

[85] Wiseman, H, & Halliwell, B. Damage to DNA by reactive oxygen and nitrogen species: role in inflammatory disease and progression to cancer. Biochem J (1996). , 313, 17-29.

[86] Cai, H, & Harrison, D. G. Endothelial dysfunction in cardiovascular diseases: the role of oxidant stress. Circ Res (2000). , 87, 840-844.

[87] Kumar, D. M, & Agarwal, N. Oxidative stress in glaucoma: a burden of evidence. J Glaucoma (2007). , 16, 334-343.

[88] Izzotti, A, Sacca, S. C, Cartiglia, C, & De Flora, S. Oxidative deoxyribonucleic acid damage in the eyes of glaucoma patients. Am J Med (2003). , 114, 638-646.

[89] Sacca, S. C, Pascotto, A, Camicione, P, Capris, P, & Izzotti, A. Oxidative DNA damage in the human trabecular meshwork: clinical correlation in patients with primary open-angle glaucoma. Arch Ophthalmol (2005). , 123, 458-463.

[90] Caballero, M, Liton, P. B, Challa, P, Epstein, D. L, & Gonzalez, P. Effects of donor age on proteasome activity and senescence in trabecular meshwork cells. Biochem Biophys Res Commun (2004). , 323, 1048-1054.

[91] Babizhayev, M. A, & Bunin, A. Y. Lipid peroxidation in open-angle glaucoma. Acta Ophthalmol (Copenh) (1989). , 67, 371-377.

[92] Fernandez-durango, R, Fernandez-martinez, A, Garcia-feijoo, J, Castillo, A, De La Casa, J. M, Garcia-bueno, B, et al. Expression of nitrotyrosine and oxidative consequences in the trabecular meshwork of patients with primary open-angle glaucoma. Invest Ophthalmol Vis Sci (2008). , 49, 2506-2511.

[93] Sorkhabi, R, Ghorbanihaghjo, A, Javadzadeh, A, Rashtchizadeh, N, & Moharrery, M. Oxidative DNA damage and total antioxidant status in glaucoma patients. Mol Vis (2011). , 17, 41-46.

[94] Ferreira, S. M, Lerner, S. F, Brunzini, R, Evelson, P. A, & Llesuy, S. F. Oxidative stress markers in aqueous humor of glaucoma patients. Am J Ophthalmol (2004). , 137, 62-69.

[95] Ghanem, A. A, Arafa, L. F, & Baz, A. Oxidative stress markers in patients with primary open-angle glaucoma. Curr Eye Res (2010). , 35, 295-301.

[96] Kinsey, V. E. Transfer of ascorbic acid and related compounds across the blood-aqueous barrier. Am J Ophthalmol (1947). , 30, 1262-1266.

[97] Becker, B. Chemical composition of human aqueous humor; effects of acetazoleamide. AMA Arch Ophthalmol (1957). , 57, 793-800.

[98] Reiss, G. R, Werness, P. G, Zollman, P. E, & Brubaker, R. F. Ascorbic acid levels in the aqueous humor of nocturnal and diurnal mammals. Arch Ophthalmol (1986). , 104, 753-755.

[99] Reddy, V. N, Giblin, F. J, Lin, L. R, & Chakrapani, B. The effect of aqueous humor ascorbate on ultraviolet-B-induced DNA damage in lens epithelium. Invest Ophthalmol Vis Sci (1998)., 39, 344-350.

[100] Schachtschabel, D. O, Binninger, E. A, & Rohen, J. W. In vitro cultures of trabecular meshwork cells of the human eye as a model system for the study of cellular aging. Arch Gerontol Geriatr (1989)., 9, 251-262.

[101] Guo, M. S, Wu, Y. Y, & Liang, Z. B. Hyaluronic acid increases MMP-2 and MMP-9 expressions in cultured trabecular meshwork cells from patients with primary open-angle glaucoma. Mol Vis (2012)., 18, 1175-1181.

[102] Knepper, P. A, Goossens, W, & Palmberg, P. F. Glycosaminoglycan stratification of the juxtacanalicular tissue in normal and primary open-angle glaucoma. Invest Ophthalmol Vis Sci (1996)., 37, 2414-2425.

[103] Knepper, P. A, Goossens, W, Hvizd, M, & Palmberg, P. F. Glycosaminoglycans of the human trabecular meshwork in primary open-angle glaucoma. Invest Ophthalmol Vis Sci (1996)., 37, 1360-1367.

[104] Jampel, H. D, Moon, J. I, Quigley, H. A, Barron, Y, & Lam, K. W. Aqueous humor uric acid and ascorbic acid concentrations and outcome of trabeculectomy. Arch Ophthalmol (1998)., 116, 281-285.

[105] Leite, M. T, Prata, T. S, Kera, C. Z, & Miranda, D. V. de Moraes Barros SB, Melo LA,Jr. Ascorbic acid concentration is reduced in the secondary aqueous humor of glaucomatous patients. Clin Experiment Ophthalmol (2009)., 37, 402-406.

[106] Lee, P, Lam, K. W, & Lai, M. Aqueous humor ascorbate concentration and open-angle glaucoma. Arch Ophthalmol (1977)., 95, 308-310.

[107] Govindarajan, B, Laird, J, Salomon, R. G, & Bhattacharya, S. K. Isolevuglandin-modified proteins, including elevated levels of inactive calpain-1, accumulate in glaucomatous trabecular meshwork. Biochemistry (2008)., 47, 817-825.

[108] Gutteridge, J. M. Lipid peroxidation and antioxidants as biomarkers of tissue damage. Clin Chem (1995)., 41, 1819-1828.

[109] Reed, T. T. Lipid peroxidation and neurodegenerative disease. Free Radic Biol Med (2011)., 51, 1302-1319.

[110] Subbarao, K. V, Richardson, J. S, & Ang, L. C. Autopsy samples of Alzheimer's cortex show increased peroxidation in vitro. J Neurochem (1990)., 55, 342-345.

[111] Tsang, A. H, & Chung, K. K. Oxidative and nitrosative stress in Parkinson's disease. Biochim Biophys Acta (2009)., 1792, 643-650.

[112] De Nadal, E, Ammerer, G, & Posas, F. Controlling gene expression in response to stress. Nat Rev Genet (2011)., 12, 833-845.

[113] Irnaten, M, Barry, R. C, Quill, B, Clark, A. F, Harvey, B. J, & Brien, O. CJ. Activation of stretch-activated channels and maxi-K+ channels by membrane stress of human lamina cribrosa cells. Invest Ophthalmol Vis Sci (2009). , 50, 194-202.

[114] Clark, A. F. The cell and molecular biology of glaucoma: biomechanical factors in glaucoma. Invest Ophthalmol Vis Sci (2012). , 53, 2473-2475.

[115] Zhou, B. B, & Elledge, S. J. The DNA damage response: putting checkpoints in perspective. Nature (2000). , 408, 433-439.

[116] Vittitow, J, & Borras, T. Genes expressed in the human trabecular meshwork during pressure-induced homeostatic response. J Cell Physiol (2004). , 201, 126-137.

[117] Vittal, V, Rose, A, Gregory, K. E, Kelley, M. J, & Acott, T. S. Changes in gene expression by trabecular meshwork cells in response to mechanical stretching. Invest Ophthalmol Vis Sci (2005). Aug;, 46(8), 2857-2868.

[118] Gonzalez, P, Epstein, D. L, & Borras, T. Genes upregulated in the human trabecular meshwork in response to elevated intraocular pressure. Invest Ophthalmol Vis Sci (2000). , 41, 352-361.

[119] Borras, T. Gene expression in the trabecular meshwork and the influence of intraocular pressure. Prog Retin Eye Res (2003). , 22, 435-463.

[120] Okada, Y, Matsuo, T, & Ohtsuki, H. Bovine trabecular cells produce TIMP-1 and MMP-2 in response to mechanical stretching. Jpn J Ophthalmol (1998). , 42, 90-94.

[121] Kim, C. Y, Kim, S. S, Koh, H. J, You, Y. S, Seong, G. J, & Hong, Y. J. Effect of IOP elevation on matrix metalloproteinase-2 in rabbit anterior chamber. Korean J Ophthalmol (2000). , 14, 27-31.

[122] Bradley, J. M, Kelley, M. J, Zhu, X, Anderssohn, A. M, Alexander, J. P, & Acott, T. S. Effects of mechanical stretching on trabecular matrix metalloproteinases. Invest Ophthalmol Vis Sci (2001). , 42, 1505-1513.

[123] Bradley, J. M, Kelley, M. J, Rose, A, & Acott, T. S. Signaling pathways used in trabecular matrix metalloproteinase response to mechanical stretch. Invest Ophthalmol Vis Sci (2003). , 44, 5174-5181.

[124] George, J, Castellazzi, M, & Buttin, G. Prophage induction and cell division in E. coli. III. Mutations sfiA and sfiB restore division in tif and lon strains and permit the expression of mutator properties of tif. Mol Gen Genet (1975). , 140, 309-332.

[125] Lopez-maury, L, Marguerat, S, & Bahler, J. Tuning gene expression to changing environments: from rapid responses to evolutionary adaptation. Nat Rev Genet (2008). , 9, 583-593.

[126] Johnson, D. H, & Tschumper, R. C. Human trabecular meshwork organ culture. A new method. Invest Ophthalmol Vis Sci (1987). , 28, 945-953.

[127] Keller, K. E, Bradley, J. M, & Acott, T. S. Differential effects of ADAMTS-1,-4, and-5 in the trabecular meshwork. Invest Ophthalmol Vis Sci (2009). , 50, 5769-5777.

[128] Gasch, A. P, Spellman, P. T, Kao, C. M, Carmel-harel, O, Eisen, M. B, Storz, G, et al. Genomic expression programs in the response of yeast cells to environmental changes. Mol Biol Cell (2000). , 11, 4241-4257.

[129] Boehm, A. K, Saunders, A, Werner, J, & Lis, J. T. Transcription factor and polymerase recruitment, modification, and movement on dhsp70 in vivo in the minutes following heat shock. Mol Cell Biol (2003). , 23, 7628-7637.

[130] Tumminia, S. J, Mitton, K. P, Arora, J, Zelenka, P, Epstein, D. L, & Russell, P. Mechanical stretch alters the actin cytoskeletal network and signal transduction in human trabecular meshwork cells. Invest Ophthalmol Vis Sci (1998). , 39, 1361-1371.

[131] Liton, P. B, Li, G, Luna, C, Gonzalez, P, & Epstein, D. L. Cross-talk between TGF-beta1 and IL-6 in human trabecular meshwork cells. Mol Vis (2009). , 15, 326-334.

[132] Zhang, X, Schroeder, A, Callahan, E. M, Coyle, B. M, Wang, N, Erickson, K. A, et al. Constitutive signalling pathway activity in trabecular meshwork cells from glaucomatous eyes. Exp Eye Res (2006). , 82, 968-973.

[133] Porter, K. M, Epstein, D. L, & Liton, P. B. Up-regulated expression of extracellular matrix remodeling genes in phagocytically challenged trabecular meshwork cells. PLoS One (2012). e34792.

[134] Kultz, D. Molecular and evolutionary basis of the cellular stress response. Annu Rev Physiol (2005). , 67, 225-257.

[135] Wang, N, Chintala, S. K, Fini, M. E, & Schuman, J. S. Activation of a tissue-specific stress response in the aqueous outflow pathway of the eye defines the glaucoma disease phenotype. Nat Med (2001). , 7, 304-309.

[136] Zhou, Q, Liu, Y. Q, Zhao, J. L, & Zhang, H. Effects of oxidative stress on the expression of endothelial-leukocyte adhesion molecule-1 in porcine trabecular meshwork cells. Zhongguo Yi Xue Ke Xue Yuan Xue Bao (2007). , 29, 394-397.

[137] Liton, P. B, Luna, C, Challa, P, Epstein, D. L, & Gonzalez, P. Genome-wide expression profile of human trabecular meshwork cultured cells, nonglaucomatous and primary open angle glaucoma tissue. Mol Vis (2006). , 12, 774-790.

[138] Giaever, G, Chu, A. M, Ni, L, Connelly, C, Riles, L, Veronneau, S, et al. Functional profiling of the Saccharomyces cerevisiae genome. Nature (2002). , 418, 387-391.

[139] Thorpe, G. W, Fong, C. S, Alic, N, Higgins, V. J, & Dawes, I. W. Cells have distinct mechanisms to maintain protection against different reactive oxygen species: oxidative-stress-response genes. Proc Natl Acad Sci U S A (2004). , 101, 6564-6569.

[140] Warringer, J, Ericson, E, Fernandez, L, Nerman, O, & Blomberg, A. High-resolution yeast phenomics resolves different physiological features in the saline response. Proc Natl Acad Sci U S A (2003). , 100, 15724-15729.

[141] Koonin, E. V. Chance and necessity in cellular response to challenge. Mol Syst Biol (2007).

[142] Stern, S, Dror, T, Stolovicki, E, Brenner, N, & Braun, E. Genome-wide transcriptional plasticity underlies cellular adaptation to novel challenge. Mol Syst Biol (2007).

[143] Hugo Gene Nomenclature CommitteeAvailable at: http://www.genenames.org/index.html.Accessed 08/14, (2012).

[144] Fingert, J. H. Primary open-angle glaucoma genes. Eye (Lond) (2011). , 25, 587-595.

[145] Nishimura, D. Y, Swiderski, R. E, Alward, W. L, Searby, C. C, Patil, S. R, Bennet, S. R, et al. The forkhead transcription factor gene FKHL7 is responsible for glaucoma phenotypes which map to 6Nat Genet (1998). , 25.

[146] Mears, A. J, Jordan, T, Mirzayans, F, Dubois, S, Kume, T, Parlee, M, et al. Mutations of the forkhead/winged-helix gene, FKHL7, in patients with Axenfeld-Rieger anomaly. Am J Hum Genet (1998). , 63, 1316-1328.

[147] Semina, E. V, Reiter, R, Leysens, N. J, Alward, W. L, Small, K. W, Datson, N. A, et al. Cloning and characterization of a novel bicoid-related homeobox transcription factor gene, RIEG, involved in Rieger syndrome. Nat Genet (1996). , 14, 392-399.

[148] Berry, F. B, Skarie, J. M, Mirzayans, F, Fortin, Y, Hudson, T. J, Raymond, V, et al. FOXC1 is required for cell viability and resistance to oxidative stress in the eye through the transcriptional regulation of FOXO1A. Hum Mol Genet 200815;, 17, 490-505.

[149] Strungaru, M. H, Footz, T, Liu, Y, Berry, F. B, Belleau, P, Semina, E. V, et al. PITX2 is involved in stress response in cultured human trabecular meshwork cells through regulation of SLC13A3. Invest Ophthalmol Vis Sci (2011). , 52, 7625-7633.

[150] Morissette, J, Cote, G, Anctil, J. L, Plante, M, Amyot, M, Heon, E, et al. A common gene for juvenile and adult-onset primary open-angle glaucomas confined on chromosome 1q. Am J Hum Genet (1995). , 56, 1431-1442.

[151] Sheffield, V. C, Stone, E. M, Alward, W. L, Drack, A. V, Johnson, A. T, Streb, L. M, et al. Genetic linkage of familial open angle glaucoma to chromosome 1q21-q31. Nat Genet (1993). , 4, 47-50.

[152] Stone, E. M, Fingert, J. H, Alward, W. L, Nguyen, T. D, Polansky, J. R, Sunden, S. L, et al. Identification of a gene that causes primary open angle glaucoma. Science (1997). , 275, 668-670.

[153] Karali, A, Russell, P, Stefani, F. H, & Tamm, E. R. Localization of myocilin/trabecular meshwork--inducible glucocorticoid response protein in the human eye. Invest Ophthalmol Vis Sci (2000)., 41, 729-740.

[154] Resch, Z. T, & Fautsch, M. P. Glaucoma-associated myocilin: a better understanding but much more to learn. Exp Eye Res (2009)., 88, 704-712.

[155] Resch, Z. T, Hann, C. R, Cook, K. A, & Fautsch, M. P. Aqueous humor rapidly stimulates myocilin secretion from human trabecular meshwork cells. Exp Eye Res 201;, 91, 901-908.

[156] Hardy, K. M, Hoffman, E. A, Gonzalez, P, Mckay, B. S, & Stamer, W. D. Extracellular trafficking of myocilin in human trabecular meshwork cells. J Biol Chem (2005)., 280, 28917-28926.

[157] Joe, M. K, & Tomarev, S. I. Expression of myocilin mutants sensitizes cells to oxidative stress-induced apoptosis: implication for glaucoma pathogenesis. Am J Pathol (2010)., 176, 2880-2890.

[158] Alward, W. L. Axenfeld-Rieger syndrome in the age of molecular genetics. Am J Ophthalmol (2000)., 130, 107-115.

[159] Sowden, J. C. Molecular and developmental mechanisms of anterior segment dysgenesis. Eye (Lond) (2007)., 21, 1310-1318.

[160] Reis, L. M, & Semina, E. V. Genetics of anterior segment dysgenesis disorders. Curr Opin Ophthalmol (2011)., 22, 314-324.

[161] Strungaru, M. H, Dinu, I, & Walter, M. A. Genotype-phenotype correlations in Axenfeld-Rieger malformation and glaucoma patients with FOXC1 and PITX2 mutations. Invest Ophthalmol Vis Sci (2007)., 48, 228-237.

Permissions

All chapters in this book were first published by InTech Open; hereby published with permission under the Creative Commons Attribution License or equivalent. Every chapter published in this book has been scrutinized by our experts. Their significance has been extensively debated. The topics covered herein carry significant findings which will fuel the growth of the discipline. They may even be implemented as practical applications or may be referred to as a beginning point for another development.

The contributors of this book come from diverse backgrounds, making this book a truly international effort. This book will bring forth new frontiers with its revolutionizing research information and detailed analysis of the nascent developments around the world.

We would like to thank all the contributing authors for lending their expertise to make the book truly unique. They have played a crucial role in the development of this book. Without their invaluable contributions this book wouldn't have been possible. They have made vital efforts to compile up to date information on the varied aspects of this subject to make this book a valuable addition to the collection of many professionals and students.

This book was conceptualized with the vision of imparting up-to-date information and advanced data in this field. To ensure the same, a matchless editorial board was set up. Every individual on the board went through rigorous rounds of assessment to prove their worth. After which they invested a large part of their time researching and compiling the most relevant data for our readers.

The editorial board has been involved in producing this book since its inception. They have spent rigorous hours researching and exploring the diverse topics which have resulted in the successful publishing of this book. They have passed on their knowledge of decades through this book. To expedite this challenging task, the publisher supported the team at every step. A small team of assistant editors was also appointed to further simplify the editing procedure and attain best results for the readers.

Apart from the editorial board, the designing team has also invested a significant amount of their time in understanding the subject and creating the most relevant covers. They scrutinized every image to scout for the most suitable representation of the subject and create an appropriate cover for the book.

The publishing team has been an ardent support to the editorial, designing and production team. Their endless efforts to recruit the best for this project, has resulted in the accomplishment of this book. They are a veteran in the field of academics and their pool of knowledge is as vast as their experience in printing. Their expertise and guidance has proved useful at every step. Their uncompromising quality standards have made this book an exceptional effort. Their encouragement from time to time has been an inspiration for everyone.

The publisher and the editorial board hope that this book will prove to be a valuable piece of knowledge for researchers, students, practitioners and scholars across the globe.

List of Contributors

Magdalena Zdybel and Barbara Pilawa
Medical University of Silesia in Katowice, School of Pharmacy with the Division of Laboratory Medicine, Department of Biophysics, Sosnowiec, Poland

Hannah Timlin and Roshini Sanders
Cataract Unit, Queen Margaret Hospital, Dunfermline, NHS Fife, UK

Vikas Tah and Farihah Tariq
Stoke Mandeville Hospital, UK

Walid Sharif, Dev Mukhey and Zuhair Sharif
UCL Institute of Ophthalmology, UK

Imran Yusuf
Oxford, UK

Marcus Posner
Royal Free Hospital, UK

Louise Ramskold
East and North Hertfordshire NHS Trust, UK

Pinakin Gunvant Davey
Western University of Health Sciences, College of Optometry, Pomona, CA, USA

Makoto Ishikawa and Takeshi Yoshitomi
Department of Ophthalmology, Akita Graduate University Faculty of Medicine, Akita, Japan

Yukitoshi Izumi
Department of Psychiatry, Washington University School of Medicine, St. Louis, M.O., USA

Retno Supriyanti
Faculty of Science and Engineering, Jenderal Soedirman University, Indonesia

Hitoshi Habe and Masatsugu Kidode
Graduate School of Information Science, Nara Institute of Science and Technology, Japan

Covadonga Pañeda, Tamara Martínez, Natalia Wright and Ana Isabel Jimenez
Sylentis SAU, R&D department, PCM c/ Santiago Grisolía, Madrid, Spain

Emina Alimanović Halilović
University Clinical Center Sarajevo, Sarajevo, Bosnia and Herzegovina

Ana Lilia Pérez-Balbuena, David Arturo Ancona-Lezama and Lorena Gutiérrez-Sánchez
Cornea Service, Asociación para Evitar la Ceguera en México I.A.P. "Hospital Dr. Luis Sánchez Bulnes", Vicente García Torres, México D.F., México

Virginia Vanzzini-Zago
Laboratory of Microbiology, Asociación para Evitar la Ceguera en México I.A.P. "Hospital Dr. Luis Sánchez Bulnes", Vicente García Torres, México D.F., México

Yoko A. Ito and Michael A. Walter
Department of Medical Genetics, University of Alberta, Edmonton, AB, Canada

Index

A

Aneurysms, 87

Anterior Segment, 26-27, 30-31, 42-43, 164, 199, 202, 207, 212, 214-216, 228

Antibiotic Therapy, 187, 189, 191-193

Artery Occlusion, 99-100

B

Blepharitis, 26-27

Bowman Layer, 24

C

Cataract, 42-43, 81, 110-112, 114, 117-121, 126-127, 159-161, 167-168, 170-172, 175, 180, 192-193, 196-197, 209-210, 221

Cell Membrane, 143, 147, 211

Cellular Level, 140

Central Retina, 132

Chalazia, 26-27

Choroid, 2-5, 25, 174-175

Ciliary Body, 2-3, 144, 161, 201

Cobalt Blue Filter, 30-31

Conjunctivitis, 154, 195

Contact Lens, 136, 162, 165, 180, 184, 187, 196

Corneal Epithelium, 81, 84-85, 164

Crystalline Lens, 67-68, 81

Cytokines, 139, 143, 154, 205, 212

D

Diabetes, 44-45, 105-106, 130, 134-135, 152, 185

Diabetes Mellitus, 130, 134, 185

Diabetic Retinopathy, 34-35, 44-45, 91-92, 99-100, 134-136, 142, 152, 170

Diffuse Illumination, 28-29

Dry Eye, 86-89, 136, 142, 152

Dry Eyes, 82-87

E

Endothelium, 24, 30-31, 167, 218, 221

Extracellular Matrix, 147, 202, 219, 226

F

Fluorescein Angiography, 63-64, 167-168

Fundus Camera, 34-35, 42-45

Fundus Image, 30-31, 36-41

G

Ganglion Cells, 90, 93-100, 103-104, 107-108, 130, 140, 199

Glaucoma, 24, 30-33, 42-43, 82-85, 88-109, 130-131, 142, 149-150, 160, 164, 169, 172, 175, 192-193, 199-201, 203-206, 208-210, 213-221, 223

Glaucoma Surgery, 218

H

Hemorrhages, 171

Hexagonal Cells, 24

I

Imaging Systems, 59-60

Inflammatory Cytokines, 205

Inner Retina, 97-100

Intraocular Pressure, 24, 30-33, 93-94, 99-100, 130, 137, 162, 164, 166-167, 169, 171-172, 200-201, 206, 219-221, 225

Ischemic Optic Neuropathy, 131, 139-140, 154

K

Keratitis, 139, 154, 174, 176-177, 179-189, 192-198

M

Macular Degeneration, 26-27, 34-37, 42-45, 63-66, 131, 147, 149-151

Macular Disease, 150

Macular Edema, 135

Macular Oedema, 36-37, 63-64, 164, 166-167

Matrix Metalloproteinases, 202, 219, 225

Meibomian Glands, 136

Molecular Weight, 146

Mycobacterium, 174-178, 181, 183-184, 186, 193-197

Myopia, 61-64, 67-68, 75-76, 130, 166

O
Ocular Disease, 24, 152

Ocular Hypertension, 91-92, 103-104, 149-150

Ocular Structures, 24, 175

Ocular Surface, 82-83, 136, 150

Ophthalmology, 1-23, 25-45, 48, 50, 52, 54, 56, 58, 60, 62, 64, 66-80, 83, 85, 87, 89, 92, 94, 96-109, 144, 150-152, 158-160, 171-172, 174, 194-197, 220

Ophthalmoscope, 32-35, 38-39, 42-45, 59-60, 110-111, 114

Optic Nerve, 24-25, 93-94, 99-101, 130-131, 135, 139-140, 149, 155, 174-175, 178, 199

Optical Coherence Tomography, 25, 34-37

Optometrist, 26-27, 30-33, 36-37, 40-41

Oscillatory Potentials, 91-92

Oxidative Stress, 204, 206-211, 213, 215-216, 222-223, 226-227

R
Retinal Ganglion Cells, 93-100, 103-104, 107-108, 130, 140, 199

Retinal Image, 73-74

Retinal Pigment Epithelium, 2-3, 132, 141, 168

Retinal Vein, 26-27, 36-37, 63-64

Retinitis Pigmentosa, 140, 155

S
Scanning Laser Ophthalmoscope, 34-35, 38-39, 44-45

Skin Lesions, 28

T
Tonometry, 24, 229, 231, 233-234, 236, 238, 245-247

Tumor Necrosis Factor, 139, 153-154

U
Uveitis, 138, 168

V
Vascular Endothelial Growth Factor, 36-37, 133, 150-154

Vision Loss, 34-35, 131-133, 139-140, 150

Visual Acuity, 61-62, 67-68, 79-80, 84-85, 133, 139-141, 161-162, 165-168, 178-179, 185, 189-190

Visual Field Loss, 63-64, 149, 199

Visual Impairment, 47, 152

www.ingramcontent.com/pod-product-compliance
Lightning Source LLC
LaVergne TN
LVHW062235200926
848484LV00006B/1548

9798887403533